INTERNATIONAL SERIES OF MONOGRAPHS IN

NATURAL PHILOSOPHY

GENERAL EDITOR: D. TER HAAR

VOLUME 33

THEORY OF EXPERIMENTS IN PARAMAGNETIC RESONANCE

THEORY OF EXPERIMENTS IN PARAMAGNETIC RESONANCE

JAN TALPE
Escola Polytécnica da Universidade de São Paulo
Now of the Instituut voor Lage Temperaturen
en Technische Fysica, Leuven, Belgium

PERGAMON PRESS
OXFORD · NEW YORK · TORONTO
SYDNEY · BRAUNSCHWEIG

Pergamon Press Ltd., Headington Hill Hall, Oxford
Pergamon Press Inc., Maxwell House, Fairview Park, Elmsford, New York 10523
Pergamon of Canada Ltd., 207 Queen's Quay West, Toronto 1
Pergamon Press (Aust.) Pty. Ltd., 19a Boundary Street, Rushcutters Bay, N.S.W. 2011, Australia
Vieweg & Sohn GmbH, Burgplatz 1, Braunschweig

First edition 1971
Library of Congress Catalog Card No. 79-137411

Printed in Germany

08 016157 X

To my people in Brazil

É difícil defender,
só com palavras, a vida,
ainda mais quando ela é
esta que vê, severina;
mas se responder não pude
à pergunta que fazia,
ela, a vida, a respondeu
com sua presença viva.
(*Morte e Vida Severina*, CABRAL)

It's difficult to defend
life only by words,
especially when it's that life
one sees, the severe one;
but if I couldn't answer
your question,
life has given the answer
with his life presence.

Contents

Contents

Contents

Errata

TALPE: Theory of Experiments in Paramagnetic Resonance
Fig. 5.1, facing page 80, is upside down

CHAPTER 1

General Introduction

One important way of examining matter is to apply a magnetic field to it and to see what happens. One looks for the magnetization. A certain time after applying a constant magnetic field $\boldsymbol{B}_s$ one may observe that the magnetization becomes time independent, attaining a certain value $\boldsymbol{M}_s$. And in the first approximation, i.e. for weak magnetic fields, one usually finds that the magnetization $\boldsymbol{M}_s$ is proportional to the field $\boldsymbol{B}_s$. Therefore we define a static susceptibility tensor χ_s by†

$$\boldsymbol{M}_s = \varepsilon_0 c^2 \chi_s \boldsymbol{B}_s = \frac{10^7}{4\pi} \chi_s \boldsymbol{B}_s. \tag{1}$$

χ_s can eventually still depend on $\boldsymbol{B}_s$ of course.

We may also be interested in how the magnetization behaves immediately after applying the field. If the field $\boldsymbol{b}(t)$ is a step function, raising from zero to $\boldsymbol{B}_s$ at the instant $t = t_0$, the magnetization $\boldsymbol{m}(t)$ will vary in time after $t = t_0$ until attaining the final value $\boldsymbol{M}_s$. In the first approximation $\boldsymbol{m}(t)$ may still be supposed proportional to the excitation $\boldsymbol{B}_s$ and therefore we define a relaxation function $\varphi(t)$ by

$$\boldsymbol{m}(t) = \frac{10^7}{4\pi} \varphi(t - t_0)\, \boldsymbol{B}_s. \tag{2}$$

† We use SI units. We do not use μ_0, writing $1/\varepsilon_0 c^2$ for it, and we define magnetic susceptibilities as functions of the $\boldsymbol{B}$-field, not of the $\boldsymbol{H}$-field. A good article about units has been written by Cornelius (1964).

Observe that φ is also a tensor just as χ is. φ can in principle depend, for example, on $\boldsymbol{m}(t_0)$ and on $\boldsymbol{B}_s$. It is assumed, however, that $\boldsymbol{m}$ was time independent just before the instant t_0.†

Finally we can also apply an alternating induction, say‡

$$\boldsymbol{b}_1 = \mathscr{R}(2\boldsymbol{B}_1\, e^{i\omega t}). \tag{3}$$

After a certain time, the variation of the magnetization $\boldsymbol{m}_1(t)$ will be in the first approximation a stationary oscillation with the same frequency, but eventually with retarded phase and with some amplitude dependent on the frequency. Therefore we define a complex transfer function, the *high-frequency susceptibility*

$$\chi(\omega) \equiv \chi'(\omega) - i\chi''(\omega), \tag{4}$$

by

$$\boldsymbol{m}_1(t) \equiv \frac{10^7}{4\pi}\, \mathscr{R}[\chi(\omega) \,.\, 2\boldsymbol{B}_1\, e^{i\omega t}]. \tag{5}$$

Of course there exists a relation between the relaxation function, the transfer function and the static susceptibility. It is evident, for instance, by their definition that

$$\chi_s = \lim_{t\to\infty} \varphi(t) = \lim_{\omega\to 0} \chi(\omega). \tag{6}$$

There even exist some general relations between the real and imaginary part and the phase of $\chi(\omega)$.

In fact such a relaxation function and transfer function appear in many problems of physics where one is interested in the time-dependent behaviour of a system. And according to the magnitude of the times involved—compared to the times that can be handled by laboratory equipment—one will examine the behaviour of the system by a relaxation function or by a transfer function. In problems of heat conduction, for

† In general χ_s as well as φ may depend on the past history of the sample. But we consider samples with different past history as different paramagnetic systems.

‡ The operator $\mathscr{R}(\ldots)$ means "the real part of ...". In the same way $\mathscr{I}(\ldots)$ selects the imaginary part of an expression. For the factor 2, see eq. (4.14) of Chapter 2 below.

instance, a relaxation function is convenient. On the other hand, in optics and X-ray spectroscopy one uses the transfer function.

In the field of paramagnetism, relaxation functions as well as transfer functions are investigated experimentally. The relaxation function $\varphi(t)$ can be measured directly by pulse techniques. However, in practice, only nuclear magnetism presents times long enough to be convenient for such measurements.†

In studying the time-dependent behaviour of electronic paramagnetic systems one has to examine a transfer function, the high-frequency susceptibility $\chi(\omega)$. An example is the Faraday effect where the quantity of interest is the phase of the transfer function. But this concerns mainly incoherent radiation at light frequency. In studies with coherent radiation, principally at radio and microwave frequencies, rather scarcely has attention been paid to the phase of the transfer function (Altschuler and Kosyrev, 1963, p. 13; Kastler, 1949; Servant, 1967). The important quantities are the real part, the dispersion, and the imaginary part, the absorption, of the high-frequency susceptibility.

Here we state a first limitation on the subject of this book. We shall only deal with *electron* paramagnetic *absorption* and *dispersion* measurements.

We said absorption *and dispersion*. As a matter of fact, one usually uses absorption unless saturation makes it necessary to use the dispersion. The technique of dispersion measurements at saturation, useful in nuclear magnetic resonance (Solomon and Ezratty, 1962), has also been used with electronic systems (Lhôte *et al.*, 1963, 1964), although it is more difficult to saturate electronic paramagnetic systems than nuclear ones. The use of dispersion in the absence of saturation is rarely mentioned in the literature (Mays *et al.*, 1958; Reimann, 1963; Nagasawa, 1964; Altschuler and Kosyrev, 1963, p. 218). We shall, however, stress its importance and possibilities in this book (Talpe and Van Gerven, 1966).

The relaxation of paramagnetic systems was originally studied by thermodynamical means, principally by the group of Gorter in Leiden. When Gorter and Kronig (1936) defined the complex HF susceptibility

† Experiments with pulse techniques in e.s.r. have been realized by Kaplan *et al.* (1961) and by Cutler and Powles (1962). See also Gentzsch (1966) and Sprinz (1965).

$\chi(\omega)$, in analogy with the complex dielectric constant, this quantity was related to spin temperatures (Casimir and Dupré, 1938) and relaxation times by thermodynamical theories. It was not by accident that cooling by adiabatic demagnetization was realized with paramagnetic salts. And the fact that until very recently this was the only means for obtaining temperatures below 0·9°K perhaps partly explains the continual interest in the study of the paramagnetic behaviour of these salts.

In 1944 Zavoisky (1944) discovered paramagnetic resonance. It was already known by Gorter (1936) that, apart from relaxation, a paramagnetic system in a static magnetic field has its own internal frequency, an "eigenfrequency", just as an LC circuit has one. This means that the relaxation function $\varphi(t)$ of the system has an oscillating character, or that the transfer function $\chi(\omega)$ is enhanced around a certain non-zero value on the frequency axis. This discovery has two important consequences for the study of systems by means of paramagnetic properties:

1. First, the eigenfrequency of the system itself yields important information. In fact, there can be different eigenfrequencies in a system, and hence different oscillation-frequencies in $\varphi(t)$ or different "resonance lines" in $\chi(\omega)$. This "structure" of $\chi(\omega)$ reveals the inner structure of matter.

2. On the other hand, this is some kind of "frequency conversion" and the relaxation of the system can now be studied at very high frequencies, yielding tremendous gain in sensitivity, together with an interesting selectivity, since one can study separately that part of the system which has a certain eigenfrequency in a given field. For instance, until very recently it was only by means of resonance techniques that it was possible to study paramagnetic relaxation of nuclear systems above 1°K.

So we have to state a second limitation on our objective. We shall only deal with electron paramagnetic *resonance* dispersion and absorption measurements at *high field*. Within this framework we are concerned with the following problem: when we perform a paramagnetic resonance measurement, what does a measured line, i.e. a line in red or black ink recorded on a sheet of paper or a photograph of an oscilloscope screen, tell us about matter?

In the following chapter we analyse the paramagnetic resonance line, i.e. the HF susceptibility as a function of certain parameters, in order to see what it tells us about matter. The third chapter will then deal with the electronic signal that gives us this HF susceptibility. And the fourth chapter will be dedicated to the enhancement of this signal above noise.

For a general survey of the field of paramagnetic resonance, the *Resource Letter* NMR-EPR-1 published by R. E. Norberg (1965) may be very useful.

References

ALTSCHULER, S. A. and KOSYREV, B. M. (1963), *Paramagnetische Elektronenresonanz*, Teubner, Leipzig (Russian original: Moscow, 1961).
CASIMIR, H. B. G. and DUPRÉ, F. M. (1938), *Physica* **5**, 507.
CORNELIUS, P. (1964), *Physica* **30**, 1446.
CUTLER, D. and POWLES, J. G. (1962), *Proc. Phys. Soc.* **80**, 130.
GENTZSCH, F. (1966), *Hochfrequenztechnik und Elektroakustik* **75**, 109.
GORTER, C. J. (1936), *Physica* **3**, 995.
GORTER, C. J. and KRONIG, R. DE L. (1936), *Physica* **3**, 1009.
KAPLAN, D. E., BROWNE, M. E., and COWEN, J. A. (1961), *Rev. Sci. Instr.* **32**, 1182.
KASTLER, A. (1949), *C.R. Acad. Sci.* **228**, 1640.
LHÔTE, G., MOTCHANE, J. L., and THEOBALD, J. G. (1963, 1964), *C.R. Acad. Sci.* **257**, 630; **258**, 2771.
MAYS, J. M., MOORE, H. R., and SCHILMAN, R. G. (1958), *Rev. Sci. Instr.* **29**, 300.
NAGASAWA, H. (1964), *Japan. J. of Appl. Phys.* **3**, 560.
NORBERG, R. E. (1965), *Am. J. Phys.* **33**, 71.
REIMANN, R. (1963), *C.R. Acad. Sci.* **257**, 3863.
SERVANT, Y. (1967), *C.R. Acad. Sci.* **265**B, 60.
SOLOMON, I. and EZRATTY, J. (1962), *Phys. Rev.* **127**, 78.
SPRINZ, H. (1965), *Wiss. Zeitschr. der Karl-Marx-Univ. Leipzig* **14**, 935.
TALPE, J. and VAN GERVEN, L. (1966), *Phys. Rev.* **145**, 718.
ZAVOISKY, J. K. (1944), Thesis, Phys. Inst. Acad. Sci., Moscow.

CHAPTER 2

The Paramagnetic Resonance Line

1. Introduction

The *system* under study in a paramagnetic resonance experiment may be considered as a collection of monads (nuclei, atoms, ions, molecules, unit cells in a crystal, ...) having a magnetic dipole moment and situated in some environment. Indeed our observation is only about the macroscopic magnetic field. And this field interacts only with—i.e. we get direct information from—the magnetic dipole moments which in turn get information from (interact with) their environment.

If the monad is a nucleus, its properties such as spin, magnetic moment, quadrupole and higher moments can be considered to a high degree of approximation as independent of the situation of the nucleus in atoms or molecules. On the contrary, the properties of an electronic monad (an ion for instance) depend highly on its situation in matter. For instance, the angular momentum of a sodium atom, due to the spin of the unpaired electron, is $\frac{1}{2}\hbar$. But a molecule of sodium chloride has no angular momentum, because the unpaired electron of sodium is now paired in the unfilled shell of the seven chloride electrons. Moreover, a sodium atom in a magnetic field has a different behaviour, according to the orientation of the spin of its nucleus in that field. We shall call the monad with which our external field interacts, as it is embedded in a given environment, a "*spin*". We use quotation marks to distinguish this from the well-known property of many elementary particles.

In our system we can now have "spins" in *different situations*. For instance, "spins" of our system can be in different magnetic fields, because of the inhomogeneity of the applied field. Or various microcrystals in a powder sample can have different orientations in the external field, and hence different "spins" have their crystal axes in different directions with respect to the static field. Another kind of situation is less obvious: if two "spins" have nuclei in different states, the "spins" are to be considered in different situations (even when the nuclei belong, for example, to the ion which constitutes the "spin"). This results in hyperfine splitting. We suppose, however, that this state of the nucleus is maintained during a time long compared to the time required for a "spin" transition (the time during which the "spin" remains in its state). Of course "spins" with different Larmor frequencies are also considered as being in different situations.

All the "spins" of our system which are in the same average situation form a *"spin" packet*. The average is taken over a time corresponding to that required for a "spin" transition. Such "spins" of the same packet interact with each other and this causes a line to have a certain width. One speaks of relaxation. If some "spins" are precessing in phase with each other, this coherence will be disturbed after a certain time, the relaxation time.

This relaxation which conserves the energy in the system, the packet, and only introduces disorder (raises the entropy), is called *spin–spin relaxation*. It maintains the "spins" of the packet in equilibrium. On the other hand, there is the interaction of these "spins" with the lattice and with the HF field. The HF field energy is distributed equally among the "spins" of a "spin" packet, since they are in the same situation. And this energy is transferred from this "spin" to the lattice, requiring the so-called *"spin"-lattice relaxation* time. Spins of different packets may also interact. This is cross-relaxation.

The *relaxation* of the "spins" of a packet in our system will give us our first information about matter. Kubo and Tomita (1954), in an excellent general theory, showed how the relaxation function of a spin system can be related to a correlation function among "spins", which in turn is accessible to theoretical calculations from other data about this average situation. Hence we shall analyse in detail what information about the relaxation function is contained in a dispersion or absorption line. Unfortunately this scheme only works if our system is linear, precluding any saturation. Therefore we shall need some complement. Sometimes we shall use the Bloch phenomenological equations.

The *different situations*, in which the various "spin" packets are, reveal of course something about the *structure of matter*. Each situation is an energy level for the "spin" and the structure may be described by a hamiltonian. Solving the Schrödinger equation, one gets the transition rates and the transition frequencies. This can then be compared with the experiment, and we shall have to analyse how transition frequencies and transition rates are given by the dispersion or absorption line. Of course the resonance lines due to the different "spin" packets will be superposed and it may be a difficult task to disentangle the line. The "different situation" may, for example, be a function of a continuous parameter which makes the narrow elementary lines glue together into a single broad line. This is called inhomogeneous broadening, to be distinguished from the broadening by relaxation.

Our intention in the second chapter is thus to analyse how a paramagnetic resonance line provides information about matter. For clarity, we shall first consider an idealized system. The system has the fundamental properties of a real system, and it avoids dealing with all the complications at once. We deal with only one "spin" packet, analysing its relaxation function, transition frequency and transition rate. The system is linear, etc. This will be helpful in deducing some general properties of paramagnetic resonance lines. Of course, after this, real experimental conditions have to be taken into account. The most important are: the fact that the line is not properly resolved in isolated contributions from different "spin" packets and the fact that the system is not completely linear and stationary (there is some saturation and some parameters must be varied with time in order to measure as functions of these parameters).

2. The Paramagnetic Resonance Line of an Idealized System

2.1. A LINEAR STATIONARY SYSTEM

As is usually done in physics, we first assume a magnetic system to be *linear*. This is because we prefer to try first the simplest mathematical formalism. And indeed, in magnetism we arrive at many satisfactory results, which eventually need "correcting" by a second-order approximation. We also assume that the properties of our system do not change while we are studying it: we assume it to be *stationary*. This is another approximation. Both conditions together make it possible to compare different types of responses of a system. We shall deduce a relation between the *transient* response and *stationary* response (both of a stationary system).

Consider a sample to which we apply magnetic fields and let us study the magnetization. We first apply a field $\boldsymbol{b}_{\text{pulse}}$, equal to $\boldsymbol{B}_s$ during a time interval from t' to $t' + dt'$ and zero otherwise:

$$\boldsymbol{b}_{\text{pulse}}(t) = \boldsymbol{B}_s \quad \text{for} \quad t' \leqq t \leqq t' + dt'$$

$$\boldsymbol{b}_{\text{pulse}}(t) = 0 \quad \text{for} \quad t < t' \quad \text{and} \quad t' + dt' < t. \tag{1}$$

This pulse is represented in Fig. 2.1 (a). The fact that the system is *linear* may be stated as follows. The magnetization produced in the sample by a field is independent of the magnetization produced in the same sample by another field at the same or another time. The two magnetizations are simply added. In this case the magnetization produced by $\boldsymbol{b}_{\text{pulse}}$ is proportional to $\boldsymbol{B}_s$ and proportional to dt'—at least for a time delay $(t - t')$, long compared to dt'. Eventually we *consider* a system as *linear* in the first approximation for weak fields. If the properties of the system itself do not depend on time, we say the system is *stationary*. Then the magnetization produced by $\boldsymbol{b}_{\text{pulse}}$ does not depend on t' but only on $(t - t')$. Eventually we *consider* a system as *stationary* by coarse graining the time, i.e. by not considering details in a time interval less than a certain minimum. In fact such a coarse graining is always necessary for considering a real physical system as stationary.

For a linear stationary system, the magnetization $\boldsymbol{m}(t)$ produced by $\boldsymbol{b}_{\text{pulse}}$ may be expressed as a *tensor* $\alpha(t - t')$ which is independent of $\boldsymbol{B}_s$ and t':

$$d\boldsymbol{m}(t) = \frac{10^7}{4\pi}\alpha(t - t')\,\boldsymbol{B}_s\,dt'. \tag{2}$$

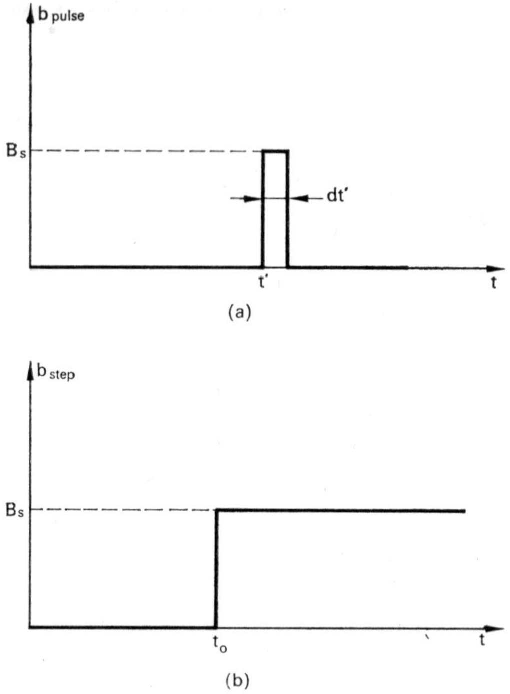

FIG. 2.1. (a) A constant field applied during an infinitesimal time interval. If $(\boldsymbol{B}_s\, dt')$ is unity, the magnetization due to this pulse will be:

$$\frac{10^7}{4\pi}\,\alpha(t-t').$$

(b) A step function field. If $\boldsymbol{B}_s$ is unity, the magnetization due to this field will be:

$$\frac{10^7}{4\pi}\,\varphi(t-t_0).$$

$(10^7/4\pi)\,\alpha(t - t')$ is the magnetization due to an infinitely short field pulse of unit integrated value.†

† Such an infinitely short pulse of unit integrated value may be represented by the delta function of Dirac. Here we consider it as the limit of $\boldsymbol{b}_{\text{pulse}}$ for $dt' \to 0$ and $\boldsymbol{B}_s$ increasing in the limit so that $\boldsymbol{B}_s dt'$ remains constant, equal to unity.

The magnetization due to an arbitrary field $\boldsymbol{b}(t')$ in a linear stationary system can be given by

$$\boldsymbol{m}(t) = \frac{10^7}{4\pi} \int_{-\infty}^{\infty} \alpha(t - t')\, \boldsymbol{b}(t')\, dt'. \tag{3}$$

Two special cases are to be considered for $\boldsymbol{b}(t')$. First, let $\boldsymbol{b}(t')$ be a step function raising from zero to $\boldsymbol{B}_s$ at $t' = t_0$. This is shown in Fig. 2.1 (b). Now

$$\boldsymbol{m}(t) = \frac{10^7}{4\pi} \int_{t_0}^{\infty} \alpha(t - t')\, dt' \,.\, \boldsymbol{B}_s \tag{4}$$

and comparing this with the definition of the *relaxation function* $\varphi(t - t_0)$, eq. (2) of Chapter 1, we find

$$\varphi(t - t_0) = \int_{t_0}^{\infty} \alpha(t - t')\, dt'. \tag{5}$$

Hence

$$\alpha(t) = \frac{d\varphi(t)}{dt} \tag{6}$$

and we shall call $\alpha(t)$ the *derived relaxation function*. Another important function is a monochromatic alternating field,

$$\boldsymbol{b}(t') = \mathscr{R}\, 2\boldsymbol{B}_1\, e^{i\omega t'}. \tag{7}$$

Since $\alpha(t)$ is defined as a real quantity [eq. (2)], we get

$$\boldsymbol{m}(t) = \frac{10^7}{4\pi} \mathscr{R} \int_{-\infty}^{\infty} \alpha(t - t')\, 2\boldsymbol{B} \,.\, e^{i\omega t'}\, dt'$$

$$= \frac{10^7}{4\pi} \mathscr{R} \left\{ \int_{-\infty}^{\infty} \alpha(t'')\, e^{-i\omega t''}\, dt'' \right\} 2\boldsymbol{B} \,.\, e^{i\omega t}. \tag{8}$$

If we compare this with the definition of the high-frequency susceptibility, eq. (5) of Chapter 1, we obtain

$$\chi(\omega) = \int_{-\infty}^{\infty} \alpha(t)\, e^{-i\omega t}\, dt = \int_{-\infty}^{\infty} (d\varphi/dt)\, e^{-i\omega t}\, dt. \tag{9}$$

$\chi(\omega)$ is the response to a unit amplitude monochromatic excitation of frequency $\omega/2\pi$. Equation (9) is a valuable relation between the relaxation function and the transfer function of a linear stationary system. (The relation is not restricted to magnetic systems, of course.)

2.2. A CAUSAL PASSIVE SYSTEM

In the preceding section we imposed on a system two conditions: it must be *linear* and *stationary*. These form the basis for defining any general relation between different types of response (here the transient and the stationary response). They also guarantee the time independence of $\chi(\omega)$, or the fact that a monochromatic excitation provides a monochromatic response (Abragam, 1961, p. 94). These are in fact two conditions that are never strictly realized but can often be assumed as valid in a first approximation. They imply a severe limitation from a practical point of view.

In order to say more about our system, we shall now also assume two other conditions that seem rather trivial. The first is that a finite excitation of the system must induce a finite response. It seems only a general precaution to exclude, for example, a system that would oscillate indefinitely in response to a triggering pulse. Therefore we say the system has to be *passive*. We do not enter into the ample philosophical discussion, e.g. in relation to cosmogenetic theories. The mathematical formulation is that the tensor $\alpha(\tau)$ has a finite Lebesgue square integrated value†

$$\int_{-\infty}^{\infty} [\alpha(t)]^2\, dt < \infty. \tag{10}$$

† In section 3.2 we shall give some comments on the mathematics we are using.

Another restriction is for the response (the magnetization) not to precede the cause (the exciting field). We say that our system is *causal.* Such a condition also does not seem to be a restriction. One naturally feels that no effect can precede the cause. This "natural feeling", however, is based on an overwhelming quantity of observations on a coarse scale, but one could ask if the principle of causality is still valid in some microscopic processes, e.g. of elementary particle physics. There exists much discussion on the subject and—apart from the many purely philosophical considerations—one generally tries to state sentences that are equivalent to the causality principle and that, on the other hand, are accessible to experiment, e.g. with elementary particles. If we define causality (Hilgevoord, 1962) as the existence of an ordering in time for cause and effect, or in general for any two events between which we consider a relation, then the mathematical expression will be

$$[\alpha(t) = 0 \quad \text{for } t < -\theta] \quad \text{or} \quad [\alpha(t) = 0 \quad \text{for } t > \theta]; \qquad \theta \text{ finite}. \tag{11}$$

This very general definition already leads to interesting consequences. However, our aim is not to prove causality by experiment but to use the consequences of a causality principle—admitted without proof—in order to deduce useful information for the quantities we are studying. Therefore, let us use a more familiar definition of causality, distinguishing cause and effect as so and taking $\theta = 0$. It will not be difficult to introduce a $\theta \neq 0$ in most formulas. We state:

$$\alpha(t) = 0 \quad \text{for} \quad t < 0. \tag{12}$$

2.3. The dispersion relation

We shall now prove a purely mathematical result based on the restrictions quoted in eq. (10) (passive system) and eq. (12) (causal system). If a real function $\alpha(t)$ is Lebesgue square integrable and vanishes for $t < 0$, then the real and imaginary parts of its Fourier transform

$\chi(\omega) = \chi'(\omega) - i\chi''(\omega)$ are Hilbert transforms of each other:

$$\chi'(\omega) = 2P_\omega \int_{-\infty}^{\infty} \frac{\chi''(\omega')}{\omega' - \omega} d\omega'/2\pi, \tag{13a}$$

$$\chi''(\omega) = -2P_\omega \int_{-\infty}^{\infty} \frac{\chi'(\omega')}{\omega' - \omega} d\omega'/2\pi, \tag{13b}$$

or in complex form

$$\chi(\omega) = 2iP_\omega \int_{-\infty}^{\infty} \frac{\chi(\omega')}{\omega' - \omega} d\omega'/2\pi. \tag{13c}$$

The operator P_ω is defined as

$$P_\omega \int_{-\infty}^{\infty} = \lim_{\varepsilon \to 0} \left\{ \int_{-\infty}^{\omega-\varepsilon} + \int_{\omega+\varepsilon}^{\infty} \right\}. \tag{14}$$

This statement is a part of Titchmarsh's theorem as given by Hilgevoord (1962). It is usually called the dispersion relation, and in practice it gives a relation between the real part ("dispersion") and the imaginary part ("absorption") of the response to a monochromatic excitation of a linear stationary causal and passive system. Such a relation between dispersion and absorption of light was long since verified experimentally by Roschdestwensky (1912). The relation as it is now known was deduced on theoretical grounds simultaneously and independently by Kramers [1927, $\chi'' = f(\chi')$] and by Kronig [1926, $\chi' = f(\chi'')$]. We may consider the transfer function $\chi(\omega)$ and the relaxation function $\alpha(t)$ as two equivalent ways of describing a *linear stationary* system. Observe that only for such a system may a transfer function and a relaxation function be defined. Then the dispersion relation is for the transfer function what the relation ($\alpha = 0$ for $t < 0$) together with $\left(\int |\alpha|^2 \, dt < \infty\right)$ is for the relaxation function, namely the expression of the fact that the *system* itself is causal and passive.

The proof of eq. (13) is as follows. $\chi(\omega)$ is defined as

$$\chi(\omega) \equiv \int_{-\infty}^{\infty} \alpha(t)\, e^{-i\omega t}\, dt \tag{15}$$

and this may be written as

$$\chi(\omega) = \int_{0}^{\infty} \alpha(t)\, e^{-i\omega t}\, dt \tag{16}$$

since $\alpha(t) = 0$ for $t < 0$. We have written eq. (15) like eq. (9). However, now we *define* $\chi(\omega)$ by eq. (15). Equation (9) then shows that $\chi(\omega)$ is the same as the transfer function defined by eq. (5) of Chapter 1.

The function

$$\chi(z) \equiv \int_{0}^{\infty} \alpha(t)\, e^{-izt}\, dt \tag{17}$$

of the complex variable $z = x + iy$ is analytic, since $\partial\chi/\partial x = \partial\chi/\partial iy$ (Cauchy–Riemann derivative test). Indeed, we may invert the order of integration and differentiation in calculating $\partial\chi/\partial x$ and $\partial\chi/\partial iy$ because $\alpha(t)$ is square integrable. Moreover, the limit of $\chi(z)$ for $|z| \to \infty$ and $y < 0$ is zero. Note that it is essential here for the integration of eq. (17) not to extend toward $-\infty$ (causality!). And $\chi(\infty + 0i) = \chi(-\infty + 0i) = 0$ because of the Lebesgue integrability of $\alpha(t)$ and hence of its Fourier transform. Consider now the integration path of Fig. 2.2. The function $\chi(z)/(z - z_0)$ is still analytic inside and on this path and hence the contour integral is zero. We may write

$$\lim_{\varrho\to 0} \left\{ \int_{-\infty}^{z_0-\varrho} + \int_{z_0+\varrho}^{\infty} \right\} \frac{\chi(z)}{z - z_0}\, dz + \lim_{R\to\infty} \int_{0}^{-\pi} \frac{\chi(z)}{\mathscr{R}^{i\varphi} - z_0}\, i\mathscr{R}^{i\varphi}\, d\varphi$$
$$+ \lim_{\varrho\to 0} \int_{-\pi}^{0} \frac{\chi(z)}{\varrho\, e^{i\varphi'}}\, i\varrho\, e^{i\varphi'}\, d\varphi' = 0. \tag{18}$$

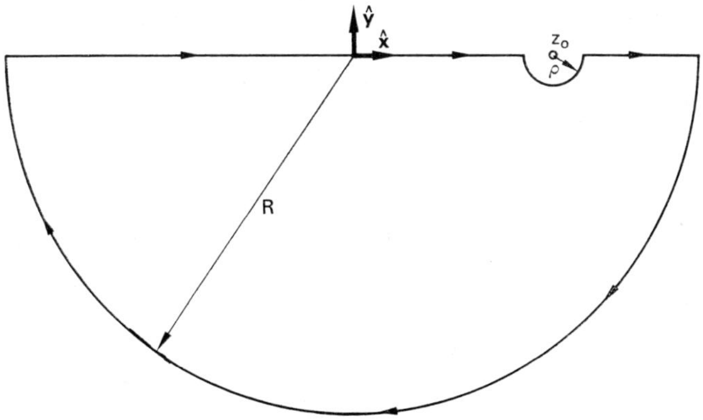

FIG. 2.2. An integration path in the complex plane $z = x + iy$.

Since $\chi(z)$ is zero at infinity and $\chi(z) = \chi(z_0)$ in the last integral, we shall obtain eq. (13c) by again puting ω' for z on the real axis and ω for z_0.

In eq. (13) we have negative values for ω. If ω represents a frequency this may be undesirable. Later we shall give a physical meaning to values of $\omega < 0$ (§ 4.2c). But here this is not necessary. Indeed, from eq. (16) we may deduce

$$\chi'(\omega) = \chi'(-\omega) \quad \text{and} \quad \chi''(\omega) = -\chi''(-\omega) \quad \text{or} \quad \chi(\omega) = \chi^*(-\omega) \tag{19}$$

since $\alpha(t)$ is real. If we introduce this in eqs. (13) we obtain

$$\chi'(\omega) = 4P_\omega \int_0^\infty \frac{\omega'\chi''(\omega')}{\omega'^2 - \omega^2} d\omega'/2\pi, \tag{20a}$$

$$\chi''(\omega) = -4\omega P_\omega \int_0^\infty \frac{\chi'(\omega')}{\omega'^2 - \omega^2} d\omega'/2\pi. \tag{20b}$$

2.4. Resonance and Drag

For any linear stationary causal and passive magnetic system we now have a relation between the dispersion $\chi'(\omega)$ and the absorption $\chi''(\omega)$. We also have a relation between the high-frequency susceptibility $\chi = \chi' - i\chi''$ and the relaxation function, eq. (9), which we now write again, taking into account that $\alpha(t) = 0$ for $t < 0$

$$\chi(\omega) = \int_0^\infty \alpha(t)\, e^{-i\omega t}\, dt = \int_0^\infty (d\varphi/dt)\, e^{-i\omega t}\, dt. \tag{21}$$

Knowing the function $\alpha(t)$ or $\varphi(t)$ completely, i.e. for any time, we can deduce $\chi'(\omega)$ and $\chi''(\omega)$ for any frequency. On the other hand we may invert eq. (9), writing the inverse transform

$$\alpha(t) = \int_{-\infty}^\infty \chi(\omega)\, e^{i\omega t}\, d\omega/2\pi \tag{22}$$

or with $\chi(\omega) = \chi^*(-\omega)$, eq. (19),

$$\alpha(t) = \int_0^\infty \chi(\omega)\, e^{i\omega t}\, d\omega/2\pi + \left[\int_0^\infty \chi(\omega')\, e^{i\omega' t}\, d\omega'/2\pi\right]^*$$

$$= 2\mathscr{R} \int_0^\infty \chi(\omega)\, e^{i\omega t}\, d\omega/2\pi. \tag{23}$$

Hence from the knowledge of $\chi'(\omega)$ or $\chi''(\omega)$ at any frequency we can deduce the complete $\chi(\omega)$ [using eqs. (13)] and thus the function $\alpha(t)$ and $\varphi(t)$ at any time. Incidentally, eq. (21) may be separated into

$$\chi' = \int_0^\infty \alpha(t) \cos \omega t\, dt, \tag{24a}$$

$$\chi'' = \int_0^\infty \alpha(t) \sin \omega t\, dt \tag{24b}$$

with inverse transforms

$$\alpha(t) = 4 \int_0^\infty \chi'(\omega) \cos \omega t\, d\omega/2\pi = 4 \int_0^\infty \chi''(\omega) \sin \omega t\, d\omega/2\pi. \tag{24c}$$

The last equality is, of course, a consequence of the dispersion relation. Equation (24c) is more explicit than eq. (23).

Unfortunately it is impossible to know $\alpha(t)$ or $\chi(\omega)$ over the whole time range or frequency range with infinite precision. And even a small error, e.g. in $\alpha(t)$ over a large time interval, gives an important error in $\chi(\omega)$ (Grant, 1964). We shall give an example in eq. (50) below. We can nevertheless try to deduce *some* information about $\alpha(t)$ or $\varphi(t)$ from a partial knowledge of $\chi(\omega)$, or vice versa. We can, for instance, develop $\alpha(t)$ in a Taylor expansion

$$\alpha(t) = \alpha(0) + t\alpha'(0) + t^2\alpha''(0)/2 + \cdots \tag{25}$$

and deduce $\alpha^{(n)}(0)$ by successive derivation of eq. (23) followed by a transition to the limit for $t \to 0$. The resulting integrals should then be derived from experiments on $\chi(\omega)$. However, we do not use this procedure.

The reason is that the results would be completely useless if the system had some definite eigenfrequency, as is the case for paramagnetic resonance in high fields. We shall make this clear by an example, which will also show us an alternative possibility.

An example

Let us consider a simple linear stationary causal passive system, a LR circuit [Fig. 2.3 (a)].

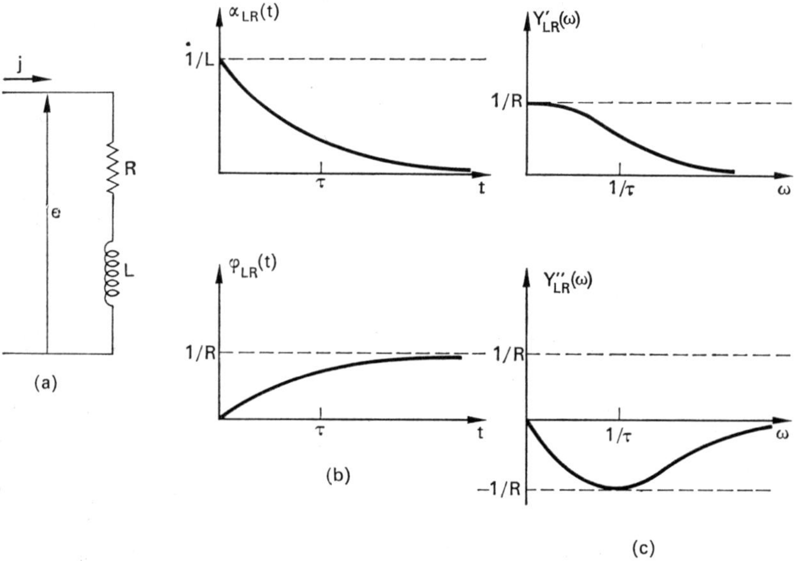

FIG. 2.3. (a) A LR circuit, a simple non-resonant linear system.
(b) Relaxation functions $\alpha(t)$ and $\varphi(t)$. The characteristic time is τ for both.

$$\alpha_{LR}(t) = L^{-1}\,e^{-t/\tau};\quad \varphi_{LR}(t) = R^{-1}(1 - e^{-t/\tau}).$$

(c) Transfer functions $Y'(\omega)$ and $Y''(\omega)$ of the LR circuit. The range over which both are important is $1/\tau$. $Y' = R^{-1}/(1+\omega^2\tau^2)$; $Y'' = -R^{-1}\omega\tau/(1+\omega^2\tau^2)$.

If we apply a voltage step to this circuit

$$e = 0 \quad \text{for} \quad t < 0, \tag{26}$$
$$e = E \quad \text{for} \quad t \geqq 0,$$

we obtain as a response a certain time-dependent current $j(t)$ which is proportional to the amplitude E of the step. Defining

$$\tau \equiv L/R \tag{27}$$

we get for $t > 0$

$$\tau \frac{\partial j}{\partial t} + j = \frac{E}{R} \qquad [t > 0] \tag{28}$$

and hence

$$j = \frac{E}{R}(1 - e^{-t/\tau}) \qquad [t > 0]. \tag{29}$$

Let us write the response to a *unit step* as $\varphi_{\text{LR}}(t)$

$$\varphi_{\text{LR}}(t) \equiv j(t)/E = \frac{1}{R}(1 - e^{-t/\tau}) \tag{30}$$

or

$$\varphi_{\text{LR}}(t) - \varphi_{\text{LR}}(\infty) = \frac{-1}{R} e^{-t/\tau}. \tag{31}$$

The response to a *unit pulse* is given by eq. (6)

$$\alpha_{\text{LR}}(t) = \frac{d\varphi_{\text{LR}}}{dt} = \frac{1}{\tau R} e^{-t/\tau} = \frac{1}{L} e^{-t/\tau}. \tag{32}$$

The transfer function of the system is called admittance in circuit theory. From eq. (21) we obtain

$$Y_{\text{LR}}(\omega) = Y'_{\text{LR}}(\omega) + iY''_{\text{LR}}(\omega) = \frac{1}{L} \int_0^\infty e^{-t/\tau} e^{-i\omega t} \, dt$$

$$= \frac{\tau}{L} \int_0^\infty e^{-(i\omega\tau + 1)t'} \, dt'$$

$$= \frac{1}{R} \frac{1}{1 + i\omega\tau} \int_0^{(i\omega\tau + 1)\infty} e^{-\sigma} \, d\sigma = \frac{1}{R} \frac{1}{1 + i\omega\tau} \int_0^\infty e^{-\sigma} \, d\sigma. \tag{33}$$

In this integration we have substituted first $t' = t/\tau$ and then $\sigma = (1 + i\omega\tau)\, t'$. The change in the integration path in the last integral is justified by Fig. 2.4. Since $e^{-\sigma}$ is analytic inside and on the contour drawn in the figure, the contour integral is zero. And the part of the contour at $|\sigma| = \infty$ contributes zero. Hence

$$Y_{LR}(\omega) = \frac{1}{R}\frac{1}{1+i\omega\tau} = \frac{1}{R}\left(\frac{1}{1+\omega^2\tau^2} - i\frac{\omega\tau}{1+\omega^2\tau^2}\right) \tag{34}$$

as expected from simple circuit theory. We have drawn this function in Fig. 2.3 (b). Observe that the relaxation function changes appreciably

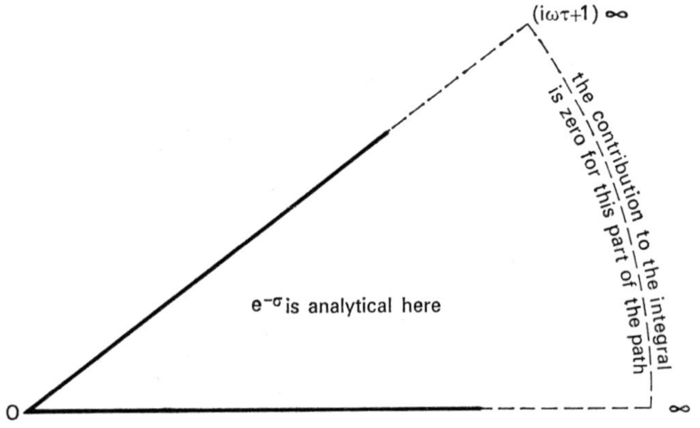

FIG. 2.4. Changing the integration path. The contour integral $\oint e^{-\sigma}\,d\sigma$ is zero, as well as the contribution to it from the path at $|\sigma| = \infty$. Hence,

$$\int_0^{(1+i\omega\tau)\infty} e^{-\sigma}\,d\sigma = \int_0^{\infty} e^{-\sigma}d\sigma + 0.$$

over a time τ and the transfer function over a frequency range of $1/\tau$. Let us call somewhat loosely τ the characteristic time of α and φ, and $1/\tau$ the line width of $Y(\omega)$.

Now let us introduce a capacitor in the circuit [Fig. 2.5 (a)]. We apply the same voltage step [(eq. (26)] and define [as in eq. (27)].

$$\tau \equiv L/R \tag{35}$$

and also now

$$\omega_0^2 = 1/(LC). \tag{36}$$

We shall use

$$\beta^2 \equiv \omega_0^2 - (2\tau)^{-2}. \tag{37}$$

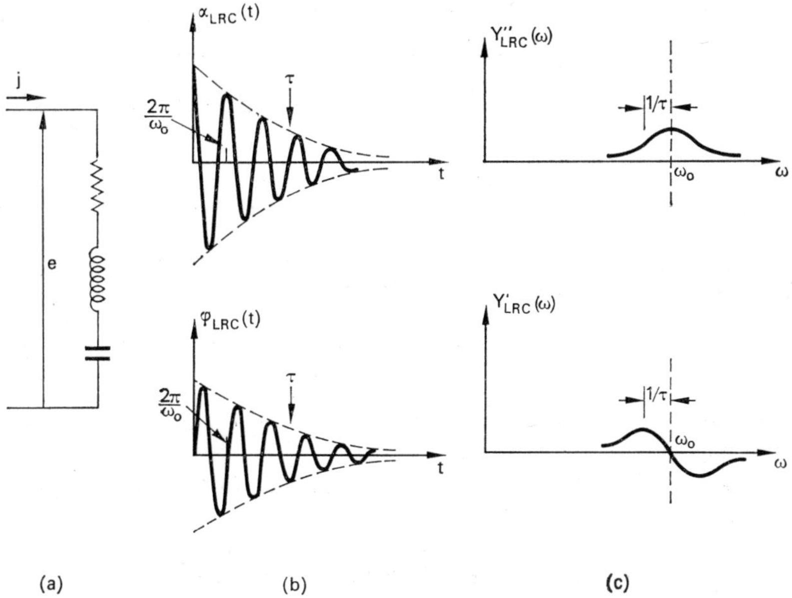

FIG. 2.5. (a) A LRC circuit, a simple resonant linear system. (b) The relaxation functions $\alpha_{LRC}(t)$ and $\varphi_{LRC}(t)$ and (c) transfer functions Y'_{LRC} and Y''_{LRC} for $\omega_0\tau \gg 1$.

For $t > 0$ we get

$$\frac{d^2j}{dt^2} + \frac{1}{\tau}\frac{dj}{dt} + \omega_0^2 j = 0 \qquad |t > 0|. \tag{38}$$

Again $\varphi_{LRC}(t) \equiv j(t)/E$. We solve the differential equation. For $\beta^2 \neq 0$ the result is:

$$\varphi_{LRC}(t) = \mathscr{R}\{A\, e^{p_+t} + B\, e^{p_-t}\} \tag{39}$$

with p_+ and p_- representing the roots of the equation $p^2 + p/\tau + \omega_0^2 = 0$ or

$$p_+ = \frac{-1}{2\tau} \pm i\beta. \tag{40}$$

Because $L\, dj/dt$ has to be finite, j must be zero for $t \to 0$. Hence $A = -B$ or

$$\varphi_{LRC}(t) = e^{-t/2\tau}\, \mathscr{R}\, A(e^{i\beta t} - e^{-i\beta t}). \tag{41}$$

And for $t \to 0$ the whole voltage E is over the inductor or $L\, d\varphi(0)/dt = 1$, from which $R\, 2i\beta A = 1/L$. The final result may be written as

$$\varphi_{\mathrm{LRC}}(t) = \frac{1}{2i\beta L}(e^{i\beta t} - e^{-i\beta t})\, e^{-t/2\tau} \tag{42a}$$

or as

$$\varphi_{\mathrm{LRC}}(t) = \frac{1}{\beta L}\, e^{-t/2\tau} \sin \beta t. \tag{42b}$$

Equation (42 a) may be more expressive for $\beta^2 < 0$ while eq. (42 b) is clearer for $\beta^2 > 0$. Incidentally, for $\beta = 0$ one has

$$\varphi_{\mathrm{LRC}}(t) = (A' + B't)\, e^{-t/2\tau} = \frac{t}{L}\, e^{-t/2\tau} \tag{43}$$

using the same condition $d\varphi_{\mathrm{LRC}}(0)/dt = 1/L$ and $\varphi_{\mathrm{LRC}}(0) = 0$ for the determination of A' and B'.

One can now calculate $\alpha_{\mathrm{LRC}}(t)$ from eq. (6), $\alpha_{\mathrm{LRC}} = d\varphi_{\mathrm{LRC}}/dt$. Together with eq. (42 b), it gives

$$\begin{aligned} \alpha_{\mathrm{LRC}}(t) &= \frac{1}{\beta L}\left(\frac{-1}{2\tau} \sin \beta t + \beta \cos \beta t\right) e^{-t/2\tau} \\ &= \frac{\omega_0}{\beta} \cos(\beta t + \eta)\, \frac{1}{L}\, e^{-t/2\tau} \end{aligned} \tag{44}$$

with

$$\tan \eta = 1/(2\beta\tau). \tag{45}$$

And from eq. (21) one may calculate $Y(\omega)$

$$Y_{\mathrm{LRC}}(\omega) = \int_0^\infty \alpha_{\mathrm{LRC}}(t)\, e^{-i\omega t}\, dt. \tag{46}$$

Here it is easier to use eq. (42 a). The calculus is straightforward (using an integration like in Fig. 2.4) and the result is

$$Y_{\mathrm{LRC}}(\omega) = \frac{1}{R}\, \frac{1}{1 + i\omega\left[1 - \dfrac{\omega_0^2}{\omega^2}\right]\tau} \tag{47}$$

as expected by ordinary circuit theory.

Consider first the case $\omega_0\tau \ll 1$. This means $C \gg L/R^2$, i.e. a very large capacitor. In the limit as $\omega_0\tau \to 0$ we must have $C \to \infty$ or a short circuit, i.e. the situation described above without the capacitor. Indeed for $\omega_0\tau \ll 1$ we have $i\beta \approx \frac{1}{2}\tau$ and $2i\beta L = R$. Equations (42) and (44) then become

$$\varphi_{\text{LRC}}(t) \approx \frac{1}{R}(1 - e^{-t/\tau}); \quad \alpha_{\text{LRC}}(t) \sim \frac{1}{L} e^{-t/\tau} \quad [\omega_0\tau \ll 1]. \tag{48}$$

On the other hand, we have for $\omega_0 \ll \omega$ [see eq. (47)]

$$Y_{\text{LRC}}(\omega) \approx \frac{1}{R} \frac{1}{1 + i\omega\tau} \qquad [\omega_0 \ll \omega]. \tag{49}$$

We find that

$$\left.\begin{aligned} \varphi_{\text{LRC}} &\approx \varphi_{\text{LR}} \\ \alpha_{\text{LRC}} &\approx \alpha_{\text{LR}} \end{aligned}\right\} \quad \text{for} \quad \omega_0 \ll 1/\tau \tag{50a, 50b}$$

$$Y_{\text{LRC}} \approx Y_{\text{LR}} \qquad \text{for} \quad \omega_0 \ll \omega \tag{50c}$$

The condition $\omega_0\tau \ll 1$ is a restriction regarding the circuit, i.e. $C \gg L/R^2$. For this circuit φ_{LR} is a good approximation at any time, as is α_{LR}. However, the Fourier transform of α, i.e. Y_{LR}, is *not* a good approximation of the actual transfer function Y_{LRC} at any frequency! (See our comment after eq. (24).) $Y_{\text{LR}} \simeq Y_{\text{LRC}}$ only for a restricted range of the variable ω, namely for $\omega \gg \omega_0$. For example, for $\omega = \omega_0$ one has $Y_{\text{LRC}} = 1/R$ and

$$Y_{\text{LR}} = \frac{1}{R} \frac{1}{1 + i\omega_0\tau}.$$

Although $\omega_0\tau \ll 1$ there is a great difference between $Y''_{\text{LRC}} = 0$ and $Y''_{\text{LR}} = i\omega_0\tau/(R + R\omega_0^2\tau^2)$. Apart from this phase shift in Y_{LRC}, however, one may assume $Y_{\text{LRC}} \simeq Y_{\text{LR}}$ for any ω, since for $\omega \gtrsim \omega_0$ the modulus of $i\omega_0\tau$ is negligible compared with unity.

Now we turn to the case $\omega_0\tau \gg 1$. Then $\beta \approx \omega_0$ and $\beta L \approx \sqrt{L/C} \approx \omega_0 L$. Hence

$$\varphi_{\text{LRC}}(t) \approx \frac{1}{\omega_0 L} e^{-t/2\tau} \sin \omega_0 t \tag{51a}$$

$$[\omega_0\tau \gg 1]$$

$$\alpha_{\text{LRC}}(t) \approx \frac{1}{L} e^{-t/2\tau} \cos \omega_0 t. \tag{51b}$$

The small phase shift $\eta \simeq \frac{1}{2}\beta\tau \ll 1$ [eq. (45)] may be neglected. On the other hand,

$$Y_{LRC}(\omega) = \frac{1}{R}\frac{1}{1 + i(\omega - \omega_0)[1 + (\omega_0/\omega)\tau]}. \tag{51c}$$

Let us define

$$\omega_d \equiv \omega - \omega_0. \tag{52}$$

For $|\omega_d| \ll \omega_0$ we have

$$Y_{LRC}(\omega_0 + \omega_d) = \frac{1}{R}\frac{1}{1 + 2i\omega_d\tau} \qquad [\omega_0 > |\omega_d|]. \tag{53}$$

We have drawn φ_{LRC}, α_{LRC} and Y_{LRC} in Fig. 2.5 (b).

Let φ_{2LR}, α_{2LR} and Y_{2LR} refer to an LR circuit of relaxation time 2τ, just as φ_{LR}, α_{LR} and Y_{LR} refer to the LR circuit of Fig. 2.3. Then we may write

$$\left.\begin{aligned} (\omega_0\tau)\frac{[\varphi_{LRC}(t) - \varphi_{LRC}(\infty)]}{\sin\omega_0 t} &= \varphi_{2LR}(t) - \varphi_{2LR}(\infty) \\ \frac{\alpha_{LRC}}{\cos\omega_0 t} &= \alpha_{2LR} \end{aligned}\right\} \quad [\omega_0\tau \gg 1]$$

$$Y_{LRC}(\omega_0 + \omega_d) = Y_{2LR}(\omega_d) \qquad [\omega_0 \gg |\omega_d|]$$

(54)

Instead of $\varphi_{LRC}(t) - \varphi_{LRC}(\infty)$ and $\alpha_{LRC}(t)$ we may introduce envelope functions, i.e. the functions divided by $(\omega_0\tau)^{-1}\sin\omega_0 t$ and $\cos\omega_0 t$ respectively. On the other hand, we may introduce a shifted function for Y_{LRC}. The envelope relaxation functions are then related to the shifted transfer function, as the relaxation functions $\varphi_{2LR}(t)$, $\varphi_{2LR}(\infty)$ and $\alpha_{2LR}(t)$ of a non-resonant circuit of double time-constant are to its transfer function Y_{2LR}, at least for frequencies in the neighbourhood of ω_0. Comparison of Fig. 2.3 (b) and Fig. 2.5 (b) may be helpful to see what happens. Let us consider why these propositions are so useful. Return to eq. (23). In our case it is

$$\alpha(t) = 2\mathscr{R} \int_0^\infty Y(\omega)\, e^{i\omega t}\, d\omega/2\pi = 2 \int_0^\infty Y'(\omega) \cos \omega t\, d\omega/2\pi$$

$$- 2 \int_0^\infty Y''(\omega) \sin \omega t\, d\omega/2\pi. \tag{55}$$

We suggested that the sucessive derivatives, in the limit as $t \to 0$, may give a relation between a Taylor expansion of $\alpha(t)$ around $t = 0$ and certain integrals over $Y(\omega)$. But the successive derivatives of $\alpha_{\text{LRC}}(t)$ in the limit as $t \to 0$ will in practice only reveal the $\cos \omega_0 t$ of α_{LRC} if $\omega_0 \tau \gg 1$, and will tell us nothing about the shape of the *envelope* of α_{LRC}. On the other hand, we may now already see that

$$\lim_{t \to 0} \frac{\partial^{2m}}{\partial t^{2m}} 2 \int_0^\infty Y'(\omega) \cos \omega t\, d\omega/2\pi$$

$$= \lim_{t \to 0} 2 \int_0^\infty (-1)^m \omega^{2m} \cos \omega t\, Y'(\omega)\, d\omega/2\pi$$

$$= 2 \int_0^\infty (-1)^m \omega^{2m}\, Y'(\omega)\, d\omega/2\pi \tag{56}$$

at least for a well-behaved† function $Y'(\omega)$.

Now look at Fig. 2.5 (b). Since $Y'(\omega)$ is only significant around $\omega \simeq \omega_0$ we have

$$\int_0^\infty Y'(\omega)\, \omega^{2m}\, d\omega/2\pi \approx \omega_0^{2m} \int_0^\infty Y'(\omega)\, d\omega/2\pi \tag{57}$$

and the successive derivatives form a power series in ω_0, without giving any information about the shape of $Y'(\omega_0 + \omega_d)$.

† We shall be more rigorous with the mathematics later.

Now look at the eqs. (54). We may use a relation between the *envelope* of the relaxation functions and the *shifted* transfer function of our LRC circuit, similar to eq. (23), since eq. (23) holds for α_{2LR} and Y_{2LR}.

We shall not go into more details about this example. The emphasis was on the general idea just mentioned. We had better return now to paramagnetic resonance.

Resonance and drag in a paramagnetic system

The magnetization due to a field pulse in a paramagnetic sample will give us a relaxation function $\alpha(t)$ or $\varphi(t)$, similar to α_{LR} or φ_{LR}. We shall also have a characteristic time τ, to be defined more accurately below, giving the range over which $\alpha(t)$ or $\varphi(t)$ extends in time. Also, we may analyse the sample by means of a transfer function $\chi(\omega)$, the range of which, over the ω-axis, will be $1/\tau$.

It happens that, just as in our LRC circuit, a paramagnetic sample in a strong static field also has a resonance element: the Larmor precession at a frequency ω_0, proportional to the static field. Hence we must expect the functions $\alpha(t)$, $\varphi(t)$ and $\chi(\omega)$ to be somewhat like those in Fig. 2.5 (b).

With the high-frequency field parallel to the static field, one does not observe the resonance, because the Larmor precession has no vibrating component parallel to the static field. One observes a complex HF susceptibility line at zero frequency, just as in our LR circuit. The line is broadened over a region given substantially by $1/\tau$, τ being the characteristic time of the corresponding relaxation function [see Fig. 2.3(b)]. Such lines give very useful information about the relaxation of the paramagnetic centres in matter and this relaxation had been studied (principally by the Gorter group in Leiden) long before paramagnetic resonance was discovered.

With the static field normal to the analysing field, one observes resonance, i.e. the behaviour of $\alpha(t)$, $\varphi(t)$ and $\chi(\omega)$ is as in Fig. 2.5 (b), if the static field is so high that $\omega_0 \gg 1/\tau$. This means that the Larmor frequency ω_0 has to be much larger than the line width. The width of the resonance lines is also due to relaxation, just as the width of the line of Fig. 2.5 (b) is due to the resistance R in the circuit. Therefore it is incorrect to designate the non-resonance experiments about relaxation simply by "relaxation experiments" (as they were named by Gorter before the discovery of paramagnetic resonance). We shall use the name "drag" for non-resonant relaxation, following Van Gerven (1963, p. 148).

Since the Larmor frequency ω_0 in paramagnetic systems is proportional to the static field, we can of course also study the drag with the analysing HF field orthogonal to the static field, taking this static field so low that $\omega_0 \ll 1/\tau$. This case has been studied by Van Gerven (1963) for some special absorption lines. In this book we shall only be interested in high fields, but the fact that $\omega_0\tau$ is only 10 or 100 and not infinite will oblige us to make some corrections. On the other hand, we shall sometimes have to consider corrections due to longitudinal drag.

2.5. The relaxation in a single paramagnetic resonance line

Let us now return to eqs. (21) to (24)

$$\chi(\omega) = \int_0^\infty \alpha(t)\, e^{-i\omega t}\, dt = \int_0^\infty (d\varphi/dt)\, e^{-i\omega t}\, dt,$$

$$\alpha(t) = 2\mathscr{R} \int_0^\infty \chi(\omega)\, e^{i\omega t}\, d\omega/2\pi = 4 \int_0^\infty \chi' \cos \omega t\, d\omega/2\pi$$

$$= 4 \int_0^\infty \chi'' \sin \omega t\, d\omega/2\pi \qquad [t > 0].$$

The second term of eq. (21) may be integrated by parts. We write $\varphi - \varphi(\infty)$ instead of φ and find

$$\chi(\omega) = [\varphi(t) - \varphi(\infty)]\, e^{-i\omega t} \Big|_0^\infty + i\omega \int_0^\infty [\varphi(t) - \varphi(\infty)]\, e^{-i\omega t}\, dt. \qquad (58)$$

Since $\varphi(t) = 0$ for $t < 0$ and $d\varphi(t)/dt = \alpha(t)$ is finite one has

$$\varphi(0) = 0. \qquad (59)$$

On the other hand, $\varphi(\infty) = \chi_s$ from eq. (6) of Chapter 1. Hence

$$\chi(\omega) - \chi_s = i\omega \int_0^\infty [\varphi(t) - \varphi(\infty)]\, e^{-i\omega t}\, dt$$

$$= \omega \int_0^\infty [\varphi(t) - \varphi(\infty)] \sin \omega t\, dt$$

$$+ i\omega \int_0^\infty [\varphi(t) - \varphi(\infty)] \cos \omega t\, dt. \quad (60)$$

And the inverse is

$$\varphi(t) - \varphi(\infty) = 4 \int_0^\infty \frac{(\chi' - \chi_s)}{\omega} \sin \omega t\, d\omega/2\pi$$

$$= -4 \int_0^\infty \frac{\chi''}{\omega} \cos \omega t\, d\omega/2\pi$$

$$= 2\mathcal{R} \int_0^\infty \frac{[\chi(\omega) - \chi_s]}{i\omega} e^{i\omega t} d\omega/2\pi \qquad [t > 0]. \quad (61)$$

All this is subject to the condition, which we shall assume satisfied, that $\varphi(t) - \varphi(\infty)$ is Lebesgue integrable (or that $[\chi(\omega) - \chi_s]/i\omega$ is Lebesgue integrable). We may still use Dirichlet's integral,

$$\int_0^\infty \frac{\sin \omega t}{\omega} d\omega/2\pi = \frac{1}{4}$$

for $t > 0$, in eq. (61). Then, since $\chi_s = \varphi(\infty)$, one has

$$\left\{ \begin{aligned} \varphi(t) &= 4 \int_0^\infty \frac{\chi'}{\omega} \sin \omega t\, d\omega/2\pi \\ \varphi(t) - \varphi(\infty) &= -4 \int_0^\infty \frac{\chi''}{\omega} \cos \omega t\, d\omega/2\pi \end{aligned} \right. \qquad [t > 0]. \quad (62)$$

Equations (21) to (24) and (58) to (62) are exactly satisfied for linear stationary systems, without any further approximation. They are, however, useless in that form if a resonant element is present in the system. For a system with an eigenfrequency† ω_0 we define $\varphi_0(t)$ by $\varphi(\infty) - \varphi(t) = \varphi_0(t) \cos(\omega_0 t + \eta_\varphi)$. $\varphi(\infty) - \varphi(t)$ is the response to a unit step excitation *decreasing* from one to zero at $t = 0$. For $t = 0$ one has $[\varphi(\infty) - \varphi(t)]_{t\to+0} = \varphi(\infty) = \chi_s$ [see eq. (59)]. If the system has a resonant element, the response will be a decay modulated at resonance frequency. We put $\varphi_0(t)$ for the decay and $\cos(\omega_0 t + \eta_\varphi)$ for the modulation. The phase η_φ has to be adjusted to the situation at $t \to 0$. Since we suppose φ_0 maximum for $t \to 0$ we must take $\eta_\varphi = 0$, so that $\varphi_0(0) = \varphi(\infty) - \varphi(0) = \chi_s$. Hence

$$\varphi(\infty) - \varphi(t) \equiv \varphi_0(t) \cos \omega_0 t; \qquad \varphi_0(0) = \chi_s. \tag{63}$$

We also define $\alpha_0(t)$ by

$$\alpha(t) = \alpha_0(t) \sin(\omega_0 t + \eta_\alpha). \tag{64}$$

By eq. (1.6) of Chapter 1 one now has

$$\alpha_0(t) \sin(\omega_0 t + \eta_\alpha) = \frac{d\varphi}{dt} = -\frac{-d\varphi_0(t)}{dt} \cos \omega_0 t$$

$$+ \omega_0 \varphi_0(t) \sin \omega_0 t$$

$$= \sqrt{(\omega_0\varphi_0)^2 + \left(\frac{d\varphi_0(t)}{dt}\right)^2} \sin\left[\omega_0 t + \arctan \frac{-d\varphi_0/dt}{\omega_0\varphi_0}\right]. \tag{65}$$

If φ_0 is a pure exponential decay, $\varphi_0 \propto e^{-t/\tau}$, as in the case of the LRC circuit, then it follows that

$$\eta_\alpha = \arctan 1/\omega_0\tau \approx 1/\omega_0\tau \ll 1 \tag{66}$$

for a highly resonant system. And

$$\alpha_0(t) = \omega_0\varphi_0 \left(1 + \frac{1}{2} \frac{1}{(\omega_0\tau)^2} + \ldots\right) \approx \omega_0\varphi_0. \tag{67}$$

† A system may have more than one eigenfrequency. We first consider a simple system in order to deal with relaxation. Another section will deal with the problem of several eigenfrequencies.

If φ_0 is not purely exponential, η_α will be time-dependent, i.e. the decay frequency will not be constant. If fact we assumed η_φ itself to be time-independent without any justification. We only may state that η_φ and η_α are *nearly* constant for $\omega_0\tau \ll 1$, i.e. that the decay frequency is *nearly* constant and that η_φ or η_α change less than π over about $\omega_0\tau$ times the relaxation time. The argument is that for a Gaussian decay, $\varphi_0 \propto e^{-(\pi/4)t^2/\tau^2}$, $\eta_\varphi = (\arctan \pi t/2\tau)/\omega_0\tau$ and that in practice the relaxation behaves like a Gaussian or an exponential decay or something in between, as we shall explain later (§ 5.2). Incidentally, for a Gaussian shape $\eta_\alpha(0) = 0$.

We shall assume that, for $\omega_0\tau \ll 1$,

$$\eta_\varphi(t) = \eta_\varphi(0) = \eta_\alpha(t) = \eta_\alpha(0) = 0 \tag{68}$$

and

$$\alpha_0(t) = \omega_0\varphi_0(t) \tag{69}$$

and

$$\alpha(t) = \alpha_0(t) \sin \omega_0 t. \tag{70}$$

In the absence of relaxation, i.e. with $\tau \to \infty$, $\alpha(t)$ would simply be a constant times $\sin \omega_0 t$. For an actual system, the amplitude of the sine function decreases and we assume that many oscillations occur before this decrease becomes important, i.e. $\tau \gg 1/\omega_0$. τ is the relaxation time of $\alpha_0(t)$, to be defined more accurately below.

Let us now introduce the definition eq. (70) in eq. (21):

$$\chi(\omega) = \int_0^\infty \alpha_0(t) \frac{e^{i\omega_0 t} - e^{-i\omega_0 t}}{2i} e^{-i\omega t}\, dt$$

$$= \frac{1}{2i} \int_0^\infty \alpha_0(t)\, e^{-i(\omega-\omega_0)t} - \frac{1}{2i} \int_0^\infty \alpha_0(t)\, e^{-i(\omega+\omega_0)t}\, dt. \tag{71}$$

For $|\omega - \omega_0| \ll \omega_0$ the second integral of the second expression may be neglected when compared to the first term of this expression because of the rapid variations of $e^{i(\omega+\omega_0)t}$ over a range $1/(\omega + \omega_0)$ much less than τ, since $\omega_0\tau \gg 1$. On the other hand, only for $|\omega - \omega_0|$ of the order of $1/\tau$ will there be a significant contribution to $\chi(\omega)$. The function $\chi(\omega)$ will be enhanced around $\omega = \omega_0$ over a range $\omega - \omega_0 \approx \pm 1/\tau$ on the ω-axis. This fact has already been emphasized for the LRC circuit admittance Y_{LRC} in Fig. 2.5.

We have already defined ω_d in eq. (52) by

$$\omega_d = \omega - \omega_0 .$$

Now

$$\chi(\omega_0 + \omega_d) = \frac{1}{2i} \int_0^\infty \alpha_0(t)\, e^{-i\omega_d t}\, dt \qquad [\omega_d \ll \omega_0;\ \omega_0\tau \gg 1]. \quad (72)$$

If eq. (72) were strictly valid for ω_d from $-\infty$ to $+\infty$, we could write the inverse transform directly as

$$\alpha_0(t) = \mathcal{R}\, 2i \int_{-\infty}^{\infty} \chi(\omega_0 + \omega_d)\, e^{i\omega_d t}\, d\omega_d \qquad \text{[false]} \quad (73)$$

since $\chi(\omega)$ is Lebesgue square integrable. It happens, however, that eq. (72) does *not* hold for any ω_d. For example, for $\omega_d \simeq -2\omega_0$ one should retain the second integral of the second expression of eq. (71) instead of the first. Therefore eq. (73) is false. However, one may consider a truncated transfer function $\tilde{\chi}(\omega_0 + \omega_d)$ *defined* by

$$\tilde{\chi}(\omega_0 + \omega_d) = \frac{1}{2i} \int_0^\infty \alpha_0(t)\, e^{-\omega_d t}\, dt \qquad [\text{all } \omega_d;\ \omega_0\tau \gg 1]. \quad (74)$$

Now, of course,

$$\alpha_0(t) = \mathcal{R}\, 2i \int_{-\infty}^{\infty} \tilde{\chi}(\omega_0 + \omega_d)\, e^{i\omega_d t}\, d\omega_d/2\pi \quad (75)$$

$$[t > 0;\ \text{correct by definition}]$$

and on the other hand,

$$\tilde{\chi}(\omega_0 + \omega_d) \approx \chi(\omega_0 + \omega_d) \qquad [|\omega_d| \ll \omega_0]. \quad (76)$$

The distinction between χ and $\tilde{\chi}$ is important in two respects. First we shall see that χ has a meaning for $\omega \simeq -\omega_0$ as well as for $\omega \simeq \omega_0$ in most experimental arrangements (in linearly polarized HF fields). In this case $\tilde{\chi}$ is the part of χ that refers to $\omega \simeq \omega_0$, without the part for $\omega \simeq -\omega_0$. Secondly $\tilde{\chi}$ is in any case only an *approximation* of χ, even in the range $\omega > 0$, so that any claim for high accuracy in integration formulas is meaningless. We shall have to refer to these facts below. For reference purposes, we summarize them here as

$$\tilde{\chi} \approx 0 \quad (\omega \approx -\omega_0), \tag{77}$$

$$\tilde{\chi} \approx \chi \quad (\omega \approx \omega_0). \tag{78}$$

An important remark: from eq. (74) we deduce that

$$\tilde{\chi}(\omega_0 + \omega_d) = -\tilde{\chi}^*(\omega_0 - \omega_d), \tag{79}$$

i.e. $\tilde{\chi}'(\omega + \omega_d)$ is antisymmetric around ω_0 and $\tilde{\chi}''(\omega_0 + \omega_d)$ is symmetric. Such a symmetry of line is shown in Fig. 2.6. But what about

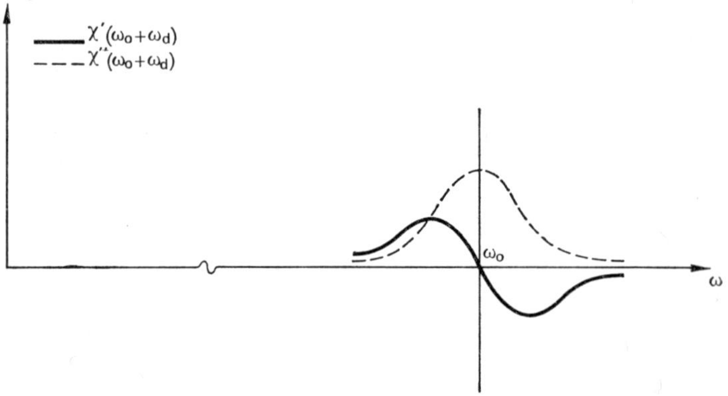

FIG. 2.6. Symmetric absorption line and antisymmetric dispersion line, with ω_0 as symmetry reference.

an asymmetric line? We must confess that we have *introduced* this symmetry somewhere in our development, namely in eq. (68). If we put $\eta_\alpha = \pi/2$ instead of zero, i.e. $\alpha(t) = \alpha_0(t) \cos \omega_0 t$, we arrive at $\tilde{\chi}(\omega_0 + \omega_d) = +\tilde{\chi}^*(\omega_0 - \omega_d)$ instead of eq. (79). The phase η_α is a property of the system under consideration. For example, for the LRC circuit in which current is measured as a function of an exciting voltage, the phase η_α is in fact $\pi/2$ and $Y(\omega_0 + \omega_d) = Y(\omega_0 - \omega_d)^*$ in Fig. 2.5 (c). The correspondence is between $i\chi$ and Y and not between χ and Y. Note that $i\chi$ is $\pi/2$ out of phase with respect to χ. It happens that for a magnetic system with a simple resonance frequency ω_0 we have $\chi''(\omega_0 + \omega_d) = \chi''(\omega_0 - \omega_d)$. This is a property of the physical system (Abragam, 1961, p. 108). It then follows that $\eta_\alpha = 0$ will give the best agreement between χ and $\tilde{\chi}$, in accordance with our former argument that $\eta_\alpha \ll 1$. (For $\varphi_0 \propto e^{-t/\tau}$, $\eta_\alpha \neq 0$ and hence χ'' could not be exactly symmetric. But there are still other reasons for which a strict Lorentzian shape is impossible in practice; see § 5.2.)

Another remark is that the dispersion relation, eqs. (13), holds for $i\tilde{\chi}(\omega_0 + \omega_d)$ *as a function of* ω_d since $\alpha_0(t)$ is Lebesgue square integrable. This is simply a matter of mathematics, as explained in § 2.3.

We may still use $\varphi(t)$ instead of $\alpha(t)$. One writes simply eq. (69)

$$\alpha_0 = \omega_0 \varphi_0(t),$$

but one could also substitute $\varphi_0(t) \cos \omega_0 t$ in eq. (60), just as we substituted $\alpha_0(t) \sin \omega_0 t$ in eq. (21). The result is the same if one makes the approximation $\omega \simeq \omega_0$ in the factor $i\omega$ before the integral of eq. (60) and if one neglects $\chi_s/i\omega$ together with $\int_{-\infty}^{\infty} \varphi_0(t)\, e^{-i(\omega+\omega_0)}\, dt$ instead of only the integral as in eq. (71). This corresponds to neglecting $d\varphi_0/dt$ in eq. (65).

For further analysis we shall no longer use the mark on $\tilde{\chi}$ as in eq. (74). One must, however, be aware of the two limitations, eqs. (77) and (78). By $\chi(\omega_0 + \omega_d)$ we mean the truncated function, unless otherwise indicated. Finally we write eq. (74) and eq. (75) separated, using eq. (79) and the fact that $\int_{-\infty}^{\infty}$ of an odd function is zero. (Remember that eq. (79) too is an approximation! It requires eq. (68).)

$$\chi'(\omega_0 + \omega_d) = -\tfrac{1}{2} \int_0^{\infty} \alpha_0(t) \sin \omega_d t\, dt, \tag{80a}$$

$$\chi''(\omega_0 + \omega_d) = +\tfrac{1}{2} \int_0^{\infty} \alpha_0(t) \cos \omega_d t\, dt, \tag{80b}$$

$$\alpha_0(t) = -8 \int_0^{\infty} \chi'(\omega_0 + \omega_d) \sin \omega_d t\, d\omega_d/2\pi \quad [t > 0], \tag{80c}$$

$$\alpha_0(t) = +8 \int_0^{\infty} \chi''(\omega_0 + \omega_d) \cos \omega_d t\, d\omega_d/2\pi \quad [t > 0]. \tag{80d}$$

2.6. The Structure of a Resolved Paramagnetic Resonance Line

We supposed in the preceding section that the paramagnetic resonance line has only one eigenfrequency. We considered only one "spin" packet. This was helpful in considering what happens with relaxation. Let us now consider various eigenfrequencies, $\omega_{01}, \omega_{02}, \omega_{03}, \ldots, \omega_{0k}$. Each corresponds to a certain "spin" packet, a collection of "spins" interacting with each other in a given average situation (see the introduction to this chapter).

If superposition holds, then the relaxation function as well as the resonance line of the whole system will be the sum of the lines due to each packet alone. And here superposition holds if there is no cross-relaxation, i.e. if what happens in one packet is independent of what happens in another packet. This may be compared with the admittance of a combination of LRC circuits, as shown in Fig. 2.7. The response

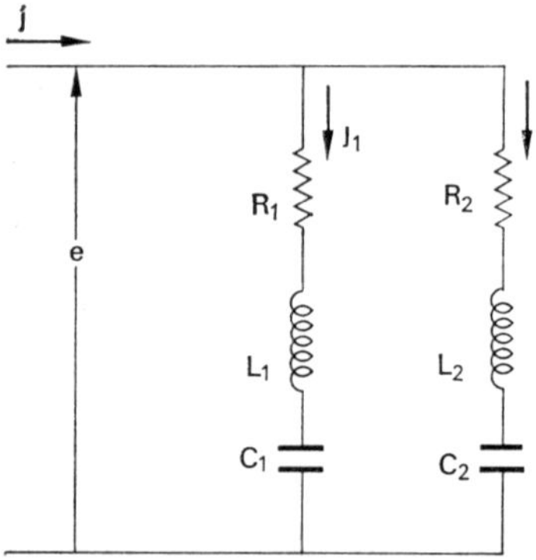

Fig. 2.7. The admittance of two circuits in parallel is the sum of the individual admittances only if no interaction occurs between the circuits.

$j(t)$ to a voltage step will be the sum of the responses $j_1(t)$ and $j_2(t)$ taken separately, unless there is, for instance, a mutual inductance between the two coils. In the case of no interaction, the total admittance is also the sum of both partial admittances, $y = y_1 + y_2$.

It happens that in an experiment we measure all the contributions of the various "spin" packets simultaneously.† We have only the sum of the lines and it may be quite a complicated problem to find the components.

However, if the width of each component resonance line is much smaller than the separation between the lines, then the contributions will be separated along the frequency axis. In the neighbourhood of each eigenfrequency the contribution of all the "spin" packets at other eigenfrequencies will be negligible. We say that we have a well-resolved line. The relaxation function, on the other hand, will last long enough to display a beat between the eigenfrequencies, since the relaxation time in this case is longer than the (difference between eigenfrequencies)$^{-1}$.

A well-resolved line reveals a spectrum of eigenfrequencies. This may be a valuable source of information about magnetic fields in matter. One incorporates, for example, nuclei of known magnetomechanical ratio in matter and investigates the field at various points in a molecule by means of the eigenfrequency spectrum due to these nuclei. This n.m.r. technique is used extensively in chemistry. In e.s.r. the situation in generally not so clear because lines are frequently not narrow compared to their separation. We shall therefore continue the discussion below in a separate section about composite lines.

3. Information about the Structure and Relaxation in the Paramagnetic Resonance Dispersion and Absorption Line

3.1. Introduction

Emphasizing the role of the eigenfrequency in a relaxation function $\alpha(t)$ or $\varphi(t)$, we could separate the information into two parts: a resonance frequency ω_0, and a relaxation $\alpha_0(t)$ or $\varphi_0(t)$. This frequency will easily be recognized in the transfer function, and we must keep in mind that there may be various eigenfrequencies. Apart from the location of these eigenfrequencies, it will be important to know how many "spins" are involved in each of them. How many "spins" are

† In some cases one may enhance or diminish artificially *some* of the contributions by multiple irradiation techniques.

there in each "spin" packet? The question about eigenfrequency and "spin" density is related to the structure of matter, the average situation in which the "spin" is embedded. On the other hand, we have already deduced a relation between our line $\chi(\omega_0 + \omega_d)$ and the envelope $\alpha_0(t)$ of the relaxation function $\alpha(t)$, which informs us about the correlation between the "spins" of the same packet, in the average situation relevant to that packet. Of course, one cannot determine completely $\chi(\omega_0 + \omega_d)$, as would be necessary in order to know $\alpha_0(t)$ completely. But we shall see how to deduce some interesting elements of $\alpha_0(t)$ from a partial knowledge of $\chi(\omega_0 + \omega_d)$.

In this section we still assume $\chi(\omega_0 + \omega_d)$ to be measured in ideal conditions, such as in a high static field ($\omega_0\tau \gg 1$), with negligible saturation (linear system), using a well-resolved line (we shall deal with only one "spin" packet), etc. In a following section our conclusions will then be adapted to more realistic conditions.

The mathematics we shall need are perhaps a little beyond what can be assumed as the normal background of a physicist. Therefore we shall first deal with some convergence problems about integrals. This will permit us to handle more easily and more clearly our specific topic, the relation between elements of $\alpha(t)$ and parameters of χ.

3.2. Some mathematics

The integrals we shall use are always supposed to be Lebesgue integrals. They behave generally as ordinary Riemann integrals, with, however, the additional feature that purely mathematical problems about infinities and discontinuities are more easily avoided. This advantage comes essentially from the fact that the Lebesgue integral deals with a curve, not point by point, but interval by interval. In this way we call a function nearly everywhere finite if it is infinite in only a finite number of points and has a finite integrated value over an interval around each of these points. An example of such a nearly everywhere finite function with two infinities is the dispersion curve associated with the rectangular absorption curve. Its shape is $\ln |(1 + x)/(1 - x)|$.

We already mentioned the fact that the Fourier transform of a square integrable function is also square integrable. Now we further recall that, for an integrable function $f(\omega, t)$,

$$\lim_{t\to 0} \int_{-\infty}^{\infty} f(\omega, t)\, d\omega/2\pi = \int_{-\infty}^{\infty} \lim_{t\to 0} f(\omega, t)\, d\omega/2\pi \tag{1}$$

if $\lim_{t\to 0} f(\omega, t)$ exists and if there exists, independent of t, an integrable function $s(\omega)$ so that

$$s(\omega) \geqq |f(\omega, t)|. \tag{2}$$

This is the Lebesgue convergence theorem for majorized functions.

An important consequence is the following statement. If $g(\omega)$ is not oscillating infinitely around zero for $\omega \to \infty$, and if the result is convergent, then

$$\lim_{t\to 0} \int_{-\infty}^{\infty} g(\omega) \cos \omega t\, d\omega/2\pi = \int_{-\infty}^{\infty} g(\omega)\, d\omega/2\pi. \tag{3}$$

This is easily proved by splitting† the integral into

$$\int_{-\infty}^{\infty} \to \int_{-\infty}^{-N} + \int_{-N}^{N} + \int_{N}^{\infty}$$

where N is such that g is either not positive or not negative for $\omega \geqq N$ and either not positive or not negative for $\omega \leqq -N$. Then the convergence of

$$\int_{N}^{\infty} g d\omega/2\pi$$

implies the convergence of

$$\int_{N}^{\infty} |g|\, d\omega/2\pi$$

† The following discussion supposes that the operator $\int_A^B$ is defined by

$$\int_A^B f d\omega/2\pi = \int_{-\infty}^{\infty} f_1\, d\omega/2\pi$$

with

$$f_1 \equiv 0 \quad \text{for} \quad \omega < A$$
$$f_1 \equiv f \quad \text{for} \quad A \leqq \omega \leqq B$$
$$f_1 \equiv 0 \quad \text{for} \quad B < \omega.$$

A or B may be infinite.

and we can apply the quoted theorem. The same holds for $\int_{-\infty}^{-N}$. And of course

$$\lim_{t\to 0} \int_{-N}^{N} = \int_{-N}^{N} \lim_{t\to 0}$$

in the assumed conditions.

For some applications, however, we shall need more refinement. We recall Dirichlet's integral:

$$\int_0^{\infty} A \frac{\sin \omega t}{\omega} d\omega/2\pi = \frac{1}{4} A \quad \text{for} \quad t > 0 \tag{4}$$

where A is a constant. Equation (1) would give zero in the limit for t going to zero but we cannot use this equation since we should have to use A/ω for $s(\omega)$ and this is not integrable. The limit is, of course, also $\frac{1}{4}A$:

$$\lim_{t\to 0} \int_0^{\infty} A \frac{\sin \omega t}{\omega} d\omega/2\pi = \frac{1}{4} A. \tag{5}$$

We shall now prove that, for finite N and for $n \geqq -1$:

$$\lim_{t\to +0} \int_0^N \omega^n g(\omega) \sin \omega t \, d\omega/2\pi = 0, \tag{6}$$

if $g(\omega)$ is nearly everywhere finite in $(0, N)$. Indeed

$$\left| \lim_{t\to +0} \int_0^N \omega^n g(\omega) \sin \omega t \, d\omega/2\pi \right| \leqq \lim_{t\to +0} \int_0^N |\omega^n g(\omega) \sin \omega t| \, d\omega/2\pi$$

$$\leqq \lim_{t\to +0} \int_0^N \omega^n \sin \omega t \, |g(\omega)| \, d\omega/2\pi \leqq \lim_{t\to +0} t \int_0^N \omega^{n+1} |g(\omega)| \, d\omega/2\pi$$

$$\leqq \lim_{t\to +0} N^{n+1} t \int_0^N |g(\omega)| \, d\omega/2\pi = 0.$$

We used the fact that

$$0 \leqq \sin \omega t < \omega t \quad \text{for} \quad 0 \leqq t \leqq 1/N.$$

A consequence is that for any fixed N:

$$\lim_{t\to +0} \int_N^{\infty} A \frac{\sin \omega t}{\omega} d\omega/2\pi = A/4. \tag{7}$$

[Use $n = -1$; $g(\omega) = A$ and combine with eq. (5).]

Further, we now state that

$$\lim_{t\to+0}\int_0^\infty f(\omega)\sin\omega t\,d\omega/2\pi=\frac{1}{4}\lim_{\omega\to\infty}\omega f \tag{8}$$

if f is nearly everywhere finite and does not oscillate infinitely and if the second limit converges:

$$\lim_{\omega\to\infty}\omega f=L<\infty. \tag{9}$$

The proof is as follows. By eq. (6) we know that the integral from zero to M vanishes for any fixed M. On the other hand, using eq. (7)

$$\lim_{t\to+0}\int_M^\infty \omega f\frac{\sin\omega t}{\omega}\,d\omega/2\pi=\lim_{t\to 0}\int_M^\infty(\omega f-L)\frac{\sin\omega t}{\omega}\,d\omega/2\pi+\frac{1}{4}L. \tag{10}$$

Let us now define I:

$$I=\lim_{t\to+0}\int_M^\infty(\omega f-L)\frac{\sin\omega t}{\omega}\,d\omega/2\pi. \tag{11}$$

The only thing to be proved is that

$$|I|\leqq\varepsilon(M), \tag{12}$$

ε being made arbitrarily small, by choosing M great enough. Because of eq. (9) we can choose M high enough to have

$$|\omega f-L|\leqq\varepsilon(M). \tag{13}$$

One might be inclined to conclude that

$$|I|\leqq\frac{1}{4}\varepsilon(M)\leqq\varepsilon(M) \tag{14}$$

by virtue of eq. (7). This is wrong because $(\omega f-L)$ could, for instance, be positive and negative alternately with $\sin\omega t$ and so disturb the convergence of the Dirichlet integral. For example,

$$\int_0^\infty\left(\frac{\sin x}{x}\right)\frac{\sin x}{x}\,dx=\pi/2.$$

One feels, however, that the inequality eq. (12) should be correct if $(\omega f-L)$ lacks any phase coherence with ωt.

Would perhaps the additional point that f is independent of t permit the proof? If, for example,

$$(\omega f-L)=(\sin\omega\tau)/\omega$$

we have no fixed phase correlation with $\sin\omega t$ but we shall have a correlation each time that $t=\tau/\pi k$ for $k=1,2,3,\ldots$. And these points accumulate when t goes to zero.

Nevertheless by direct calculation one obtains

$$\lim_{t\to+0}\int_M^\infty \frac{\sin\omega\tau}{\omega}\,\frac{\sin\omega t}{\omega}\,d\omega/2\pi = 0. \tag{15}$$

Apart from this special case, we shall only prove the theorem with the additional condition that f is of arbitrarily small total variation for $\omega > M$. This condition is fulfilled if f is not infinitely oscillating and is nearly everywhere finite.

Then let

$$\alpha(\omega) \equiv \omega f - L$$

be split up for $\omega > M$ into three parts:

$$\alpha(\omega) = \alpha(M) + P(\omega) - N(\omega)$$

with

$$0 \leqq |\alpha(M)|,\quad P(\omega),\quad N(\omega) \leqq \varepsilon(M)$$

and P and N not decreasing. ε is made arbitrarily small by choosing M great enough.

Such a splitting is possible because the total variation in f is arbitrarily small. The splitting is illustrated schematically in Fig. 3.1.

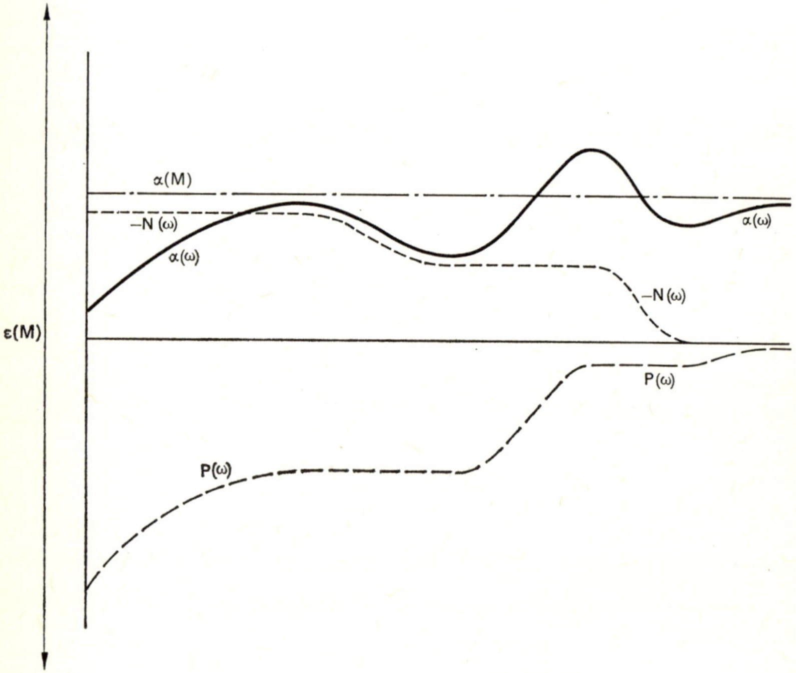

FIG. 3.1. Splitting of a function in non-negative non-decreasing parts $\alpha(M)$, $P(\omega)$ and $N(\omega)$. $\alpha(\omega) - \alpha(M) = P(\omega) - N(\omega)$.

Now we apply the theorem of Bonnet which states the following: "If $f(x)$ is positive not decreasing and $g(x)$ continuous, then

$$\int_a^b fg\,dx = f(b)\int_c^b g\,dx,\quad a \leqq c \leqq b."$$

This gives

$$I = \lim_{t\to+0}\int_M^\infty \alpha(M)\frac{\sin\omega t}{\omega}\,d\omega/2\pi + \lim_{t\to+0}\ \lim_{M_1\to\infty} P(M_1)\int_{M'(M_1)}^{M_1}\frac{\sin\omega t}{\omega}\,d\omega/2\pi$$

$$-\lim_{t\to+0}\ \lim_{M_1\to\infty} N(M_1)\int_{M''(M_1)}^{M_1}\frac{\sin\omega t}{\omega}\,d\omega/2\pi.$$

The first term is $\frac{1}{4}\alpha(M)$. Because of the dependence of M' and M'' on M_1, the two last integrals are not simply $\frac{1}{4}$ for $M_1 \to \infty$ *and then* $t \to 0$. But in any case their absolute value is not greater than $\frac{1}{4}$. Since $P(M_1) \leqq \varepsilon(M)$ and $N(M_1) \leqq \varepsilon(M)$ we finally get

$$|I| \leqq 3\varepsilon(M)/4 \leqq \varepsilon(M).$$

It may be interesting to observe that eq. (15) holds, in spite of the fact that the total variation of $(\sin\omega\tau)/\omega$ is infinite.

Another useful theorem, about inverting integration and differentiation, is the following

$$\frac{d}{dt}\int_0^\infty f(\omega)\,e^{i\omega t}\,d\omega/2\pi = \int_0^\infty i\omega f(\omega)\,e^{i\omega t}\,d\omega/2\pi \tag{16}$$

if the second member converges uniformly with respect to t. And in general

$$\frac{d^n}{dt^n}\int_0^\infty f(\omega)\,e^{i\omega t}\,d\omega/2\pi = \int_0^\infty (i\omega)^n f(\omega)\,e^{i\omega t}\,d\omega/2\pi \tag{17}$$

if the second member converges uniformly. The real and imaginary parts of this equation hold separately under the respective conditions.

In connection with the former results, eq. (3) and eq. (8), we may now write

$$\lim_{t\to+0}\frac{d}{dt}\int_0^\infty f(\omega)\sin\omega t\,d\omega/2\pi = \int_0^\infty \omega f(\omega)\,d\omega/2\pi \tag{18}$$

and

$$\lim_{t \to +0} \frac{d}{dt} \int_0^\infty f(\omega) \cos \omega t \, d\omega/2\pi = -\frac{1}{4} \lim_{\omega \to \infty} \omega^2 f \qquad (19)$$

if the result converges and if f is not oscillating infinitely.

Indeed, with the stated requirements, the uniform convergence of the second member of eq. (16) is guaranteed.

3.3. Structure: eigenfrequency (g-factor)

The first information about the structure of matter, i.e. about the average environment of the "spins" in a packet, is the *eigenfrequency*, the Larmor frequency of these "spins". We used this frequency ω_0 in the definition of α_0 and φ_0, e.g. eq. (2.70),

$$\alpha = \alpha_0 \sin \omega_0 t$$

and in the definition of ω_d, eq. (2.52),

$$\omega_d = \omega - \omega_0 .$$

This frequency ω_0 is generally proportional to the applied static field, $\boldsymbol{B}_s$, and therefore it is usual to define the relation $\omega_0/\boldsymbol{B}_s$, rather than ω_0, as a property of the "spins" in matter.

For nuclei, one defines a gyromagnetic ratio γ by

$$\boldsymbol{\mu} = \gamma \hbar \boldsymbol{I} \qquad (20)$$

where $\boldsymbol{\mu}$ is the magnetic moment of the nucleus and $\hbar \boldsymbol{I}$ the nuclear spin angular momentum. The Larmor theorem then states that

$$\boldsymbol{\omega}_0 = -\gamma \boldsymbol{B}. \qquad (21)$$

This gyromagnetic ratio γ is a constant of the nucleus, and $\boldsymbol{B}$ is the field at the nucleus. γ is a scalar and its sign determines the sense of rotation of the Larmor precession, indicated here by the *vector* $\boldsymbol{\omega}_0$, colinear with $\boldsymbol{B}$.

For electronic "spins" the question is more involved, since an electronic "spin" is not so independent of its environment as is a nucleus. A classical calculation of the Larmor frequency $\boldsymbol{\omega}$ for an electron orbiting in a field $\boldsymbol{B}$ yields (e and m are respectively the charge and the mass of the electron):

$$\boldsymbol{\omega} = -\frac{e}{m}\boldsymbol{B}. \tag{22}$$

Hence an electronic orbital gyromagnetic ratio would be $(+e/m)$. The electronic "spin" in general will also precess around a certain direction, with an eigenfrequency we denote by $\boldsymbol{\omega}_0$.

This $\boldsymbol{\omega}_0$ may still be defined phenomenologically as a function of the externally applied field $\boldsymbol{B}$. However, the orientation of $\boldsymbol{\omega}_0$ may be influenced, for example, by a crystal lattice. We therefore define a g factor g by:

$$\boldsymbol{\omega}_0 = \{g\}\left(\frac{-e}{m}\right)\boldsymbol{B}. \tag{23}$$

$\boldsymbol{B}$ is now the *externally* applied field, and $\{g\}$ is now a *tensor*, since $\boldsymbol{\omega}_0$ is not necessarily parallel to $\boldsymbol{B}$. We use $\{\}$ (only in this section) to indicate this fact. The phenomenological gyromagnetic ratio is also a tensor:

$$\{\gamma_e\} = -\{g\}\left(\frac{-e}{m}\right) \tag{24}$$

and the effective magnetic moment is

$$\boldsymbol{\mu}_e = -\{g\}\left(\frac{-e}{m}\right)\hbar\boldsymbol{S} = -\{g\}\,\beta\boldsymbol{S} \tag{25}$$

where $\hbar\boldsymbol{S}$ is the angular momentum and

$$\beta = \frac{-e\hbar}{m} \tag{26}$$

is called the Bohr magneton. Of course, experimentally we shall determine *components* of $\{g\}$. If the sample has a certain orientation (θ, ψ) with respect to the field, it will have a certain eigenfrequency $\omega_0(\theta, \psi)$ which determines the component of $\{g\}$ for this relative orientation

$$\omega_0(\theta, \psi) = g(\theta, \psi)\left(\frac{-e}{m}\right)B. \tag{27}$$

We may also define a scalar γ as

$$\omega_0 = -\gamma(\theta, \psi)\, B \tag{28}$$

for this particular situation of sample and field.

Let us now see how to determine the eigenfrequency ω_0 of a sample in a certain field, in a certain orientation. As a matter of fact we shall determine ω_0 by looking for the zero of $\chi'(\omega_0 + \omega_d)$ or the maximum of $\chi''(\omega_0 + \omega_d)$. Hence we define ω_0 so that

$$\lim_{\omega_d \to 0} \chi'(\omega_0 + \omega_d) = -\lim_{\omega_d \to 0} \frac{1}{2} \int_0^\infty \alpha_0(t) \sin \omega_d t\, dt = 0 \tag{29}$$

or

$$\lim_{\omega_d \to 0} d\chi''(\omega_0 + \omega_d)/d\omega = -\lim_{\omega_d \to 0} \frac{1}{2} \int_0^\infty t\, \alpha_0(t) \sin \omega_d t\, dt = 0. \tag{30}$$

We have used eq. (2.80) and also eq. (16). By eq. (8) we know that this is equivalent respectively to

$$\lim_{t \to \infty} t\alpha_0(t) = 0 \tag{31}$$

and

$$\lim_{t \to \infty} t^2\alpha_0(t) = 0 \tag{32}$$

with $\alpha_0(t)$ not infinitely oscillating. [The parts played by ω and t are inverted with respect to eq. (8).] These conditions are indeed verified if we eliminate correctly the oscillation by means of eq. (2.70):

$$\alpha = \alpha_0 \sin \omega_0 t.$$

And this supposes the oscillation of $\alpha(t)$ to have the same frequency throughout the decay. Such an approximation is allowed for negligible damping, i.e. for $\omega_0\tau \gg 1$. For $\omega_0\tau \not\gg 1$ the oscillation frequency may be slightly different from ω_0, and the maximum of χ'' or the zero of χ' will not coincide exactly with the Larmor frequency. Observe, however, that the requirements are stronger for the absorption ($t^2\alpha$ in eq. (32)) than for the dispersion ($t\alpha$ in eq. (31)). Other advantages of the use of dispersion will appear later.

3.4. STRUCTURE: "SPIN" DENSITY (STATIC SUSCEPTIBILITY)

Further information about structure is given by the number of "spins" in each "spin" packet. As a matter of fact, the interaction between our macroscopic field and these "spins" is only effective to a certain extent. Only the interaction with some excess "spins" has a net macroscopic effect. The percentage of "spins" which are in excess depends on the temperature according to the well-known Boltzmann distribution. The number of "spins" in excess per unit volume represents a certain magnetization $\boldsymbol{M}$ which in turn is proportional to the field $\boldsymbol{B}$. In this way we defined static susceptibility by [eq. (1) of Chapter 1]

$$\boldsymbol{M} = \frac{10^7}{4\pi} \chi_s \boldsymbol{B}_s .$$

In fact, when speaking about *number of "spins"* we always mean the number in excess.

For a single line with one eigenfrequency eqs. (2.63) and (2.69) give us the static susceptibility of the sample,

$$\chi_s = \varphi_0(0) = \frac{1}{\omega_0} \alpha_0(0) \tag{33}$$

and hence the number of "spins". We shall first see how to determine χ_s from χ' or χ'' and then we shall make some remarks about lines with various eigenfrequencies.

Let us first look at eq. (2.80 d).

$$\chi_s = \alpha_0(0)/\omega_0 = \frac{8}{\omega_0} \lim_{t \to 0} \int_0^\infty \chi''(\omega_0 + \omega_d) \cos \omega_d t \, d\omega_d/2\pi . \tag{34}$$

We know on physical grounds that an absorption curve $\chi''(\omega_0 + \omega_d)$ is positive for $\omega_0 > 0$, since $\omega\chi''(\omega)$ is proportional to an absorbed energy, and $\chi'' < 0$ at some $\omega > 0$ would be contrary to the principle of conversation of energy. Hence by eq. (3), and using eq. (2.79),

$$\boxed{\chi_s = \frac{8}{\omega_0} \int_0^\infty \chi''(\omega_0 + \omega_d) \, d\omega_d/2\pi = \frac{4}{\omega_0} \int_{-\infty}^\infty \chi''(\omega_0 + \omega_d) \, d\omega_d/2\pi} \tag{35}$$

if the integral is convergent. Remember that χ'' is truncated, eqs. (2.77) and (2.78). This result is frequently used for determining χ_s from $\chi''(\omega_0 + \omega_d)$.

We can, however, also use eq. (2.80c) and determine χ_s from the dispersion curve:

$$\chi_s = \alpha_0(0)/\omega_0 = -8 \lim_{t\to 0} \frac{1}{\omega_0} \int_0^\infty \chi'(\omega_0 + \omega_d) \sin \omega_d t \, d\omega_d/2\pi \tag{36}$$

and from eq. (8):

$$\boxed{\chi_s = -2 \lim_{\omega_d\to\infty} \frac{\omega_d}{\omega_0} \chi'(\omega_0 + \omega_d)} \tag{37}$$

if the limit converges. The use of eq. (37) instead of eq. (35) has many advantages (Talpe and Van Gerven, 1966).

If the line is not single but has various (well separated) eigenfrequencies we may consider the experimental line as a superposition of elementary lines. In most cases we may assume the same type of relaxation for the different lines, eventually giving a different relaxation time. In this case the shapes of the lines are all equal (see below, § 3.5 and § 3.6) and it is evident from eqs. (35) and (37) that χ_s for each "spin" packet is then proportional to a product like $\chi''_{\max} . \delta''_\omega$ or $(\partial\chi'/\partial\omega)_{\max} . \delta'^2_\omega$ of the corresponding line.

$$\chi_{s,i} = K''\chi''_{\max,i}\,\delta''_{\omega,i} = K'(\partial\chi'/\partial\omega)_{\max,i}\,\delta'^2_{\omega,i} \tag{38}$$

the factors K' and K'' depending only on the common line shape. δ''_ω and δ'_ω are line widths, to be defined in the following section. Thus we can estimate the relative "spin" density by the relative value of $\chi''_{\max} . \delta''_\omega$ or of $(d\chi'/d\omega)_{\max} . \delta'^2_\omega$ or of some other convenient product. Such a product is a better indication of the *relative* "spin" density than the value of eqs. (35) and (37) since it is less affected by the neighbour lines. Of course, the total number of "spins" is still given by the integral of χ'' over the whole line. It is still given too by the tails of χ' over the whole line. This makes possible the determination of the constants K' and K''.

3.5. Relaxation: characteristic time (line width)

After studying how the structure of matter is expressed by the eigen-frequency and number of "spins" of each packet, we shall now consider the correlation of "spins" in the same packet. First, we shall deal with the most elementary parameter, the characteristic time or relaxation time. This is the time during which the relaxation function is important, compared to its maximum. We need, of course, a more quantitative definition of this relaxation time τ. We could, for instance, define this time by the instant at which $\varphi_0(t)$ or $\alpha_0(t)$ is one half or $1/e$ of its maximum. We shall adopt a more general definition:

$$\tau = \frac{\int_0^\infty \varphi_0(t)\,dt}{\varphi_0(0)} = \frac{\int_0^\infty \alpha_0(t)\,dt}{\alpha_0(t)}\,. \tag{39}$$

The last expression is added by virtue of eq. (2.69). $\varphi_0(0)$ as well as $\alpha_0(0)$ are the maximum values. Since α_0 and φ_0 are not oscillating infinitely we have from eq. (2.80b)

$$\chi''(\omega_0) = \lim_{\omega_d \to 0} \tfrac{1}{2} \int_0^\infty \alpha_0(t) \cos \omega_d t\, dt = \tfrac{1}{2} \int_0^\infty \alpha_0(t)\, dt, \tag{40}$$

at least if the result is convergent [eq. (3), with ω_d for t and t for ω]. Hence by eq. (39) and eq. (33)

$$\chi''(\omega_0) = \tfrac{1}{2}\,\alpha_0(0)\,\tau = \tfrac{1}{2}\,\omega_0 \tau \chi_s. \tag{41}$$

And with eq. (35)

$$\frac{1}{\tau} = \frac{2\int_{-\infty}^{\infty} \chi''(\omega_0 + \omega_d)\, d\omega_d/2\pi}{\chi''(\omega_0)}\,. \tag{42}$$

Equation (42) obviously represents the width of the line $\chi''(\omega_0 + \omega_d)$. In this way we *define* the width of the line $\chi''(\omega_0 + \omega_d)$ on the ω_d-axis as

$$\delta \equiv 1/\tau. \tag{43a}$$

In practice one also uses some other parameters which characterize the width of a resonance line. We define here

$$\left.\begin{array}{l}\delta' \equiv \text{half width between maximum and minimum of} \\ \qquad \chi'(\omega_0 + \omega_d)\end{array}\right\} \qquad (43\,b)$$

$$\left.\begin{array}{l}\delta'' \equiv \text{half width between the points where } \chi''(\omega_0 + \omega_d) \\ \qquad \text{is half its maximum value}\end{array}\right\} \qquad (43\,c)$$

$$\left.\begin{array}{l}\delta^* \equiv \text{half width between maximum and minimum of} \\ \qquad \partial\chi''(\omega_0 + \omega_d)/\partial\omega_d \text{ (inflexion points).}\end{array}\right\} \qquad (43\,d)$$

For an asymmetric line, we may consider the width between the centre of the line ($\chi' = 0$ or $\partial\chi''/\partial\omega_d = 0$) and the points where χ' is maximum or minimum or χ'' is at half height or $\partial^2\chi''/\partial^2\omega_d = 0$. We indicate these values by

$$\delta'^{+}, \delta''^{+}, \delta^{*+}, \delta'^{-}, \delta''^{-}, \delta^{*-}$$

using + or − for $\omega_d > 0$ or $\omega_d < 0$ respectively (assuming $\omega_0 > 0$). For a symmetric line, of course, $\delta' = \delta'^{+} = \delta'^{-}$ and similarly for δ'' and δ^*. For a given line shape there exists a constant relation between all these line widths, e.g. for a Lorentzian line $\delta' = \delta'' = \sqrt{3}\delta^* = \delta$. As an illustration of eq. (38) we may use eq. (43) in eq. (41) and obtain $\chi_s = (2/\omega_0)\,\delta\chi''_{\max}$. For a Lorentzian line, then, $\chi_s = (2/\omega_0)\,\delta''\,\chi''_{\max}$.

3.6. Relaxation: correlation (moments and asymptotic expansion)

Finally, for any complementary information about the correlation, we now have to look more carefully at the shape of $\alpha_0(t)$. How can we get any information about the shape of $\alpha_0(t)$, by analysing χ' or χ''? The trick is to expand $\alpha_0(t)$ in a Taylor series. Fortunately it happens that what can be calculated, from other information about the physical system, is generally not $\alpha_0(t)$ directly but just the terms of this expansion, at least the lowest order ones. We write $\alpha_0(t)$ as

$$\alpha_0(t) = \alpha_0(0) + \dot{\alpha}_0(0)\,t + \ddot{\alpha}_0(0)\,t^2/2! + \ldots + \alpha_0^{(n)}(0)t^n/n! + \ldots \qquad (44)$$

Let us first try the absorption curve and then the dispersion curve.

The relations between $\alpha^0_{(n)}(0)$ and $\chi''(\omega_d)$ are deduced easily by successive differentiations of eq. (2.80d)

$$\dot{\alpha}(0) \equiv \lim_{t\to 0} d\alpha(t)/dt = -\lim_{t\to 0} 8 \int_0^\infty \omega_d \chi''(\omega_0 + \omega_d) \sin \omega_d t \, d\omega_d/2\pi$$

$$= -\lim_{\omega_d\to\infty} 2\omega_d^2 \chi''(\omega_0 + \omega_d) \tag{45}$$

if the limit converges [eq. (8)]. The second derivative is given by:

$$\ddot{\alpha}(0) = -\lim_{t\to 0} 8 \int_0^\infty \omega_d^2 \chi''(\omega_0 + \omega_d) \cos \omega_d t \, d\omega_d/2\pi$$

$$= -8 \int_0^\infty \omega_d^2 \chi'' \, d\omega_d/2\pi \tag{46}$$

if the last integral is convergent [eq. (3)]. We assume that $\chi''(\omega_0 + \omega_d)$ cannot oscillate indefinitely and also that it is even. The integral of eq. (46) is essentially what we call the second moment of the line. More precisely, we define the *n*th moment of a line as

$$M_n = 4 \int_{-\infty}^{\infty} \omega_d^n \chi''(\omega_0 + \omega_d) \, d\omega_d/2\pi. \tag{47}$$

Once again, χ'' is the truncated line, eqs. (2.77), (2.78). Of course

$$\alpha_0(0) = \omega_0 \chi_s = M_0. \tag{48}$$

And now

$$\ddot{\varphi}_0(0)/\varphi_0(0) = \ddot{\alpha}''(0)/\alpha(0) = -M_2/M_0. \tag{49}$$

For a symmetric line shape, the odd moments are zero.† On the other hand, if the second moment is convergent then necessarily $\dot{\alpha}(0) = 0$, from eq. (45). With the same convergence requirements, we have finally

$$\alpha_0^{(2n)}(0) = (-1)^n M_{2n}. \tag{50}$$

† The third moment has been used to analyse asymmetric line shapes (Van Tiggelen, 1964; Svare, 1965).

And in general convergence of M_{2n} implies that $\alpha_0^{(2n-1)}(0)$ vanishes,

$$(M_{2n} < \infty) \rightarrow [\alpha^{(2n-1)}(0) = 0]. \tag{51}$$

The first coefficient of the Taylor expansion of $\alpha_0(t)$, the static susceptibility, could be related to χ'' as well as to χ'. The same is true for the other coefficients and similar advantages appear. The formulas connecting $\alpha^{(n)}(0)$ to $\chi'(\omega)$ are, however, not derived so straightforwardly. We suppose that $\chi'(\omega_0 + \omega_d)$ has an *asymptotic expansion.*† We define the coefficients as follows:

$$-2\omega_d\chi'(\omega_0 + \omega_d) = a_0 + a_2\omega_d^{-2} + a_4\omega_d^{-4} + \ldots + a_{2p}\omega^{-2p} + R_{2p}. \tag{52}$$

We have dropped the odd terms, since χ' is odd, and hence $\omega_d\chi'$ even. Although eventually the series does not converge for $p \rightarrow \infty$, we have for any finite p

$$\lim_{\omega_d \to \infty} R_{2p}\omega_d^{2p} = 0. \tag{53}$$

Now, of course,

$$\alpha_0(0) = \omega_0\chi_s = a_0 \tag{54}$$

since the convergence conditions are amply fulfilled [eq. (53), $p = 0$]. But we shall also prove that

$$\alpha^{(2n)}(0) = (-1)^n a_{2n}. \tag{55}$$

We insert eq. (52) in eq. (2.80c) taking $p = n$

$$\begin{aligned} \alpha_0(t) &= 4\int_0^\infty (-2\omega_d\chi')\frac{\sin\omega_d t}{\omega_d}\,d\omega_d/2\pi \\ &= 4\sum_{k=0}\int_{-0}^\infty a_{2k}\omega_d^{-2k}\frac{\sin\omega_d t}{\omega_d}\,d\omega_d/2\pi \\ &\quad + 4\int_0^\infty R_{2n}\frac{\sin\omega_d t}{\omega_d}\,d\omega_d/2\pi \end{aligned} \tag{56}$$

† One can consult Angot (1961) for this mathematical technique introduced by Poincaré (1886).

and we apply eq. (17)

$$\alpha_0(t)^{(2n)} = 4 \sum_{k=0}^{n} (-1)^n \int_0^\infty a_{2k}\omega_d^{2(n-k)} \frac{\sin \omega_d t}{\omega_d}\, d\omega_d/2\pi$$

$$+ 4 \int_0^\infty R_{2n}\omega_d^{2n} \frac{\sin \omega_d t}{\omega_d}\, d\omega_d/2\pi. \tag{57}$$

Now we use eq. (4) for the last but one and eqs. (8) and (53) for the last term of the second member:

$$\alpha^{(2n)}(0) = (-1)^{(n)} 4 \sum_{k=0}^{n-1} \lim_{t\to 0} \int_{-0}^{\infty} a_{2k}\omega_d^{2(n-k)} \frac{\sin \omega_d t}{\omega_d}\, d\omega_d/2\pi$$

$$+ (-1)^n a_{2n} + 0. \tag{58}$$

Hence we obtain eq. (55) if we prove that

$$\lim_{t\to 0} \int_0^\infty a_{2k}\omega_d^{2(n-k)} \frac{\sin \omega_d t}{\omega_d}\, d\omega_d/2\pi = 0 \qquad \text{for } 0 \leqq k < n \tag{59}$$

or that

$$\lim_{t\to +0} \int_0^\infty \omega_d^{s-1} \sin \omega_d t\, d\omega_d/2\pi = 0 \qquad \text{for } s > 0 \tag{60}$$

or, using eq. (6), that

$$\lim_{t\to +0} \lim_{N_1\to\infty} \int_N^{N_1} \omega_d^{s} \frac{\sin \omega_d t}{\omega_d}\, d\omega_d/2\pi = 0 \quad \text{for } s > 0. \tag{61}$$

The integral is an oscillating function of N_1. Its value is determined by the phase of $N_1 t$ in the sine and hence the frequency is of the order of N_1. The amplitude is of the order of N_1^{2k}. But for t less than a given value t_1, the term with R_{2p} in eq. (57) is negligible with respect to $\alpha^{(2n)}(t)$ and α_{2n}. Therefore if the asymptotic expansion exists, the limit of the integral for $N_1 \to \infty$ has to be taken in an unambiguous way and must become independent of t for $t \to 0$. The only way to realize these conditions is for the whole expression to be zero.

Let us now also consider $\dot{\alpha}(0)$. Using again eq. (2.80c) and applying eq. (18), we should find

$$\dot{\alpha}(0) = 4 \int_0^\infty -2\chi'\omega_a \, d\omega_a/2\pi \tag{62}$$

but the result diverges, since $\chi'\omega_a$ converges to a non-zero limit. This does not mean, however, that the result is infinite but only that the way of calculating it was erroneous. In fact $\dot{\alpha}_0(0)$ is generally zero and, even for the Lorentz line, finite. We knew this already by considering χ''. Therefore we do not insist on calculating the integral more rigorously. The trouble comes from

$$\frac{d}{dt}\int \neq \int \frac{d}{dt}.$$

Let us only emphasize the second derivative:

$$\ddot{\alpha}(0) = -2a_2. \tag{63}$$

Some remarks about moments and asymptotic expansion are still in order. Compare eq. (50) with eq. (55). We get

$$M_{2n} = a_{2n}. \tag{64}$$

In fact, eq. (64) was demonstrated by Stieltjes (1894, 1895) for two functions χ' and χ'' which are related by what we now call the dispersion relation. The theory in its actual form, as it is applied to paramagnetic resonance, has recently been developed by Hervé (1957, 1960) and independently by Talpe and Van Gerven (1966). Stieltjes used the cumbersome technique of continuous fractions. However, even with the refinements of Hamburger (1920), this famous theorem of moments is only valid for finite moments. The statement of eq. (55) holds also, for instance, for a Lorentzian line, where M_{2n} is infinite for $n \geqslant 1$ (see below, § 5.2). The asymptotic expansion is then even convergent [with respect to p, eq. (52)]. That eq. (50) breaks down for a Lorentzian line is due to the fact that χ'' does not vanish quickly enough under the initial part of $\cos \omega_a t$. This, however, does not impede χ' being convergently mixed with a sine. Observe that the a_{2k} of a Lorentz line have alternate signs, incompatible with eq. (64). We may say that for a Lorentz line shape χ'' deviates from "convergent" integrals to "divergent" ones while χ' deviates from a divergent asymptotic expansion to a convergent one.

Theoretically this analysis of moments and asymptotic expansion seems to furnish detailed information about $\alpha_0(t)$ from χ'' or χ'. However, one has to be aware of the limitations in its applicability. First of all if the second moment or $\ddot{\alpha}_0(0)$ is accessible to calculations from properties of matter, the computation of $\alpha_0^{(4)}(0)$ is rather complicated and very seldom are the calculations made for a sixth moment. On the other hand, Grant (1964) has pointed out that functions that seem very similar can give a very different collection of zeroth, second and fourth moments. And the knowledge of even the first hundred moments of a line is not sufficient to get a idea of what its shape is. The reason is that small variations at the extremities of the line cause an important variation in the moments. Grant gives a whole collection of curves with the same M_0, M_2 and M_4 as for a Gaussian curve, but with very different shapes, including some very similar to a Lorentzian curve. These observations are, of course, also valid for χ' and the *a*-coefficients, e.g. the knowledge of the coefficients a_{2k} does not permit us to determine the central part of a dispersion curve. In general, however, one has some idea about what the curve should be, and then one can make a test by measuring M_{2n} or a_{2n} and calculating $\alpha^{(2n)}(0)$, at least, for example, for $n = 0, 1, 2$. The measurement of a_{2n} or of M_{2n} is yet another problem. A technique for the measurement of a_0 is described by Talpe and Van Gerven (1966). See also Hervé (1957).

4. A Single Paramagnetic Resonance Line in Experimental Conditions

4.1. Introduction

Until now we have supposed the system under study to be linear, stationary, causal and passive with a single symmetric narrow resonance line, or at least a well-resolved spectrum of such lines, displayed as a function of the frequency of excitation and in the presence of a very strong static magnetic field. This was important for understanding the basic principles, but we now have to deal with more realistic experimental conditions.

(a) The HF susceptibility χ is a tensor and experimentally we do not measure a tensor but only its components. Therefore we shall first consider the various components of χ, including some components unusual in tensor analysis. Namely, we shall deal with rotating fields, considering first the mathematical presentation of such fields.

(b) For technical reasons one usually does not measure $\chi(\omega)$ as a function of ω, the excitation frequency, but function of the resonance frequency ω_0 of the system—which is proportional to the applied (and scanned) static field. This will make a certain transformation necessary in our formulas. The main trouble arises for low static field. We shall then have to consider whether any correction is needed.

(c) As to the relaxation, problems may arise when the system is no longer linear. We shall have to discuss saturation, and the main difficulty is that our relaxation-function theory is no longer valid.

(d) The system is not only not linear, but in principle also not stationary. We have to vary the magnetic field or the frequency, and the question is how this influences the line. We must analyse at what speeds any correction becomes necessary.

(e) For the description of an experimental line shape, two *models* are often used, the Lorentzian and the Gaussian shapes. We shall discuss these briefly.

4.2. The components of the susceptibility tensor

(a) *Static susceptibility*

It is well known that the susceptibility is in general a tensor, since it relates two vectorial quantities ***m*** and ***b*** which are not necessarily parallel. If the magnetic properties of a sample are anisotropic, the magnetization in a certain direction can depend on the field in another direction. Observe that an isotropic sample can have an anisotropic property due to an external field. For example, the Larmor precession due to a static field is such an anisotropic property. In order to be practical we shall limit ourselves to the situation met in paramagnetic studies. Let us have a certain static field $\boldsymbol{B}_s$ and a HF field. We first consider the magnetization $\boldsymbol{M}_s$ due to the field $\boldsymbol{B}_s$ and assume $\Delta\boldsymbol{M}_s$ proportional to $\Delta\boldsymbol{B}_s$ in the small region of interest. We assume the system to be "statically linear". Superposed on $\boldsymbol{M}_s$, we consider a HF magnetization, due to the HF field, and which can be not linear. This HF magnetization may depend on $\boldsymbol{B}_s$, but if so $\boldsymbol{B}_s$ is considered as a parameter.

Tensors and vectors are specified by components in a right-turning orthogonal coordinate system with unit vectors $\hat{\boldsymbol{x}}$, $\hat{\boldsymbol{y}}$ and $\hat{\boldsymbol{z}}$, always oriented with $\hat{\boldsymbol{z}}$ along $\boldsymbol{B}_s$

$$\boldsymbol{B}_s = B_s\hat{\boldsymbol{z}}. \tag{1}$$

As for the static field, if the sample is isotropic, the static magnetization $\boldsymbol{M}_s$ is parallel to $\boldsymbol{B}_s$ defining a scalar static susceptibility χ_s. More generally χ_s is a tensor but has only three non-vanishing components since $\boldsymbol{B}_s = B_s\hat{\boldsymbol{z}}$ or $B_{sx} = B_{sy} = 0$. Thus:

$$\boldsymbol{M}_s = \frac{10^7}{4\pi}\chi_s\boldsymbol{B}_s \tag{2}$$

or

$$M_{sx} = \frac{10^7}{4\pi}\chi_{sxz}B_s; \quad M_{sy} = \frac{10^7}{4\pi}\chi_{syz}B_s; \quad M_{sz} = \frac{10^7}{4\pi}\chi_{szz}B_s.$$

The notation

$$M_s = \frac{10^7}{4\pi}\chi_s B_s \tag{3}$$

(without vectors) means that the sample is "statically" isotropic and hence χ_s is scalar.

We shall always designate the *static* magnetization and susceptibility by a leading subscript *s*. As to the static field, we shall later consider a variation of its value around a centre value. The centre value is B_{s0} and the actual value $B_s = B_{s0} + B_d$. Since $|B_d| \ll B_{s0}$ one has $B_s, B_{s0} > 0$ and B_d positive or negative or zero, according to eq. (1).

(b) *HF susceptibility in a linearly polarized field*

The fact that the susceptibility is a tensor is perhaps most important for the HF magnetization. Indeed, because of the Larmor precession, there appear normal components of the HF magnetization, as important as the colinear components if the HF field is orthogonal to the static field. In addition, the value of a static field $\boldsymbol{B}_s$ is of the greatest importance for the magnetization along an orthogonal HF field. We shall, however, consider this influence of $\boldsymbol{B}_s$ as represented by a parameter.

Let us first assume a linear monochromatic alternating field

$$\boldsymbol{b}_1 = 2\boldsymbol{B}_1 \cos \omega t = \mathscr{R}\, 2\boldsymbol{B}_1\, e^{i\omega t}. \tag{4}$$

This produces a HF magnetization and, since we wish to include non-linearity, we must introduce in its expression terms proportional to $b_1^2, b_1^3, b_1^4, b_1^n \ldots$ However, it will be more convenient to introduce terms proportional to $\mathscr{R}(2B_1\, e^{i\omega t})^n$ rather than terms proportional to $(\mathscr{R}2B_1\, e^{i\omega t})^n$. This is a question of arrangement of terms. We now get the successive harmonics of the HF magnetization, which we shall label by a (first) numerical subscript (generalized by $n, m, l, k \ldots$ but not by s, x, y, z). Observe that we also define a zeroth order term, a static component due to b_1 and to be distinguished from $\boldsymbol{M}_s$. Let the HF magnetization be

$$\begin{aligned} m &= \boldsymbol{M}_0 + \boldsymbol{M}_1' \cos \omega t + \boldsymbol{M}_1'' \sin \omega t + \boldsymbol{M}_2' \cos 2\omega t + \boldsymbol{M}_2'' \sin 2\omega t + \\ \ldots &= \sum_{n=0}^{\infty} (\boldsymbol{M}_n' \cos n\omega t + \boldsymbol{M}_n'' \sin n\omega t) = \sum_{n=0}^{\infty} \mathscr{R}(\boldsymbol{M}_n' - i\boldsymbol{M}_n'')\, e^{in\omega t} \\ &= \sum_{n=0}^{\infty} \mathscr{R} M_n\, e^{in\omega t}. \end{aligned} \tag{5}$$

We define the HF susceptibility tensor by

$$\boldsymbol{M}_n = \frac{10^7}{4\pi} \chi_n 2\boldsymbol{B}_1 (2B_1/B_s)^{n-1}. \tag{6}$$

The parameter B_s is introduced for consistency. We emphasize the difference between, for example, χ_{1xx} and χ_{1zz}. The former component is due to $\boldsymbol{b}_1$, orthogonal to $\boldsymbol{B}_s$, while the latter is a HF drag component for parallel fields. So, for example, in a stationary state $\chi_{1xz} = \chi_{1yz} = 0$. (Remember our convention $\boldsymbol{B}_s = B_s z$, eq. (1).) If we consider only the first harmonic χ_1, we make this clear by dropping the numerical subscript, leaving the tensor χ without a subscript.

$$\boldsymbol{M} = \frac{10^7}{4\pi}\chi 2\boldsymbol{B}_1 . \tag{7}$$

If we consider only χ_{xx} we use simply χ to designate the tensor and the component.

(c) *Rotating fields*

Until now we have only considered a linear alternating field, a linearly polarized HF magnetic field:

$$\boldsymbol{b}_1 = 2\boldsymbol{B}_1 \cos \omega t . \tag{8}$$

However, the fact that the Larmor precession is a rotating magnetic moment may suggest the use of rotating magnetic fields. This was indeed done in Bloch's original theory on magnetic induction and it is a common technique to deal with the Bloch theory by using rotating magnetic fields. Moreover, their ample use in the geometrical representation of paramagnetic resonance is fruitful, not only in connection with the phenomenological theory of Bloch. Recent techniques, e.g. concerning adiabatic demagnetization in the rotating frame, are imagined and discussed using rotating fields. In fact, the very use of a rotating frame is intimately connected with the consideration of rotating fields.

On the contrary, in experimental arrangements, rotating fields are hardly ever used. The reason is that, on the one hand it is technically easier by far to obtain a linear oscillating field or a linearly polarized HF field, and on the other hand, each linear oscillating field can be decomposed into the sum of two circularly polarized (rotating) fields, one right-handed and one left-handed. Hence if the theory is restricted to cases where one of the two circular components has negligible effect, one can easily use a linear field for experiments and a circularly polarized field for the theory. In general this will happen when the condition $\omega_0\tau \gg 1$ of section 2.4 is fulfilled. $\omega_0\tau \gg 1$ was indeed the condition assumed in order to "reduce" the line $\chi(\omega)$ to $\tilde{\chi}(\omega_0 + \omega_d)$ by dropping the "counter-turning" component [eqs. (2.77) and 2.78)].

If, however, $\omega_0\tau \ll 1$, one must be careful in considering a right- and a left-handed component in the theory and summing the results for comparison with experiment. This is allowed only if one restricts oneself to the linear theory, excluding any saturation. If some saturation is present, even this "summing" method is no longer exact. Then one has either to formulate the theory with linear fields or the experiments with rotating fields. The Bloch theory has indeed been studied to some extent for linear fields (Van Gerven, 1963) and, on the other hand, experiments in rotating fields have been done (Manus *et al.*, 1954).

We shall now analyse the question of how to describe a rotating field, emphasizing the connection it has with linearly polarized fields. One can describe rotating fields by specifying the axes $\hat{\boldsymbol{x}}$ and $\hat{\boldsymbol{y}}$ in a coordinate system and write, for example,

$$\boldsymbol{b}_{1c}(\text{right}, \omega) = B_1(\cos \omega t\, \hat{\boldsymbol{x}} + \sin \omega t\, \hat{\boldsymbol{y}}). \tag{9}$$

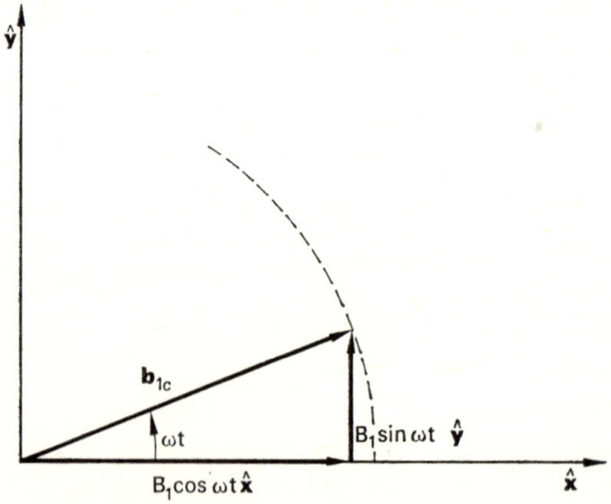

FIG. 4.1. A rotating field $\boldsymbol{b}_{1c}$, turning right-handed around $\hat{z}$, described with the axes $\hat{\boldsymbol{x}}$ and $\hat{\boldsymbol{y}}$:

$$\boldsymbol{b}_{1c}(\text{right}, \omega) = B_1(\cos \omega t\, \hat{\boldsymbol{x}} + \sin \omega t\, \hat{\boldsymbol{y}}).$$

The $\hat{z}$-axis (and $\boldsymbol{\omega}$) comes out of the paper.

This field will turn right-handed around the z-axis (see Fig. 4.1). It is evidently composed of two linearly polarized fields, orthogonal and out of phase with each other. A left-handed field is given by changing the phase relationship:

$$\boldsymbol{b}_{1c}(\text{left}, \omega) = B_1(\cos \omega t\, \hat{\boldsymbol{x}} - \sin \omega t\, \hat{\ }) = B_1 [\cos(-\omega t)\hat{\boldsymbol{x}} + \sin(-\omega t)\hat{\boldsymbol{y}}], \tag{10}$$

or

$$\boldsymbol{b}_{1c}(\text{left}, \omega) = \boldsymbol{b}_{1c}(\text{right}, -\omega). \tag{11}$$

One can also write this in complex form

$$\boldsymbol{b}_{1c}(\text{right}, \omega) = \mathscr{R}[B_1\, e^{i\omega t}(\hat{x} - i\hat{y})],$$

$$\boldsymbol{b}_{1c}(\text{left}, \omega) = \mathscr{R}[B_1\, e^{i\omega t}(\hat{x} + i\hat{y})] = \mathscr{R}B_1\, e^{-i\omega t}(\hat{x} - i\hat{y}) = b_{1c}(\text{right}, -\omega). \tag{12}$$

We observe that we can specify any rotating field around $\hat{z}$ right-handed as well as left-handed, by

$$b_{1c}(\omega) = B_1(\cos \omega t\,.\,\hat{x} + \sin \omega t\,.\,\hat{y}) = \mathscr{R}[B_1\, e^{i\omega t}(\hat{x} - i\hat{y})] \tag{13}$$

since for $\omega > 0$ this is a right-handed field and for $\omega < 0$ this is a left-handed field. ω can be considered as the component along $\hat{z}$ of the vector $\boldsymbol{\omega}$ which represents the rotation in orientation, sense and amplitude. It is evident that

$$b_{1c}(\omega) + b_{1c}(-\omega) = 2B_1 \cos \omega t\,.\,\hat{x} = b_1 \tag{14}$$

which shows the decomposition of a linearly polarized field b_1 into two rotating fields. Equation (14) also gives the historical reason for the factor 2 in the definition, eq. (8) and eq. (3) of Chapter 1.

Here we have a physical significance of a sign of ω, unlike in the case of linearly polarized fields where a sign on ω is only a matter of mathematical symmetry convenience. Nevertheless, by virtue of the foregoing discussion, we may consider ω positive or negative for linearly polarized fields. One "considers" respectively the right-handed or the left-handed component as effective. The Larmor frequency can be given by $\omega_s = -\gamma B_s$ and ω_s will be positive or negative according to $\gamma(B_s \geqq 0$ by definition, eq. (1)). For protons ($\gamma > 0$) the frequency is negative, the precession turning negatively around the field ($\boldsymbol{\omega} \cdot \boldsymbol{B}_s < 0$). For electrons the frequency is positive, and only the positive component of a linearly polarized field will be effective in a high field resonance experiment.

Until now we were only able to discuss rotating fields in a certain given coordinate system. Indeed b_x is a vector with time-dependent orientation and this fact is not expressed unambiguously unless one uses $\hat{x}$ and $\hat{y}$. We could make a convention and write, for instance, $\boldsymbol{b}_{1c} = (\boldsymbol{B}_1; \boldsymbol{\omega} t)$ or something like this, so describing a vector equal to $\boldsymbol{B}_1$ rotated over an angle $\boldsymbol{\omega} t$. We shall now use a formalism (Talpe, 1967a) which is much more expressive, introducing no new notation, and entering easily into the scheme of vector calculus by using cross products and dot products. The procedure is somewhat like the method of introducing the curl in vector calculus.

The rotation through an angle α about a certain direction and in a certain sense is commonly expressed by a vector $\boldsymbol{\alpha}$. The rotation of an arbitrary vector $\boldsymbol{v}$ through an infinitesimal angle ε about a direction $\hat{\varepsilon}$, or "about $\boldsymbol{\varepsilon}$", is given by

$$R_{\boldsymbol{\varepsilon}} \boldsymbol{v} = \boldsymbol{v} + \boldsymbol{\varepsilon} \wedge \boldsymbol{v} = (1 + \boldsymbol{\varepsilon} \wedge) \boldsymbol{v} \tag{15}$$

whence the operator equation

$$R_{\boldsymbol{\varepsilon}} = 1 + \boldsymbol{\varepsilon} \wedge . \tag{16}$$

Clearly a rotation through $2\boldsymbol{\varepsilon}$ involves two successive applications of this operator and in general

$$R_{n\varepsilon} = (1 + \varepsilon \wedge)^n = (R_\varepsilon)^n. \tag{17}$$

Let us now consider the rotation through a finite angle $\boldsymbol{\alpha}$. Decomposing it into n rotations over $\boldsymbol{\alpha}/n$, and increasing n to infinity, one obtains

$$R_{\boldsymbol{\alpha}} = \lim_{n \to \infty} (R_{\boldsymbol{\alpha}/n})^n = \lim_{n \to \infty} (1 + n^{-1} \boldsymbol{\alpha} \wedge)^{-n}. \qquad 18)$$

This last expression is generally abbreviated as:

$$R_{\boldsymbol{\alpha}} = \exp (\boldsymbol{\alpha} \wedge). \tag{19}$$

It is easily verified by vector calculation that indeed

$$\exp(\boldsymbol{\alpha}\wedge) = 1 + \boldsymbol{\alpha}\wedge + (\boldsymbol{\alpha}\wedge)^2/2! + (\boldsymbol{\alpha}\wedge)^3/3! + \ldots \tag{20}$$

This series expansion is illustrated in Fig. 4.2 for $\alpha = 1$ ($\boldsymbol{\alpha}$ normal to the plane of the figure) and applied to a vector $\boldsymbol{v}$ orthogonal to $\boldsymbol{\alpha}$ (the operator

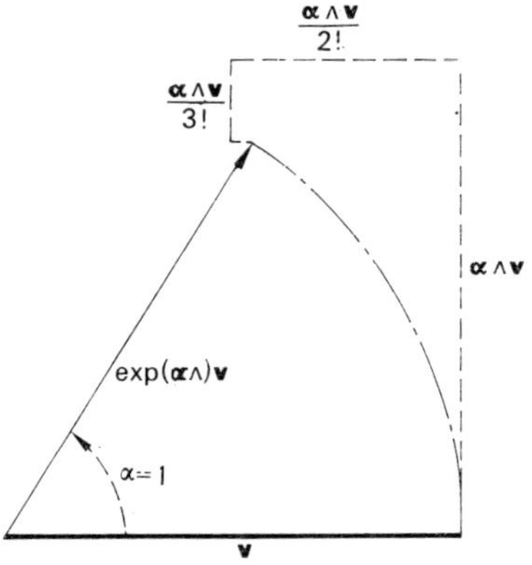

FIG. 4.2. Series expansion of the rotation operator $\exp(\alpha\wedge)$. α comes out of the paper.

leaves any vector parallel to $\boldsymbol{\alpha}$ invariant). An useful relation, which we call the exchange relation, is

$$\boldsymbol{a} \,.\, \exp(\boldsymbol{\alpha}\wedge)\,\boldsymbol{b} = \boldsymbol{b} \,.\, \exp(-\boldsymbol{\alpha}\wedge)\,\boldsymbol{a}, \tag{21}$$

since the dot product of a vector $\boldsymbol{a}$ with the rotated vector $\boldsymbol{b}$ equals the dot product of the inversely rotated vector $\boldsymbol{a}$ with the vector $\boldsymbol{b}$. Often the vector $\boldsymbol{\alpha}$ is time-dependent. We easily verify the operator equation

$$d/dt[\exp(\boldsymbol{\omega}t\wedge)] = \boldsymbol{\omega}\wedge\exp(\boldsymbol{\omega}t\wedge) \tag{22}$$

and, in general,

$$(d^n/dt^n)\,[\exp(\boldsymbol{\omega}t\wedge)] = (\boldsymbol{\omega}\wedge)^n\exp(\boldsymbol{\omega}t\wedge). \tag{23}$$

We recall that for $\boldsymbol{v} \,.\, \boldsymbol{\omega} = 0$ we have

$$(\boldsymbol{\omega}\wedge)^{2n}\,\boldsymbol{v} = (-\omega^2)^n\,\boldsymbol{v}. \tag{24}$$

For our purpose now

$$\boldsymbol{b}_{1c} = \exp(\omega t\wedge)\,\boldsymbol{B}_1 \tag{25}$$

represents a field of amplitude B_1, turning right-handed about the direction of $\hat{\boldsymbol{\omega}}$ with frequency ω, and initially oriented along $\boldsymbol{B}_1$. Of course a field turning left-handed about the same direction is given by $\exp(-\boldsymbol{\omega}t \wedge)\, \boldsymbol{B}_1$. Equation (25) is also meaningful when $\boldsymbol{B}_1$ is not orthogonal to $\boldsymbol{\omega}$. For example, if $\boldsymbol{B}_1$ is normal to $\boldsymbol{\omega}$ $(\boldsymbol{B}_1 . \boldsymbol{\omega} = 0)$ and $\boldsymbol{B}_s$ parallel to $\boldsymbol{\omega}(\boldsymbol{B}_s \wedge \boldsymbol{\omega} = 0)$ one can write the total field as

$$\boldsymbol{b} = \boldsymbol{B}_s + \boldsymbol{b}_{1c} = \exp(\boldsymbol{\omega}t \wedge)(\boldsymbol{B}_1 + \boldsymbol{B}_s) \tag{26}$$

since the operator $\exp(\boldsymbol{\omega}t \wedge)$ has no effect on a vector parallel to $\boldsymbol{\omega}$. A special case usually encountered is that of $\boldsymbol{\omega}$ colinear with $\boldsymbol{B}_s$ (and hence, in our convention, with $\hat{\boldsymbol{z}}$). Then we take $\boldsymbol{B}_1$ as parallel to $\hat{\boldsymbol{x}}$, since any $\hat{\boldsymbol{z}}$ component can be handled by redefining $\boldsymbol{B}_s$ and any $\hat{\boldsymbol{y}}$ component by redefining the time origin. We state

$$\boldsymbol{\omega} = \omega\hat{\boldsymbol{z}} \quad \text{and} \quad \boldsymbol{B}_1 = B_1 . \hat{\boldsymbol{x}} \tag{27}$$

and then we have

$$\boldsymbol{b}_{1c} = \exp(\boldsymbol{\omega}t \wedge)\, \boldsymbol{B}_1 = \mathscr{R} B_1 \exp(i\omega t)(\hat{\boldsymbol{x}} - i\hat{\boldsymbol{y}}). \tag{28}$$

(d) *Circular susceptibility component*

Let us now consider the magnetization due to $\boldsymbol{b}_{1c}$. We assume the special case mentioned above, $\boldsymbol{\omega}$ parallel to $\boldsymbol{B}_s$, or $\boldsymbol{\omega} \wedge \boldsymbol{B}_s = 0 = \boldsymbol{B}_1 \wedge \hat{\boldsymbol{x}}$ $\boldsymbol{b}_{1c}$ is given by eq. (28). If the system is linear, the total magnetization is found by adding the effects of the component along $\hat{\boldsymbol{x}}$ and of the component along $\hat{\boldsymbol{y}}$. Hence

$$\boldsymbol{m}(\omega) = \frac{10^7}{4\pi} \mathscr{R}(\chi\hat{\boldsymbol{x}} - i\chi\hat{\boldsymbol{y}})\, B_1\, e^{i\omega t}$$

or, in components,

$$m_x(\omega) = \frac{10^7}{4\pi} \mathscr{R}(\chi_{xx} - i\chi_{xy})\, B_1\, e^{i\omega t},$$

$$m_y(\omega) = \frac{10^7}{4\pi} \mathscr{R}(\chi_{yx} - i\chi_{yy})\, B_1\, e^{i\omega t}, \tag{29}$$

$$m_z(\omega) = \frac{10^7}{4\pi} \mathscr{R}(\chi_{zx} - i\chi_{zy})\, B_1\, e^{i\omega t}.$$

If the material is isotropic, there is no preferential direction in the plane orthogonal to $\boldsymbol{B}_s$ and hence the magnetization component along $\hat{\boldsymbol{y}}$, due to $B_1\hat{\boldsymbol{x}}$, equals the component along $-\hat{\boldsymbol{x}}$, due to $B_1\hat{\boldsymbol{y}}$. We get

$$\chi_{xy} = -\chi_{yx} \tag{30}$$

and of course

$$\chi_{xx} = \chi_{yy} \tag{31}$$

and

$$\chi_{zx} = \chi_{zy}. \tag{32}$$

Then eq. (29) becomes

$$\boldsymbol{m} = \frac{10^7}{4\pi} \mathscr{R}(\chi_{xx} + i\chi_{yx})\, B_1\, e^{i\omega t}(\hat{\boldsymbol{x}} - i\hat{\boldsymbol{y}})$$

$$+ \frac{10^7}{4\pi} \mathscr{R}\, \chi_{zx}\, B_1\, e^{i\omega t}(1 - i)\,\hat{\boldsymbol{z}}. \tag{33}$$

On the other hand, the magnetization due to the rotating field $\boldsymbol{b}_{1c}$ is also a rotating vector, apart from a z component:

$$\boldsymbol{m} = \boldsymbol{m}_c + \boldsymbol{m}_z. \tag{34}$$

The vector $\boldsymbol{m}_c$ has a certain phase lag:

$$\boldsymbol{m}_c = \mathscr{R}|M_c|\, e^{i(\omega t - \varphi_c)}\,(\hat{\boldsymbol{x}} - i\hat{\boldsymbol{y}}) = \mathscr{R}\,|M_c|\, e^{-i\varphi_c} \,.\, e^{i\omega t}(\hat{\boldsymbol{x}} - i\hat{\boldsymbol{y}})$$

$$= \mathscr{R}(M_c' - iM_c'')\, e^{i\omega t}(\hat{\boldsymbol{x}} - i\hat{\boldsymbol{y}}) = \mathscr{R} M_c\, e^{i\omega t}(\hat{\boldsymbol{x}} - i\hat{\boldsymbol{y}}). \tag{35}$$

We now define a circular susceptibility component by

$$M_c = \frac{10^7}{4\pi} \chi_c\, B_1. \tag{36}$$

Comparison with eq. (33) yields

$$\chi_c = \chi_{xx} + i\chi_{yx}. \tag{37}$$

The term χ_{xx} is the same for a left-handed as for a right-handed field, as may be seen by rotating the coordinate system around the x-axis, $\chi_{xx}(\omega) = \chi_{xx}(-\omega)$. But the same operation shows that $\chi_{yx}(\omega) = \chi_{xy}(-\omega) = -\chi_{yx}(-\omega)$. Hence

$$\chi_c(\omega) = \chi_c^*(-\omega). \tag{38}$$

Stating it another way:

$$\begin{aligned} 2\chi_{xx}(\omega) &= \chi_c(\omega) + \chi_c(-\omega), \\ 2i\chi_{yx}(\omega) &= \chi_c(\omega) - \chi_c(-\omega). \end{aligned} \tag{39}$$

If the system is not linear, we cannot simply assume the total magnetization to be the sum of the magnetization due to $\boldsymbol{b}_{1c} \cdot \hat{x}$ and that due to $\boldsymbol{b}_{1c} \cdot \hat{y}$, nor the magnetization due to the linear field $\boldsymbol{b}_1$ to be the sum of the magnetizations due to $\boldsymbol{b}_{1c}(\omega)$ and $\boldsymbol{b}_{1c}(-\omega)$. Nevertheless, in the Bloch theory the linear experimental field is considered as a sum of two circularly polarized fields $\boldsymbol{b}_{1c}(\omega)$ and $\boldsymbol{b}_{1c}(-\omega)$. This is because one component is negligible in high static fields ($\omega_0\tau \gg 1$). One can then assume a non-linearity in the system with respect to the remaining component—as is done by Bloch, who considers a dependence of χ on the amplitude $\boldsymbol{B}_1$. This is, however, not valid when $\omega_0\tau \gtrsim 1$. We draw attention to the fact that the non-linearity in the Bloch equations is merely a dependence on the amplitude of B_1 in the first harmonic of $\boldsymbol{m}$ and hence in χ, not taking into account higher harmonics. Hence this approach of Bloch can only give some information about the first-order component of $\boldsymbol{m}$ due to influences proportional to $(\mathcal{R}B_1 \exp i\omega t)^n$. One must be very careful in comparing Bloch's final equations with solutions of the Bloch differential equation for linear fields in which the non-linearity is dealt with as before [eq. (5)]. By forgetting this, confusion has sometimes spread in the literature. For example, $(\cos \omega t)^2$ does not contain $\cos \omega t$, while $(\cos \omega t)^3$ contains $\cos \omega t$.

4.3. Resonance line as a function of the static field

(a) *High static field*

Until now we assumed that the static field $\boldsymbol{B}$ applied to the sample was fixed and we looked for the quantity $\chi(\omega_0 + \omega_d)$ as a function of the frequency of the applied HF field. However, for high fields ($\omega_d\tau \gg 1$), the resonance line is only important for ω in the neighbourhood of ω_0 and we may suppose that the line as a function of $(\omega - \omega_0)$ will be exactly the same if, for example, ω_0 is 1 per cent higher or lower. I.e. if $\omega_0\tau \gg 1$, we may consider the line as a function of the applied frequency ω as well as considering it as a function of the Larmor frequency ω_0. In fact, it will be technically much more convenient during an experiment to vary the static field, to which ω_0 is proportional, than to vary the frequency of the HF field. We shall establish the relation between field scanning and frequency scanning. The only problem in using high fields is to be careful about signs and to have a good notation for the quantities involved.

Let us write χ explicitly as a function of the frequency of the HF field and of the Larmor frequency actually present. By *convention* we first write the applied frequency and then the Larmor frequency, i.e. the applied static field strength. We write:

$$\chi(\omega_{\mathrm{HF}}, \omega_{\mathrm{Larmor}}). \tag{40}$$

The fact that the line depends only on $\omega - \omega_0$ and not on ω_0, in the range of interest, may be written as

$$\chi(\omega_{\mathrm{HF}}, \omega_{\mathrm{Larmor}}) = \chi(\omega_{\mathrm{HF}} + \Delta\omega, \omega_{\mathrm{Larmor}} + \Delta\omega) \tag{41}$$

for any ω_{HF} and ω_{Larmor} within a small range around ω_{Larmor}. Observe that ω_{Larmor} indicates not a frequency but a field, being the field to which a Larmor frequency equal to ω_{Larmor} corresponds. Incidentally, we may associate a field with any frequency and a frequency with any field, by the relation

$$\omega = -\gamma B, \tag{42}$$

where the gyromagnetic ratio γ is defined by eq. (3.20) or eq. (3.28). This B will in practice be the field at maximum absorption or zero dispersion for a HF field with frequency ω. Remember that γ may be positive or negative, according to the sample. In e.s.r. it will in general be negative, while for protons, $\gamma > 0$. Let us now take $\omega_0 + \omega_d$ for the actual frequency ω_{HF} of eq. (41) and ω_0 for the Larmor frequency ω_{Larmor}:

$$\chi(\omega_0 + \omega_d, \omega_0) = \chi(\omega_0 + \omega_d + \Delta\omega, \omega_0 + \Delta\omega). \tag{43}$$

We assume $\omega_{HF} > 0$ and hence $\omega_{Larmor} > 0$. If we take $\Delta\omega = -\omega_d$ this becomes

$$\chi(\omega_0 + \omega_d, \omega_0) = \chi(\omega_0, \omega_0 - \omega_d). \tag{44}$$

We may also change the notation and write the field instead of ω_{Larmor}. Then

$$\chi(\omega_0 + \omega_d, B_0) = \chi(\omega_0, B_0 - B_d). \tag{45}$$

For $\gamma > 0$ the transposition requires an inversion of the relative orientation of the $\boldsymbol{\omega}$- and $\boldsymbol{B}$-axis, because we assumed $\omega_0 + \omega_d$ of the first term, as well as $B_0 - B_d$ of the second, positive [see eq. (1)]. Let us consider the static susceptibility formulae. Equation (3.35) gives

$$\begin{aligned}\chi_s &= \frac{4}{\omega_0} \int\limits_{-\infty}^{\infty} \chi''(\omega_0 + \omega_d, B_0)\, d\omega_d/2\pi \\ &= \frac{2/\pi}{-\gamma B_0} \int\limits_{-\infty}^{\infty} \chi''(\omega_0, B_0 - B_d)\, d(-\gamma B_d) \\ &= \frac{2/\pi}{B_0} \int\limits_{-\infty}^{\infty} \chi''(\omega_0, B_0 + B_d)\, dB_d. \end{aligned} \tag{46}$$

In the same way eq. (3.37) transforms into:

$$\begin{aligned}\chi_s &= -2 \lim_{\omega_d \to \infty} \chi'(\omega_0 + \omega_d, B_0) \,.\, \omega_d/\omega_0 = -2 \lim_{B_d \to \infty} \chi'(\omega_0, B_0 - B_d)\, B_d/B_0 \\ &= 2 \lim_{B_d \to \infty} \chi'(\omega_0, B_0 + B_d) \,.\, B_d/B_0. \end{aligned} \tag{47}$$

In the last equation we have used the fact that χ' is an odd function of B_d. The moments [eq. (3.47)] are now defined as

$$M_n = (-\gamma)^n \frac{2/\pi}{B_0} \int\limits_{-\infty}^{\infty} B_d^n \chi''(\omega_0, B_0 + B_d)\, dB_d \tag{48}$$

and the coefficients of the asymptotic expansion of χ' [eq. (3.52)] by

$$2\frac{B_d}{B_0}\chi'(\omega_0, B_0 + B_d) = \sum_{k=0}^{p} (-\gamma)^{-2k} a_{2k} B_d^{-2k} + R_{2p} \tag{49}$$

assuming again χ' odd.

From now on we shall no longer use the cumbersome notation of eq. (45). We shall write $\chi(B_d)$ for $\chi(\omega_0, B_0 + B_d)$. For comparison, we finally write eqs. (46) and (47) as

$$\chi_s = \lim_{B_d \to \infty} \frac{2/\pi}{B_0} \int_{-B_d}^{B_d} \chi''(B_d') \, . \, dB_d' \tag{50a}$$

$$\chi_s = \lim_{B_d \to \infty} \frac{2}{B_0} B_d \, . \, \chi'(B_d) \tag{50b}$$

emphasizing that both equations contain a transition to limit.

A note about line widths should be useful: we defined $\delta, \delta', \delta''$, etc., in § 3.5. We may, of course, also measure the width of a line on the B_s-axis or on the B_d-axis. We use the same symbols for the corresponding definitions. For example,

$$\delta_{(\omega_d)} = |\gamma| \, \delta_{(B_d)} \tag{51}$$

and generally we do not write the subscript ω_d or B_d since the distinction is mostly evident from the dimensions of the formula. For instance, in $\tau = 1/\delta$ we mean $\delta_{(\omega_d)}$ and in $\tau = 1/|\gamma| \, \delta$ we mean $\delta_{(B_d)}$. Observe that

$$\delta'^{+}_{(\omega_d)} = \delta'^{-}_{(B_d)} \tag{52}$$

and so on, for asymmetric lines. The δ-symbols always indicate positive quantities.

(b) *Low static field*

The simple transformation from frequency scanning to field scanning discussed so far is only valid if $\omega_0 \tau \gg 1$ or $B_0 \gg B_d$. If this condition is not fulfilled, the problem turns out to be much more complicated.

A first approach is to consider directly the field scanning in the theory. The Bloch equations, for example, were originally deduced on a phenomenological basis as a function of the applied field, and, with two modifications introduced afterwards, they can be applied to low fields (Van Gerven and Talpe, 1967). A fundamental study—mainly of the absorption and the first modification—has been published by Van Gerven (1963). Unfortunately the theory is applicable only in certain cases, because of some restricting basic assumptions. A frequent case in e.s.r. is when we have some "narrowing" effect, similar to the motional narrowing in n.m.r. in liquids. One important feature, however, has to be mentioned. The Bloch equation can take into account some saturation, i.e. conditions where the r.f. field is not of negligible strength. We return to this in the next section.

A more general solution, assuming negligible saturation however, (linear system), consists in retaining the two parts of eq. (2.71) unchanged and making a supposition about $\alpha_0(t)$. As an example we take a Lorentzian line shape, as in Bloch's theory, in a field B_s. The Larmor frequency is ω_s and

$$\alpha_0(t) = \omega_s \chi_s \, e^{-t/\tau} \tag{53}$$

[with τ in accordance with eq. (3.39)]. The total line is [eq. (2.71)]

$$\chi(\omega, \omega_s) = \frac{\omega_s \chi_s}{2i} \int_0^\infty [e^{-t/\tau} \, e^{-i(\omega-\omega_s)t} - e^{-t/\tau} \, e^{-i(\omega+\omega_s)t}] \, dt \tag{54}$$

$$\chi(\omega, \omega_s) = \frac{\omega_s \chi_s}{2i} \left[\frac{1}{1 + i(\omega - \omega_s)} + \frac{1}{1 + i(\omega + \omega_s)} \right]. \tag{55}$$

Let us take ω_0 as the actual frequency, with a resonance field $B_0 = -\omega_0/\gamma$, and consider the field (or the eigenfrequency ω_s) as variable:

$$\chi(\omega_0, B_s) = \frac{-\gamma B_s \chi_s}{2i} \quad \frac{1}{1 - i(B_s - B_0)(-\gamma\tau)} + \frac{1}{1 - i(B_s + B_0)(-\gamma\tau)}. \tag{56}$$

We may still use $\delta = 1/\tau$, or in field units $\delta = 1/(-\gamma\tau)$. Then

$$\chi(\omega_0, B_s) = \frac{B_s \chi_s}{2i} \left[\frac{1}{\delta - i(B_s - B_0)} + \frac{1}{\delta - i(B_s + B_0)} \right]. \tag{57}$$

One may now introduce different values of δ and compare this function of B_s with experiment.†

† The procedure proposed by Lacroix (1954) is similar but more complicated and less exact.

4.4. Non-linear system

(a) *Criterion of linearity*

In former sections we assumed the system was linear. This is an assumption frequently made in physics. For example, Ohm's law states that the voltage across a conductor is proportional to the current through it. But, unlike the application of Ohm's law to a copper wire, where it is valid to a high approximation for any realizable current, a paramagnetic system may easily depart from linearity. The non-linearity of a paramagnetic system is characterized by a non-equilibrium value of the magnetization. Let the equilibrium value, in the direction of the static field $\boldsymbol{B}_s$, be given by M_0 and let the actual component along $\boldsymbol{B}_s$ be given by M_z. Then we define a parameter s by

$$s = \frac{M_0 - M_z}{M_0}\,. \tag{58}$$

It is evident that s is a measure of the departure from equilibrium. A strong HF field drives the system away from equilibrium, so that the response to the excitation is no longer proportional to the excitation, but depends on how much the excitation alters the system itself. On the other hand, relaxation tends to restore equilibrium, and if the influence of the HF field driving s away from zero is much less than the influence of the relaxation restoring s to zero, we say that the HF field is "small". A strong HF field results in a non-negligible s and then we say the system is *saturated* to some extent. This is because for $s \approx 1$ the system can no longer absorb HF energy, as we shall see below. Therefore s is called the *saturation parameter*. The linear theory of the former sections is valid only for

$$s \ll 1\,. \tag{59}$$

We shall first derive an expression for s as a function of the amplitude B_1 of the HF field and of a parameter τ_1 of the relaxation, for small s, in order to replace the requirement $s \ll 1$ by a requirement for B_1 and τ_1. Then we shall analyse the situation $s < 1$ since it may be of interest, e.g. for improving the signal-to-noise ratio, to use non-negligible HF fields.

Let us for simplicity represent the relaxation between "spins" and lattice by a single time constant τ_1. Then the equilibrium magnetization is restored at a rate

$$\left(\frac{dM_z}{dt}\right)_{\text{relax}} = \frac{M_0 - M_z}{\tau_1} \tag{60}$$

On the other hand, the magnetization is reduced because of the "spin" flips induced by the HF field and is proportional to the actual excess of "spins" along B_s over the "spins" antiparallel to $\boldsymbol{B}_s$,

$$\left(\frac{-dM_z}{dt}\right)_{\text{HF}} = W. \quad [M_z - (-M_z)]. \tag{61}$$

W is the probability (the number of times it happens per unit time) that a certain "spin" flips from one level to another, due to the HF field. W is proportional to the intensity B_1^2 of the HF field and so we define a constant τ_2 by

$$W = \tfrac{1}{2}(\gamma B_1)^2\,\tau_2\,. \tag{62}$$

The fact that we define a single constant τ_2 implies again that the system is simple, e.g. a single spin packet with only two energy levels. If we may simply add the relaxation and the induced transitions, we get

$$\frac{dM_z}{dt} = \frac{M_0 - M_z}{\tau_1} - 2WM_z \tag{63}$$

and in the steady state ($dM_z/dt = 0$) we readily obtain

$$s = \frac{M_0 - M_z}{M_0} = \frac{2W\tau_1}{1 + 2W\tau_1} = \frac{(\gamma B_1)^2\,\tau_1\tau_2}{1 + (\gamma B_1)^2\tau_1\tau_2} \tag{64}$$

or

$$(\gamma B_1)^2\,\tau_1\tau_2 = \frac{s}{1 - s}. \tag{65}$$

Hence $s \ll 1$ corresponds to

$$(\gamma B_1)^2\,\tau_1\tau_2 \ll 1. \tag{66}$$

The meaning of τ_1, the spin–lattice relaxation time, is obvious. Let us emphasize, still for $s \ll 1$, the meaning of τ_2. The energy the system loses per unit time by relaxation may be written as

$$B_s \frac{d\boldsymbol{M}}{dt} = B_s \frac{dM_z}{dt} = B_s \frac{M_0 - M_z}{\tau_1} = B_s M_0 s/\tau_1 = \frac{10^7}{4\pi} \chi_s B_s^2 s/\tau_1 . \tag{67}$$

This power is supplied by the HF field and hence equals the time average of $\boldsymbol{b}_1 . d\boldsymbol{m}/dt$. Thus

$$\frac{10^7}{4\pi} \chi_s B_s^2 s/\tau_1 = \langle \boldsymbol{b}_1\, d\boldsymbol{m}/dt \rangle = \frac{10^7}{4\pi} 2B_1^2\, \chi''(\omega) . \omega . \tag{68}$$

We solve for s, using $\gamma B_s = \omega$,

$$s = (\gamma B_1)^2 \tau_1 \left[\frac{2\chi''(\omega)}{\chi_s \omega} \right]. \tag{69}$$

From eq. (65) we see that the expression in brackets is τ_2 for $s \ll 1$. Hence τ_2 is the relaxation time defined in eq. (3.39) (for the linear system), or $1/\gamma\tau_2$ is the width of the unsaturated resonance line [see eq. (3.41)].

A simple comparison with the Bloch theory shows that in cases where this theory is valid, τ_1 and τ_2 are the relaxation times introduced by Bloch. The meaning of τ_1 and τ_2 introduced here is, however, more general.

(b) *Non-linear system*

If s becomes of the order of unity, we can no longer apply the simple formulae used in the former sections (for linear systems). Perhaps we might still assume the relaxation and the transition probability above, with τ_1 and τ_2 as defined. Then we should still have eq. (65)

$$(\gamma B_1)^2\, \tau_1 \tau_2 = \frac{s}{1 - s}$$

and for $(\gamma B_1)^2\, \tau_1\tau_2$ up to the order of unity, or say $s \lesssim \frac{1}{2}$, we may still hope to measure something interpretable. Therefore we must look a little closer at the parameter τ_2.

The Bloch formalism is a theory which allows for some saturation. It gives a Lorentzian line, to be considered as a broader line which is "narrowed" by some mechanism. If the interaction between spins, which broadens the line, has a width $1/\gamma\tau_{dd}$ and this broadening is averaged out to a certain extent by some random fluctuation of this interaction, with time constant $\tau_c \ll \tau_{dd}$ (e.g. due to motion of spins, or more frequently in e.s.r. due to exchange), then the line will be narrowed. The line width will be

$$\frac{1}{\gamma\tau_2} = (1/\gamma\tau_{dd})^2\,\gamma\tau_c. \tag{70}$$

Of course, since $\tau_c \ll \tau_{dd}$, it follows that

$$\frac{1}{\tau_2} \ll \frac{1}{\tau_{dd}} < \frac{1}{\tau_c}. \tag{71}$$

We may now state†: "If the physical situation is such that for $s \ll 1$ the Bloch equations are valid, then the Bloch equations are still valid for non-negligible B_1 provided

$$B_1 \ll 1/\gamma\tau_c.\text{"} \tag{72}$$

In practice, when the shape of the (elementary) line is Lorentzian, we may assume some such narrowing, since otherwise the shape will in general be rather Gaussian. In most cases the Bloch theory will then be valid for $(\gamma B_1)^2\,\tau_1\tau_2$ up to some units, say for $B_1 < 1/\gamma\tau_{dd}$, since in general

$$\frac{1}{\tau_1} \leqq \frac{1}{\tau_2} \ll \frac{1}{\tau_{dd}} < \frac{1}{\tau_c}. \tag{73}$$

Assuming now a Bloch line, one can easily deduce some of the results obtained in the previous section by direct calculation. Let the Bloch equations be given by

$$\chi' - iS\chi'' = \frac{\frac{1}{2}\chi_s B_0}{B_d + iS\delta}; \quad S^2 = 1 + \gamma^2 B_1^2 \tau_1\tau_2 = \frac{1}{1-s}. \tag{74}$$

† Quoted from Abragam (1961, p. 517).

For the calculation of χ_s we find that eq. (3.37) or eq. (47), using the dispersion, remains valid. Equations (3.35) or (46), however, using the absorption line, supposes s or S^2 to be known—which is rather inconvenient. As for the g-factor there is no problem and the line width is given by $S\delta$ instead of $\delta = 1/\gamma\tau_2$. Let us note that the determination of $M^{(2n)}$ or a_{2n} is only useful here in order to check if the line is in fact Lorentzian.

Finally we consider the case when B_1 is strong or, more precisely,

$$B_1 \not\ll \frac{1}{\gamma\tau_{dd}}. \tag{75}$$

The case $B_1 \approx 1/\gamma\tau_{dd}$ is theoretically rather difficult to deal with and one cannot draw definite conclusions. But on the other hand, in e.s.r. $1/\gamma\tau_{dd}$ is always at least about 1 mT and, from a technological point of view, there is little interest in using values of B_1 of this order of magnitude for improving the signal-to-noise ratio. Another question however, is the use of very strong high-frequency fields,

$$B_1 \gg 1/\gamma\tau_{dd}. \tag{76}$$

Although involving some technological difficulties in microwave spectroscopy, one may expect advantages similar to those obtained in the case of n.m.r. (Solomon and Ezratty, 1962). Some experiments have indeed been done in e.s.r. (Lhôte *et al.*, 1963) but we shall not discuss them.

4.5. Non-stationary system

A final topic to be discussed is the meaning of a "stationary" system. In dealing with the idealized line shape, we assumed a system excited by a HF magnetic field of fixed frequency and with time-independent properties such as eigenfrequency (or static field) and relaxation. In fact we should like to make measurements as a function of certain parameters of the system; the necessary variations of these parameters cannot be achieved infinitely slowly. Moreover, we may prefer to use a.c. measuring techniques, which oblige us to modulate the parameters of the system.

Hence the static field is no longer "static". It is time dependent and can in principle induce transitions. The eigenfrequency is no longer "fixed" but modulated and hence sidebands may appear. The system itself varies during relaxation and hence the relaxation in one state of the system may be influenced by a new, different state that appears in the meantime.

Therefore we must now express these effects quantitatively in order to establish the conditions in which we may neglect them.

(a) *Adiabatic field variation*

A time-independent static field means a time-independent coupling of the "spin" system to a magnet. This corresponds to a time-independent term in the Hamiltonian describing the system, or simply a time-independent force acting on the spins. Such a coupling cannot change the energy of the spin system. Only a time-dependent part of the Hamiltonian, such as the coupling with the HF field, can induce transitions. This is a matter of conservation of energy. A magnetic moment, a "spin", precessing freely around a magnetic field, maintains its angle with respect to the field, and hence its energy, constant.

When the field changes very slowly, this angle may still be maintained. We then say that the field changes adiabatically. The change is so slow that it does not induce transitions from one energy level to another. The magnetic moment vector simply follows the movement of the field vector. On the other hand, a sudden change in field, if fast enough, will leave the magnetic moment vector where it was. The magnetic moment vector starts precessing around the new field position from its position (under the influence of the old field) just before the change. This slow or fast change of magnetic field is the essential difference between steady state and pulse methods. We must now discover what an adiabatic change is, in order to express quantitatively that we confine ourselves to steady state measurements. For the moment, we neglect relaxation. We have here a problem of pure mechanics. It is dealt with classically by Abragam (1961, p. 35) and quantum mechanically by Messiah (1960).

Let us consider the frame rotating† with the effective (right-handed or left-handed) component of the HF field. Then in this frame $(\hat{x}, \hat{y}, \hat{z})$ the field is fixed:

$$\boldsymbol{B}_e = (B_s - \omega/\gamma)\, z + B_1 \hat{x} \tag{77}$$

and the magnetization precesses around it. "Slow changes" are changes slow compared with the precession of the magnetization around $\boldsymbol{B}_e$.

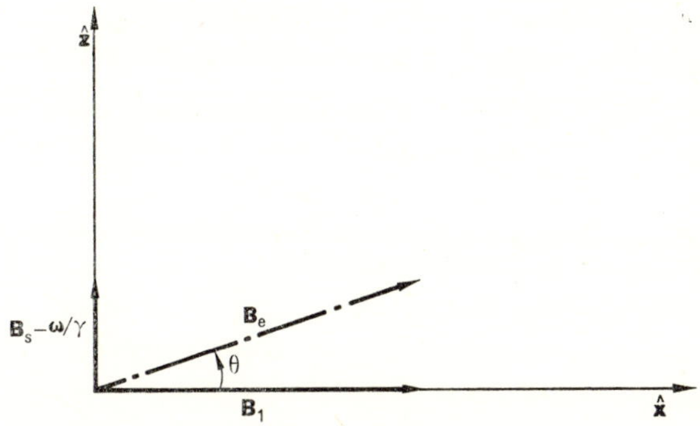

FIG. 4.3. The change in time of the field $\boldsymbol{B}_e$ in the rotating frame may be given by $\dot{\theta} = d\theta/dt$, to be compared with the precession speed γB_e of the magnetization. The adiabatic condition is $\dot{\theta} \ll \gamma B_e$.

The fields are represented in Fig. 4.3, in the $(\hat{x}, \hat{z})$ plane. We may express the field variation speed by

$$\dot{\theta} \equiv \frac{d\theta}{dt}. \tag{78}$$

The adiabatic condition is now:

$$\dot{\theta} \ll \gamma B_e. \tag{79}$$

$d\theta/dt$ is readily expressed in terms of field quantities, observing that $(B_s - \omega/\gamma)$ and B_e change with time and B_1 does not:

$$\frac{d\theta}{dt} = \cos^2\theta \, \frac{d \tan\theta}{dt} = \frac{B_1^2}{B_e^2} \cdot \frac{d(B_s - \omega/\gamma)/dt}{B_1}. \tag{80}$$

† One may consult Abragam (1961, p. 19) about the rotating frame technique.

Hence the adiabatic condition is

$$\dot{\theta} = \frac{d\theta}{dt} = B_1 \frac{d(B_s - \omega/\gamma)/dt}{B_e^2} \ll \gamma B_e. \tag{81}$$

This condition is strongest at resonance, where $B_e = B_1$:

$$\dot{\theta}_{\text{res}} = \frac{1}{B_1} d(B_s - \omega/\gamma)/dt \ll \gamma B_1. \tag{82}$$

In another section (§ 4.3), dealing with field modulation, we shall see that the restriction

$$\dot{\theta} \ll \gamma B_1 \tag{83}$$

is of no great practical importance in e.s.r. Let us only emphasize here that eventually one may take advantage of the fact that

$$\dot{\theta} \ll \gamma B_e \tag{84}$$

even when

$$\dot{\theta}_{\text{res}} \approx \gamma B_1 \tag{85}$$

by measuring on the edges of a dispersion line. An important part of the information in the dispersion line is indeed contained in the region farther than δ from resonance. Observe finally that $\dot{\theta}$ expresses the variation due to change in the eigenfrequency γB_s as well as the variation due to a change in the exciting frequency ω. It is irrelevant whether we vary the field or the applied frequency.

(b) *Sidebands*

It is well known that any modulation of a HF signal of unique constant frequency $\omega/2\pi$ produces subsidiary signals of different frequencies, called sidebands. If a wave

$$a(t) = A \sin \omega t \tag{86}$$

is sinusoidally modulated in amplitude, so that

$$A = A_0(1 + m \sin pt) \tag{87}$$

then the time dependence of $a(t)$ becomes:

$$\begin{aligned} a(t) &= A_0(1 + m \sin pt) \sin \omega t \\ &= A_0[\sin \omega t + \tfrac{1}{2} m \cos(\omega - p)\, t - \tfrac{1}{2} m \cos(\omega + p)\, t]. \end{aligned} \tag{88}$$

If the wave is frequency-modulated the function $a(t)$ becomes somewhat more complicated. (See, for example, Fagot and Magne (1961), p. 69.) In $a(t)$ the amplitude is now constant but the phase is time dependent in a non-linear way

$$a(t) = A_0 \sin[\omega t + \phi(t)]. \tag{89}$$

If

$$\phi(t) = \phi_m \sin pt$$

then

$$a(t) = A_0 \sin(\omega t + \phi_m \sin pt) \tag{90}$$

and the instantaneous frequency, the derivative of the phase, is

$$d(\omega t + \phi_m \sin pt)/dt = \omega + \phi_m p \cos pt = \omega + \Delta \cos pt \tag{91}$$

at each instant. The spectrum of $a(t)$ is now

$$a(t) = A_0 \sum_{n=-\infty}^{+\infty} J_n(\phi_m) \sin(\omega_0 + np)\, t \tag{92}$$

or [since $J_n = (-1)^n J_{-n}$]:

$$\begin{aligned} a(t)/A_0 = J_0(\phi_m) \sin \omega_0 t \\ &+ J_1(\phi_m)[\sin(\omega_0 + p)\, t - \sin(\omega_0 - p)\, t] \\ &+ J_2(\phi_m)[\sin(\omega_0 + 2p)\, t + \sin(\omega_0 - 2p)\, t] \end{aligned} \tag{93}$$

$J_n(\phi_m)$ are the Bessel functions.

If we now modulate the exciting frequency in frequency, it is clear that a whole set of exciting frequencies will be present. This is, however, also valid if we modulate the eigenfrequency in frequency. A whole set of eigenfrequencies appears. This has been shown by Karplus (1948). See also Macomber and Waugh (1965) and Gabillard and Ponchel

(1963). An amplitude modulation of the static fields is in fact a frequency modulation of the eigenfrequency. The instantaneous eigenfrequency is

$$\gamma B_s + \gamma B_m \cos \Omega t. \tag{94}$$

And therefore the spectrum of eigenfrequencies is

$$\gamma B_s, \gamma B_s \pm \Omega, \gamma B_s \pm 2\Omega, \gamma B_s \pm 3\Omega, \ldots \tag{95}$$

the amplitude of the nth eigenfrequency $\gamma B_s \pm n\Omega$ having a relative importance $J_n(\gamma B_m/\Omega)$. Since the observed signal is proportional to the square of the H.F. amplitude, the lines of the different sidebands will be proportional to $J_n^2(\gamma B_m/\Omega)$. And, of course,

$$\sum_{-\infty}^{+\infty} J_n^2 = 1.$$

The "spins" are distributed among the sidebands $\omega \pm n\Omega$ and the carrier ω.

Such sidebands have indeed been observed experimentally. But if one is interested in getting information about the sample, the simplest way of taking this effect into account is to avoid it, i.e. to impose conditions such that it becomes negligible. In fact, the nth sideband is important if its distance from the centre line exceeds the linewidth, or if

$$n\Omega/\gamma \gtrsim \delta. \tag{96}$$

But the modulation amplitude may in general not exceed the linewidth

$$\delta \gtrsim B_m. \tag{97}$$

Hence only the sidebands of order n given by

$$n\Omega/\gamma \gtrsim B_m \tag{98}$$

are important. But $J_n(\gamma B_m/\Omega)$ becomes negligible for

$$n > \frac{\gamma B_m}{\Omega}, \tag{99}$$

at least for high n.

Thus the only trouble with sidebands may arise when

$$\gamma B_m \lesssim \Omega. \tag{100}$$

For $\Omega/2\pi = 400$ Hz the condition $\gamma B_m \approx \Omega$ means that $B_m \approx 0{\cdot}014\ \mu$T so that even for the smallest lines only the 100th sideband exceeds the line. For $\Omega/2\pi = 100$ kHz, $\gamma B_m \approx \Omega$ means $B_m \approx 3\ \mu$T, and in this case one can observe sidebands. (It is even easier with, for example, $\Omega/2\pi = 2$ MHz.) The way to avoid them is to take

$$\gamma B_m/\Omega \gg 1 \tag{101}$$

since then

$$J_n \ll J_0 \tag{102}$$

for $n \neq 0$, so that the sidebands, although no longer sufficiently near the carrier, are now sufficiently weak with respect to the carrier. An interesting feature is that for $\gamma B_m/\Omega = 2{\cdot}4$ the carrier disappears since $J_0(2{\cdot}4) = 0$. One can then observe sidebands only.

(c) *Relaxation*

In order to be stationary with respect to the relaxation, the system must not change during a relaxation process. Hence the time over which the field changes from one position to a different one, expressed quantitatively by $1/\dot{\theta}$ [eq. (78)], must be long compared to the relaxation times of the system. For a linear system there is no problem:

$$\gamma B_1 < \frac{1}{\tau_1}, \frac{1}{\tau_2} \tag{103}$$

and the condition of eq. (83) then gives

$$\dot{\theta} \ll \frac{1}{\tau_1}, \frac{1}{\tau_2}. \tag{104}$$

If B_1 is of the order of $1/\gamma\tau_2$, for example, and the Bloch equations are applicable, then one must require eq. (104) explicitly.

We have already mentioned experiments in which a very strong HF field B_1 is used. Then $\dot{\theta} \ll \gamma B_1$ is easily satisfied. An interesting technique is the slow-scan–fast-modulation (Solomon and Ezratty, 1962). One uses a slow scan, i.e. $\dot{\theta}_{\text{scan}} \ll 1/\tau_1$, but at the same time a fast modulation, the frequency being $\omega_m \gg 1/\tau_1$. The modulation gives the free spin response, since the system does not relax with the bath during a period. This is called *adiabatic fast passage*. Mathematically:

$$\gamma B_1 \gg \dot{\theta}_{\text{mod}} \gg 1/\tau_1 . \tag{105}$$

The scanning is conventional, i.e. slow with respect to B_1 as well as with respect to relaxation. For the interpretation of these signals we refer to the quoted publication and to the book of Abragam (1961).

5. Composite Lines

5.1. Introduction

"Spins" from a certain "spin" packet in a static field give rise to an eigenfrequency and a relaxation function. This is brought to light in a paramagnetic resonance line. But a sample may contain various "spin" packets, i.e. "spins" in various different situations. Suppose we measure the resonance line of a powder sample of DPPH (diphenyl picryl hydrazyl). This powder is composed of many microcrystals and each of them has a certain orientation with respect to the static field $\boldsymbol{B}_s$. It happens that the resonance line of a monocrystal of DPPH depends—in its g-factor as well as in its line width – on the orientation of the crystal. Thus we may expect for the powder sample a total line that is composite. In fact it is even asymmetric, as can be seen in Fig. 5.1. In certain cases the "spins" of different packets do not interact. For example, if the "different situation" is a different applied magnetic field, due to the inhomogeneity of this field, it is evident that there is no interaction between different packets, since "spins" only interact with their neighbours. The same is true for anisotropy effects in a powder sample: spins interact with their neighbours of the same microcrystal only. If the "spins" of different packets are *mixed in space* they may interact in principle, but they are still isolated when the a "spin" *flip* in one packet does not correspond

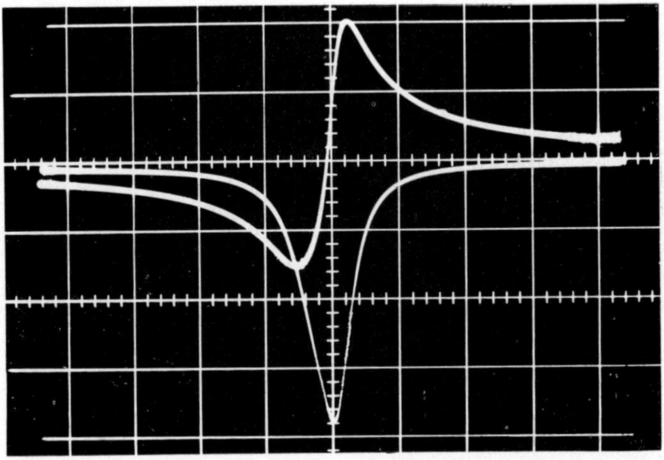

FIG. 5.1. Dual-beam oscillogram of an experimental e.s.r. dispersion and absorption line at 9 GHz from a sample of 7·38 mg DPPH powder at 291°K. Total width of the trace: 0·90 mT (= 9·0 G). Total height of the dispersion line: 0·466 mm^2. The static field increases from left to right.

energetically to a "spin" *flop* in the other packet. If the lines of different packets overlap, however, interactions between the packets may occur. Bloembergen *et al.* (1959) called this effect *cross relaxation.* A good account of this effect is given in the book by Pake (1962, pp. 129–34).

We shall deal in this section with the composition of lines from non-interacting spins, and in more detail with the two mentioned cases of "spin" packets that are not mixed in space. In this introduction, however, we shall say a little more about cross relaxation.

Let us consider the phenomenon by means of the concept of spin-temperature. In each packet of "spins" there is easy interchange of energy between the spins of the packet, which means that inside the packet the population of the energy levels is uniform. After a disturbance, equilibrium is restored in a time τ_s, the spin–spin relaxation time. So we can define for each "spin" packet a temperature which expresses the population of the levels. If two different "spin" packets, s and t, with spin–spin relaxation times, respectively τ_s and τ_t, interact, their respective temperatures can reach equilibrium, say in a time τ_{st}. If $\tau_{st} \lessgtr \tau_s, \tau_t$, then the temperature of the two packets will always be the same. In fact the situation of "spins" s and "spins" t is not a "different situation" as defined above, since the difference is not maintained during a time long compared to a "spin" flip. We only have one packet. Therefore we may state $\tau_{st} \gg \tau_s, \tau_t$. ($\tau_t > \tau_{st} > \tau_s$, for example, is impossible since "spins" t would become homogeneous in a time τ_{st} through interaction with "spins" s, hence in a time of the order of τ_{st}, if $\tau_s < \tau_{st}$.)

If the excitation of the spins is low, if there is no saturation, the "spin" temperature of all the packets is the same, equal to the lattice temperature. There is no net energy exchange between the packets. Hence the total resonance line is simply the sum of the individual lines of each packet. We measure, of course, the total line, and the problem is to extract from it the individual lines. The question is more complicated if there is some saturation. But if the "spin"–lattice relaxation time as well as the "spin"–"spin" relaxation time is the same for all "spin" packets, we may still consider the total line as the sum of the individual packet lines. The histories of the different "spin" packets run parallel. There is always the same spin temperature, even if this is different from the lattice. No net energy is transferred from one packet to the other. There is an important point, however: the relaxation time, responsible for the saturation, is related to the width of the resonance line. This means that the widths of the individual lines due to the single spin packets are much less than the width of the total composite lines.

The broadening due to the composition of narrower lines from non-interacting spin packets with different eigenfrequencies is called inhomogeneous broadening (Portis, 1953), in reference to the particular case occurring with lines in an inhomogeneous external field. This *inhomogeneous* broadening has nothing to do with relaxation—which gives rise to *homogeneous* broadening. Inhomogeneous broadening can sometimes be removed by increasing the static field, so that the line splits up or, for example, by spin echo techniques in nuclear magnetic renance (Abragam, 1961, pp. 32–34, 58–59, 542). It is an ordered effect. Homogeneous broadening is due to statistical disorder and cannot be removed. It cannot be visualized as being caused by a spread of eigenfrequencies of individual spins.

The condition quoted above that the "spin" packets relax all in the same way is of course not always fulfilled. Consider for instance two "spin" packets, s and t, with equal spin–spin relaxation times $\tau_s = \tau_t$, while the spin–lattice relaxation is different, say $\tau_{lt} \ll \tau_{ls}$. If the cross coupling is important, $\tau_{st} \ll \tau_{ls}$, then the "spins" s will relax to the lattice in a much shorter time than τ_{ls} because they will give their energy to the "spins" t and via them to the lattice. If τ_{st} is changed, e.g. by using a higher static field, the relaxation to the lattice of the "spins" s changes. Such cross coupling will influence the line width and the line shape. We cannot, however, give a general relation. Each type of cross coupling has to be examined separately, and this is outside the scope of this book. The effect of cross relaxation on inhomogeneous broadening has been studied by Kaplan (1965). We shall now consider only the superposition of single lines for the cases where it is applicable.

5.2. Line shape models

In describing relaxation processes, use is very frequently made of two models for the line shapes: the Lorentzian and the Gaussian. These models have already been presented in the early history of paramagnetic resonance, in a famous review article by Van Vleck (1957). Their use is based on the fact that they represent relatively simple mathematical expressions which are good approximations for the line shape in two limiting cases. They correspond respectively to relaxation functions of the type

$$\exp(-t/\tau) \quad \text{(Lorentzian)},$$
$$\exp\left[-\frac{\pi}{4}(t/\tau)^2\right] \quad \text{(Gaussian)}. \tag{1}$$

If a long-range coupling exists between spins, such as the dipolar coupling, so that each spin is subjected to a randomly distributed influence, we may approximate this influence by a Gaussian probability distribution of the "spins" over the field. If this distribution were completely time-independent, this would give rise to an inhomogeneous broadening. The influence, although of a rather complicated type and involving many "spins", is not a statistical distribution, and it also does not give rise to a relaxation, since it is a time-independent coupling. But if this coupling is slowly time-independent, it really becomes a statistical distribution of influences, which lacks coherence. Thus it gives rise to relaxation. As far as the coupling is really statistical without coherence, it obeys the ergodic theorem: the space distribution of the couplings at one instant is the same as the time distribution of the coupling to which one "spin" is subject in the course of time. This gives rise to a Gaussian relaxation function $\alpha_0(t)$ and hence to a Gaussian line shape. This line shape will represent the space distribution of the coupling between "spins", expressed in "local fields". The limit for infinitely slow time-dependence would be an infinitely narrow line, broadened inhomogeneously by this distribution of interaction or "local fields".

If on the other hand this long-range coupling is not only time-dependent but so fast time-dependent that it is smoothed out, then only some mean coupling will be effective in determining the relaxation. The magnetization will relax proportionally to its mean value, $dm/dt \sim -m$, which gives rise to an exponential relaxation $\exp(-t/\tau)$ and hence a Lorentzian line shape. The "local fields" are effective only by some random value, hence the line is narrowed.

The time variation of this long-range coupling may be characterized by a constant τ_c, a correlation time. We have a Gaussian or a Lorentzian line respectively if τ_c is much longer or much shorter than a Larmor period around the effective field in the rotating frame. Assuming B_1 small, this gives:

$$\tau_c \gg |\omega - \omega_s| = |1/\gamma B_d| \leftrightarrow \text{Gauss},$$

$$\tau_c \ll |1/\gamma B_d| \qquad \leftrightarrow \text{Lorentz}. \tag{2}$$

Hence any line is somewhat Gaussian well towards the wings and somewhat Lorentzian at the very centre. Or, any relaxation function is Gaussian for $t \to 0$ and Lorentzian for $t \to \infty$. But the line will have as a general characteristic shape:

$$\text{Gaussian for } \tau_c \gg 1/\delta \equiv \tau,$$

$$\text{Lorentzian for } \tau_c \ll \tau. \tag{3}$$

In fact, the Lorentzian line will generally have a "relaxation constant" τ given by

$$\tau \lesssim \tau_{dd}^2/\tau_c \tag{4}$$

where τ_{dd} is the relaxation time calculated for slow time variation. It is a "narrowed" line, the narrowing mechanism being characterized by τ_c.

Secondary effects in matter may sometimes completely distort the line. This is the case for skin depth, which influences the resonance line due to the conduction electrons in metals. Dyson showed that the line shape depends on the time it takes an electron to diffuse through the skin depth and through the sample, compared to the relaxation times. This gives rise to the so-called Dyson shape, an assymmetric shape. Poole (1967) gives an account of it, with references to literature.

Mathematically the Lorentzian and Gaussian absorption line shapes are two special cases of the class of self-folding line shapes, i.e. line shapes which folded by an identical shape yield again this same shape.† The relaxation function corresponding to a self-folding line shape is given by

$$\alpha_0(t) = \alpha_0(0) \exp[-(a_n t/\tau)^n]. \tag{5}$$

† For more details see, for example, the article of Hughes and McDonnald (1961). In the next section we shall explain what is meant by the "*folding*" of lines.

and a_n may be chosen for consistency with eq. (3.39). Integration of this equation gives a gamma function for a_n:

$$a_n = \Gamma(1 + n^{-1}). \tag{6}$$

For example, $a_1 = 1$ and $a_2 = \sqrt{\pi}/2$, as in eq. (1). [For $n \geqq 1$ and with a precision of 1 per cent one has $a_n = 1 - 0{\cdot}455(n^{-1} - n^{-2})$.] For calculating the moments or asymptotic expansion coefficients we may use

$$\begin{aligned}\lim_{t\to 0} \alpha_0(t)^{(k)}/\alpha_0(0) &= \lim_{t\to 0} [\exp -(a_n t/\tau)^n]^{(k)} = \lim_{t\to 0} [\exp - (a_n t/\tau)^n] [D - D(a_n t/\tau)^n]^k . 1 \\ &= (a_n/\tau)^k \lim_{t\to 0} [D - Dt^n]^k . 1,\end{aligned} \tag{7}$$

D being considered as a non-commutative operator $\partial/\partial t$. (The number 1 is introduced because $\partial/\partial t$ is meaningless while $(\partial/\partial t) . 1$ is zero.)

The first derivative gives

$$(a_n/\tau) \lim_{t\to 0} (D - Dt^n) . 1 = -a_n\, nt^{n-1}/\tau \tag{8}$$

$$\text{which is} \begin{cases} \text{zero} & \text{for } n > 1 \quad \text{(e.g. Gaussian)} \\ -1/\tau & \text{for } n = 1 \quad \text{(Lorentzian)} \\ \infty & \text{for } n < 1. \end{cases} \tag{9}$$

The second derivative gives

$$(a_n/\tau)^2 \lim_{t\to 0} [D^2 - D^2 t^n - Dt^n D + (Dt^n)^2]\, 1 = (a_n/\tau)^2\, [(nt^{n-1})^2 - n(n-1)\, t^{n-2}] \tag{10}$$

$$\text{which is} \begin{cases} \text{zero,} & \text{for } n < 2 \\ -2(a_2/\tau)^2, & \text{for } n = 2 \qquad \text{(Gaussian shape)} \\ \infty, & \text{for } n < 2,\ n = 1 \\ (1/\tau)^2, & \text{for } n = 1 \qquad \text{(Lorentzian shape).} \end{cases} \tag{11}$$

Here we see the very special kind of shapes the Lorentzian ($n = 1$) and Gaussian ($n = 2$) are. In general for $n < 1$ all derivatives for $t \to 0$ are infinite, a fact which is incompatible with relaxation. It corresponds to infinite moments of the absorption line. The line approaches zero too slowly. In fact the Lorentzian shape itself also has its even moments infinite (the odd ones are zero). (Remember, however, that the relation between derivatives of α_0 and moments supposes the moments finite.) Even for $1 < n < 2$ the derivatives are infinite. It seems an accident that for $n = 1$ (Lorentzian shape) all the derivatives are finite. Only for $n = 2$ are the derivatives and moments comfortably defined. The Gaussian shape appears to be a very special one.

In fact, the point is that the description of resonance lines by Gaussian or Lorentzian shapes is to be considered as a qualitative indication. Convergence problems are in practice more easily avoided than when considering, for example, a Lorentzian shape. Indeed no relaxation is exponential ($\exp(-t/\tau)$) at the very beginning (for $t \to 0$) so that $\alpha(0)$ is in practice always zero. This means that, for example, an experimental absorption line approaches zero at the wings faster than a Lorentzian curve, so that the moments are finite. This fact is sometimes investigated by using a cut-off Lorentzian shape. The cut-off parameter is, however, a rather undefined quantity, a fact that makes the whole procedure of reduced interest. An account of this cut-off Lorentzian line shape is given in Poole's book (1967).

5.3. Superposition of lines

(a) *Finite number of lines*

There may be a few distinct different "spin" packets, as, for example, may be the case for hyperfine structure. "Spins" are located in the neighbourhood of different nuclei of a complex structure, or one may simply have nuclei in different magnetic energy levels. Of course, since cross relaxation is not considered, the total line will be a superposition of the elementary lines, even if each subsystem is not linear, i.e. even when some saturation is present. If these elementary lines are well separated, i.e. if each line is much narrower than the separation between the lines, one can easily determine the various eigenfrequencies without substantial error. Also the relative intensities can be determined, using some product of amplitude times width. The shape may be more distorted, but in general one can still make a check, comparing the shape, for example, with the Lorentzian shape or with the Gaussian shape, using some relevant parameters. In order to disentangle a poorly resolved line one can try to resolve the line better, either by increasing the splitting (e.g. by using a higher field $\boldsymbol{B}_s$, if the splitting is proportional to it) or by decreasing the line width of the elementary lines (e.g. by dilution of the sample, decreasing the *d–d* coupling). Another, more drastic—and usually more effective—method is sometimes applicable: the use of double resonance. It is, however, out of the scope of this book to deal in detail with this feature.

When it is impossible to resolve the splitting satisfactorily, one can still make an assumption about the elementary line, compute a certain composition of lines and compare this composite line with the experimental one. This is the work for an electronic computer. The results for the Lorentzian or Gaussian elementary line shapes and for variable combinations of up to nine different lines with various intensity ratios have been tabulated in an atlas for e.s.r. (Lebedev *et al.*, 1963). Only the case of identical relaxation for all packets is considered. Unfortunately, this atlas deals only with absorption lines. A complete collection of graphs has been published for two cases not dealt with by the atlas mentioned: it considers the composition of two Lorentzian lines of equal widths but with arbitrary different amplitudes and arbitrary spacing, and of nine Gaussian lines of equal width and amplitude grouped in three triplets with arbitrary inter- and intratriplet spacing (Rotaru *et al.*, 1964).

(b) *Folding of lines*

When the "different situations" of the various "spin" packets depend on a continuous parameter, then of course a separation of the lines is impossible. Such different situations may, for example, be the orientations of a crystal in the static field. But some hyperfine interaction may also represent a continuous parameter. This was actually the case in the example studied by Portis (1953) where he introduced the idea of inhomogeneous broadening. Portis considers a continuous distribution of hyperfine fields to which a spin can be subjected. The total line is now the *folding* of the individual lines with the function which gives the different situations.

If we suppose that all the individual lines have the same relaxation, we can obtain some interesting general results. The "different situation" is then a variable eigenfrequency. So one defines dN as the number of "spins" with eigenfrequency between $\omega_0 + \varepsilon$ and $\omega_0 + \varepsilon + d\varepsilon$. The density of the "spin" distribution over the eigenfrequencies, conveniently normalized, is then:

$$f(\varepsilon) = \frac{1}{N}\,\frac{dN(\varepsilon)}{d\varepsilon/2\pi}; \qquad \int_{-\infty}^{\infty} f(\varepsilon)\, d\varepsilon/2\pi = 1. \tag{12}$$

And the total resonance line as a function of the eigenfrequency ω_0 is the sum of lines with eigenfrequency $\omega_0 + \varepsilon$, each multiplied by its weighting factor dN/N:

$$\chi_{\text{total}}(\omega_0) = \int_{-\infty}^{\infty} \chi(\omega_0 + \varepsilon) \, . \, f(\varepsilon) \, d\varepsilon/2\pi. \tag{13}$$

We say that χ_{total} is the *folding* of χ with the folding function f. Given the experimental line, one can now make some assumptions about the individual lines and *unfold* the *experimental* line. The theory of the unfolding procedure has been studied by Stokes (1948). See also Moore (1968).

A further assumption about the folding function which we shall make from the beginning is that $f(\varepsilon)$ is symmetric. This will in general be so and will, on the other hand, permit us to use the powerful tool of the Fourier transforms. Indeed, since f is real, its Fourier transform will be real only if $f(\varepsilon)$ is symmetric. From eqs. (2.75) and (2.76) we have $\alpha_0(t)$ as the Fourier transform of $2i\chi(\omega_0 + \omega_d)$

$$\alpha_0(t) = \int_{-\infty}^{\infty} 2i\chi(\omega_0 + \omega_d) \, e^{i\omega_d t} \, d\omega_d/2\pi. \tag{14}$$

Let now $\psi(t)$ be the Fourier transform of $f(\varepsilon)$, the symmetric real function giving the "spin" distribution function over the different situations:

$$\psi(t) = \int_{-\infty}^{\infty} f(\varepsilon) \, e^{i\varepsilon t} \, d\varepsilon/2. \tag{15}$$

The experimental line is

$$\chi_{\text{exp}} = \int_{-\infty}^{\infty} \chi(\omega + \varepsilon) \, f(\varepsilon) \, d\varepsilon/2\pi$$

and we shall prove that

$$\alpha_{\text{exp}} = \alpha_0 \, . \, \psi \tag{16}$$

where α_{exp} is the Fourier transform of $2i\chi_{\text{exp}}$, defined as in eq. (14). We write the definitions of α_0 and ψ

$$\alpha_0 \, . \, \psi = \left[2i \int_{-\infty}^{\infty} \chi(\omega) \, e^{i\omega t} \, d\omega/2\pi \right] \left[\int_{-\infty}^{\infty} f(\varepsilon) \, e^{i\varepsilon t} \, d\varepsilon/2\pi \right]$$

$$= 2i \int_{-\infty}^{\infty} \chi(\omega) \, e^{i\omega t} \, d\omega/2\pi \int_{-\infty}^{\infty} f(\varepsilon) \, e^{-i\varepsilon t} \, d\varepsilon/2\pi. \tag{17}$$

The last equation holds because f is symmetric. Hence

$$\alpha_0 \,.\, \psi = 2i \int_{-\infty}^{\infty} \left[\int_{-\infty}^{\infty} \chi(\omega)\, f(\varepsilon)\, e^{i(\omega-\varepsilon)t}\, d\varepsilon/2\pi \right] d\omega/2\pi. \tag{18}$$

Substituting first $\omega = \omega' + \varepsilon$ and then inverting the order of integration, we find

$$\alpha_0 \,.\, \psi = 2i \int_{-\infty}^{\infty} \left[\int_{-\infty}^{\infty} \chi(\omega' + \omega)\, f(\varepsilon)\, d\varepsilon/2\pi \right] e^{i\omega' t}\, d\omega'/2\pi$$

$$= 2i \int_{-\infty}^{\infty} \chi_{\text{exp}}(\omega')\, e^{i\omega' t}\, d\omega'/2\pi \tag{19}$$

which is indeed α_{exp}, by definition.

$\alpha_0(t)$ is the relaxation function of the individual line, and $\alpha_{\text{exp}}(t)$ gives in the same way the experimental relaxation function, since it is derived from χ_{exp} and the system is linear. Hence the result expressed by eq. (16) separates formally the relaxation and the structure of the line. It will behave as an inverse transform of the function that gives the spin density over different situations multiplying the relaxation function. A good example is the fluor nuclear magnetic resonance in CaF_2 (see Abragam, 1961, p. 115). The experimental relaxation function α_{exp} is

$$\alpha_{\text{exp}} = \alpha_0(0)\, e^{-\pi t^2/2\tau_1{}^2} \,.\, \psi(0)\, (\sin t/\tau_2)/(t/\pi_2) = \alpha \,.\, \psi. \tag{20}$$

This can be interpreted as a Gaussian relaxation for each spin packet,

$$\alpha_0 = \alpha_0(0)\, e^{-\pi t^2/\tau_1{}^2}, \tag{21}$$

giving a Gaussian line, and a rectangular spin density function,

$$\psi = \psi(0) \sin (t/\tau_2)/(t/\tau_2). \tag{22}$$

Indeed, $\psi = \psi(0)\, (\sin t/\tau_2)/(t/\tau_2)$ is the Fourier transform of a rectangular symmetric function, $2/\tau_2$ broad. One can then try to find a model for the CaF_2 molecule which gives this rather uncommon field distribution.

The saturation behaviour of a line, i.e. the variations of the line width and of the line shape as a function of the amplitude of the HF field, yields important information as to how to separate the relaxation part α_0 from the structural part ψ in the folded line. One can determine $\alpha_{\text{exp}} = \alpha_0 \,.\, \psi$ in negligible saturation conditions, but one does not know what part of α_{exp} is α_0. However, the presence of saturation changes only the effect of α_0 in the line and not the effect of ψ. All spin packets are indeed assumed to have the same relaxation behaviour, so that the saturated total line remains the folding of the individual saturated lines by the same folding function f. In practice, one can only measure some parameters of χ_{exp} and hence of α_{exp}. But one has some idea of what form α_0 or even ψ has to take. Measurement of these parameters as a function of the HF field amplitude can therefore give valuable information. Another method of separating α from ψ, at least in the line width, is given by Motchane *et al.* (1963): if one modulates faster than the spin–lattice relaxation, then, in many cases, the relaxation time of α can be deduced.

A straightforward result is obtained by differentiation of eq. (16). Let a superscript (k) indicate the kth derivative with respect to time. Then

$$\alpha_{\text{exp}}^{(n)} = (\alpha_0 \,.\, \psi)^{(n)} = (\alpha_0 + \psi)^{\{n\}} \tag{23}$$

where the superscript $\{k\}$ is to be considered first as an exponent and, after the binomial expansion has been made, as a (k) (Leibnitz's formula). Equation (23) holds in the limit $t \to 0$ and then it gives a relation between the moments of the experimental and the elementary absorption lines. Let us, according to eq. (3.47) and observing the difference between eq. (14) and eq. (15), define the moments of the function $f(t)$ as

$$M_{f,n} = 2 \int_{-\infty}^{\infty} \varepsilon^n \,.\, f(\varepsilon)\, d\varepsilon/2\pi . \tag{24}$$

The nth moment of χ''_{exp} is given, according to eq. (3.50) and eq. (23), by

$$M_{\text{exp},n} = (M + M_f)^{[n]} \tag{25}$$

where $[n]$ is now first an exponent n and then a subscript n. This becomes a very simple relation for the second moment since f is symmetric and hence $M_{f,1} = 0$:

$$M_{\text{exp},2} = M_2 + M_{f,2} . \tag{26}$$

Similar relations between the asymptotic expansion coefficients of the experimental and elementary dispersion lines may be obtained using the Hilbert transform of the distribution function $f(\varepsilon)$.

One might also like to find some relations between line widths. This is, however, a hopeless problem, because line width is a parameter which has a precise meaning only for a given line shape. Its definition is always somewhat arbitrary and one can only meaningfully compare line widths of lines which have the same shape.

5.4. Inhomogeneous applied fields

(a) *Inhomogeneous static field. The problem in general*

It is clear that an inhomogeneity of the static field $\boldsymbol{B}_s$ will broaden the resonance line. Let the field be given as a function of the position in the sample by

$$\boldsymbol{B}_s(\boldsymbol{r}) = \langle \boldsymbol{B}_s \rangle + \boldsymbol{\Delta}(\boldsymbol{r}) \tag{27}$$

with $\langle \boldsymbol{B}_s \rangle$ representing the average field over the sample:

$$\langle \boldsymbol{B}_s \rangle = \frac{1}{V} \int_{V\text{sample}} \boldsymbol{B}_s \, dv. \tag{28}$$

Of course, $\boldsymbol{\Delta}$ is not necessarily parallel to $\langle \boldsymbol{B}_s \rangle$ and in fact must not be parallel to it, since an inhomogeneous colinear field is contradictory to curl $\boldsymbol{B}_s = \boldsymbol{0}$. (For example, if $\boldsymbol{B}_s // \hat{z}$ in $z = x = 0$, then curl $\boldsymbol{B}_s = \boldsymbol{0}$ means that $\partial B_{sx}/\partial z \neq 0$ if $\partial B_{sz}/\partial x \neq 0$.) The direction of $\boldsymbol{B}_s$ is important on the one hand with respect to the orientation of the crystalline axes (for anisotropic samples) and on the other hand with respect to the orientation of the HF field $\boldsymbol{b}_1$. Referring now to the anisotropy of the samples, one can in general obtain a sufficiently homogeneous field in order that the deviations in orientation of $\boldsymbol{B}_s$ are less important than the uncertainty in orientation of the crystal as a whole. In relative measurements with two samples, it is better to put the anisotropic sample to be studied in the centre (the most homogeneous region) and the isotropic reference sample away from it, than to put both samples in symmetric situation in the static field. As for the orientation with respect to the HF field $\boldsymbol{b}_1$, the deviation from colinearity will in general be much more important in $\boldsymbol{b}_1$ itself, and this effect will be considered in a discussion about $\boldsymbol{b}_1$ inhomogeneity. For the present purpose we consider only the magnitude of the vector $\boldsymbol{B}_s$, composing

$$B_s = \langle B_s \rangle + \Delta(\boldsymbol{r}). \tag{29}$$

Typical inhomogeneities are proportional to the field itself and are less than $\approx 10^{-3}$. On the other hand, considerations about inhomogeneous fields are only important if the elementary line width is not much greater than the maximum inhomogeneity. Hence the part of the field scan over which one deals with the same inhomogeneity problem is always less than about 1 per cent of the total field and we may consider $\Delta(\boldsymbol{r})$ as being independent of $\langle B_s \rangle$. Therefore, in scanning through a line, we consider only the average field $\langle B_s \rangle$ as time-dependent:

$$\langle B_s \rangle = \langle B_0 \rangle + \langle B_d(t) \rangle. \tag{30}$$

Hence we definitely start our considerations with

$$B_s = \langle B_0 \rangle + \langle B_d(t) \rangle + \Delta(\boldsymbol{r}), \tag{31}$$

i.e. we separate the time-dependence from the space-dependence.

We may now consider the problem using the mathematical tool of folding lines, as discussed in a previous paragraph. Let $dN(\Delta)$ be the number of "spins" for which B_s lies between

$$\langle B_0 \rangle + \langle B_d(t) \rangle + \Delta(\boldsymbol{r}) \quad \text{and} \quad \langle B_0 \rangle + \langle B_d(t) \rangle + \Delta(\boldsymbol{r}) + d\Delta(\boldsymbol{r}). \tag{32}$$

Then the normalized† density of the "spin" distribution over a field's axis is

$$f(\Delta) = \frac{1}{N}\,\frac{dN}{d\Delta}. \tag{33}$$

† The definition differs from eq. (12) by a constant factor.

The total HF susceptibility of the spins in fields between B_s and $B_s + d\Delta$ is given by

$$\chi(B_s)\, dN \tag{34}$$

and the resultant line is the sum of these contributions:

$$\chi_{\text{exp}}(B_s) = \frac{1}{N} \int_{\text{sample}} \chi(B_s)\, dN = \int_{-\infty}^{\infty} (B_{sm} + \Delta)\, .\, f(\Delta)\, d\Delta\, . \tag{35}$$

The experimental line is the folding of the elementary line with the "line" $f(\Delta)$. Both $\chi(B_s)$ and $f(\Delta)$ have a certain width along the field axis.

If χ is much narrower than f, the problem is hopeless since χ_{exp} does not give any information about the shape of χ. Indeed χ'' is then a quasi-delta function around $B_d = 0$, with, however, an integrated value different from one [see eq. (3.35)]:

$$\chi''(B_d + \Delta) \simeq \frac{\chi_s B_0}{2/\pi}\, \delta(B_d + \Delta) \tag{36}$$

and

$$\chi''_{\text{exp}} \simeq \frac{\chi_s B_0}{2/\pi}\, f(B_d). \tag{37}$$

We find that the shape of the absorption line is exclusively determined by the shape of f.

On the other hand, the shape of the dispersion line χ' is practically given by the Hilbert transform of the delta function, or

$$\chi' = \frac{\text{constant}}{B_d + \Delta} \tag{38}$$

and we find that

$$\chi'_{\text{eff}} = \text{constant} \int_{-\infty}^{\infty} \frac{f(\Delta)}{B_d + \Delta}\, d\Delta \tag{39}$$

which is indeed the Hilbert transform of χ'' [apart from a factor π, which is a matter of definition, see eq. (2.13)].

In fact, in electron spin resonance the narrowest elementary lines are still larger than a microtesla. Using very high fields to resolve a splitting is meaningful only if one conserves at least an (absolute) homogeneity of the order of the width of the elementary lines. For narrow lines there are usually no sensitivity considerations justifying the use of extremely high fields, and for fields of the order of 0·3 T a homogeneity of the order of a microtesla over a convenient sample volume can be obtained with a common laboratory magnet. Hence the condition that χ be much narrower than f is rather academic in e.s.r.—if not used for example for determining $f(\Delta)$ (but for this rather uncommon application it is better and simpler to use n.m.r.). Some good examples of this last case are given by Von Dolega (1955).

If on the other hand χ is much broader than f, the problem is trivial, since then $f(\Delta) \approx \delta(\Delta)$ or

$$\chi_{\text{exp}} \approx \chi. \tag{40}$$

Of course if one could reduce the size of the sample and so obtain f much narrower than χ, this would be the simplest solution. But there may be sensitivity problems and other reasons (for example, boundary conditions in the crystal) which prevent this method. On the other hand, the technique of spinning the sample—as used in n.m.r.—is not only technically much more difficult in e.s.r., but is ineffective in general because of the short relaxation times encountered in e.s.r. (the spinning speed would be prohibitive). Therefore we now have to analyse the intermediate case, where χ and f are of comparable width. Here we must make some definite assumption about shapes. From the foregoing discussion we conclude that only lines that are narrowed by motion or exchange must be considered. Hence it is reasonable to restrict ourselves to the Lorentzian shape for χ. Sometimes f too is assumed to be Lorentzian, perhaps because only for similar shapes does the folding operation give a significant relation between line widths. This leads to a linear addition formula for the line widths. It is, however, completely unrealistic to assume f Lorentzian. Therefore we shall develop a new approach (Talpe, 1967b) based only on the assumptions that χ is Lorentzian and that f is not broader than χ.

(b) *Broadening of a Lorentzian resonance line, due to an inhomogeneous static field*

A Lorentzian line, as it appears in the Bloch theory, can be given by:

$$\chi'(B_d) - iS\chi''(B_d) = \frac{D}{B_d + iS\delta}. \tag{41}$$

B_d is the deviation from the resonance field $B_0 = -\omega_0/\gamma$ where χ'' is maximum and χ' zero. The factor S is introduced to take into account partial saturation

$$S^2 \equiv 1 + (\gamma B_1)^2 \tau_1 \tau_2, \tag{42}$$

and D is a constant

$$D = \tfrac{1}{2}\chi_s B_0. \tag{43}$$

δ is called the unsaturated line width. For this line, we shall consider the effect of the inhomogeneity of B_d without using the function f, but introducing directly $\Delta(\boldsymbol{r})$ into $\chi(B_d, S)$. We deal with both absorption and dispersion simultaneously.

Let the *spatial* density of "spins" be $\varrho(\boldsymbol{r})$. There are $dn = \varrho\, dv$ "spins" in a volume element. The total number of spins is N and the volume of the sample is V. We define a *mean value* as:

$$\langle \ldots \rangle \equiv N^{-1} \int_V \ldots \varrho\, dv. \tag{44}$$

For instance, the mean value of the static field at any instant is

$$\langle B_s \rangle = N^{-1} \int_V B_s \varrho\, dv. \tag{45}$$

The field at any point in the sample, at any time during the scanning, is given by

$$B_s = \langle B_s(t) \rangle + \Delta(\boldsymbol{r}) = \langle B_0 \rangle + \langle B_d(t) \rangle + \Delta(\boldsymbol{r}). \tag{46}$$

The elementary line for the "spins" situated at a certain $\boldsymbol{r}$, as a function of $\langle B_d(t) \rangle$, is now

$$[\chi'(B_d) - iS\chi''(B_d)]_r = \frac{D}{B_d + \Delta(\boldsymbol{r}) + iS\delta}. \tag{47}$$

The contribution to the total line of the $\varrho\, dv$ such "spins", contained in the volume element dv, will be

$$d[\chi'_{\text{exp}}(B_d) - iS\chi''_{\text{exp}}(B_d)] = [\chi'(B_d) - iS\chi''(B_d)]_r\, N^{-1}\, \varrho\, dv, \tag{48}$$

and the total line is the integral over the sample, i.e. with eq. (44),

$$\chi'_{\text{exp}} - iS\chi''_{\text{exp}} = \langle \chi' - iS\chi'' \rangle. \tag{49}$$

Let us introduce eq. (47) into this equation:

$$\chi'_{\text{exp}} - iS\chi''_{\text{exp}} = D \int_V \frac{\varrho\, dv/N}{B_d + \Delta(\boldsymbol{r}) + iS\delta}$$

$$= \frac{D}{B_d + iS} \int_V \frac{\varrho\, dv/N}{1 + \left(\dfrac{\Delta(\boldsymbol{r})}{B_d + iS\delta}\right)}. \tag{50}$$

We recall that

$$(1 + x)^{-1} = 1 - x + x^2 - x^3 \ldots \tag{51}$$

for $xx^* < 1$. Hence if $|\Delta(\boldsymbol{r})| < \delta S$ for all $\boldsymbol{r}$ inside V we may expand the integrand in this way. We use the definition of eq. (44),

$$\langle \Delta^n \rangle = N^{-1} \int_V \Delta^n\, \varrho\, dv, \tag{52}$$

and observe that $\langle \Delta \rangle = \langle (B_s - \langle B_s \rangle) \rangle = 0$. Now

$$\chi'_{\text{exp}} - iS\chi''_{\text{exp}} = \frac{D}{B_d + iS\delta}\left[1 + \frac{\langle \Delta^2 \rangle}{(B_d + iS\delta)^2} - \frac{\langle \Delta^3 \rangle}{(B_d + iS\delta)^3} + \ldots\right]. \tag{53}$$

For the subsequent discussion we shall put $S = 1$, since a partial saturation can always be introduced at the end of a calculation by simply multiplying δ and χ''_{exp} by S. A simple calculation gives the derivatives of χ_{exp}. Using the abbreviation

$$u_n = \langle \Delta^n \rangle / (B_d + iS\delta)^n \tag{54}$$

we finally obtain

$$\chi_{\text{exp}} = \chi_{\text{exp}\,(\Delta=0)} \cdot [1 + u_2 - u_3 + u_4 \ldots],$$
$$d\chi_{\text{exp}}/dB_d = (d\chi_{\text{exp}}/dB_d)_{(\Delta=0)} \cdot [1 + 3u_2 - 4u_3 + 5u_4 - \ldots], \quad (55)$$
$$d^p\chi_{\text{exp}}/dB_d^p = (d^p\chi_{\text{exp}}/dB_d^p)_{(\Delta=0)} \cdot \left[1 + \sum_{k=2}^{\infty} \frac{(-1)^k (k+p)!}{k!\,p!}\, u_k\right].$$

Let us now consider in more detail the second-order approximation, valid for $|\Delta| \ll \delta$.

$$\chi_{\text{exp}} = \chi_{(\Delta=0)} \cdot [1 + u_2] = \frac{D}{B_d + i\delta} + \frac{\langle \Delta^2 \rangle D}{(B_d + i\delta)^3}. \quad (56)$$

The field at which χ' is zero and χ'' maximum is B_0, just as in a homogeneous field. There will be no first- or second-order shift due to inhomogeneity if we use the mean field $\langle B_s \rangle$ as the field axis. We now calculate the line width. We consider successively: δ''_{exp}, the half width at half height of χ''_{exp}; δ'_{exp}, the half width between maximum and minimum of χ'_{exp}; and χ^*_{exp}, the half width between the inflexion points of χ''_{exp}. Since χ is Lorentzian, one has for $\Delta = 0$ (i.e. $\chi_{\text{exp}} = \chi$):

$$\delta''_{\text{exp}\,(\Delta=0)} = \delta'_{\text{exp}\,(\Delta=0)} = \sqrt{3}\,\delta^*_{\text{exp}\,(\Delta=0)} = \delta. \quad (57)$$

Making the appropriate calculation with eq. (55) we get:

$$\delta'^2_{\text{exp}} = \delta^2 + 1{\cdot}5\,\langle \Delta^2 \rangle\,[1 + 0{\cdot}75\,\langle \Delta^2 \rangle/\delta^2 + \mathcal{O}(\langle \Delta^2 \rangle^2/\delta^4)],$$
$$\delta''^2_{\text{exp}} = \delta^2 + 3\,\langle \Delta^2 \rangle\,[1 + 2\,\langle \Delta^2 \rangle/\delta^2 + \mathcal{O}(\langle \Delta^2 \rangle^2/\delta^4)], \quad (58)$$
$$3\delta^{*2}_{\text{exp}} = \delta^2 + 6\,\langle \Delta^2 \rangle\,[1 + 4\,\langle \Delta^2 \rangle/\delta^2 + \mathcal{O}(\langle \Delta^2 \rangle^2/\delta^4)].$$

Calculations to higher order in $\langle \Delta^2 \rangle/\delta^2$ first require, of course, the introduction of $\langle \Delta^3 \rangle$, $\langle \Delta^4 \rangle$, etc., which makes them rather complicated. The brackets are only intended to give an idea of the approximation.

In a realistic approach to the problem of inhomogeneity broadening, one obtains a quadratic relation for the line width. Indeed a linear relation would give

$$\delta'^2_{\text{exp}} = \delta^2 + \delta_m^2 + 2\delta\delta_m \approx \delta^2 + 2\delta\delta_m \quad (59)$$

for $\delta_m \ll \delta$, while our $\langle \Delta^2 \rangle$ does not depend on δ. Here δ_m represents the width of the function that gives the distribution of the spins over the field values. On the other hand, the fact that the influence of the inhomogeneity is different for δ' and δ'' can be used to determine in one and the same measurement the true line width and the inhomogeneity $\langle \Delta^2 \rangle$. One only has to use a spectrometer registering simultaneously δ' and δ'' and to measure δ'_{exp} and δ''_{exp} since

$$\langle \Delta^2 \rangle = \tfrac{2}{3}(\delta''^2_{\text{exp}} - \delta'^2_{\text{exp}}) \tag{60}$$

and

$$\delta^2 = 2\delta'^2_{\text{exp}} - \delta''^2_{\text{exp}}. \tag{61}$$

This technique is valid in the first approximation of u_2/δ^2 or when

$$|\delta''^2_{\text{exp}} - \delta'^2_{\text{exp}}| \ll \delta'^2_{\text{exp}}, \delta''^2_{\text{exp}}. \tag{62}$$

(c) *Broadening due to inhomogeneous HF fields*

Inhomogeneity in the HF field $\boldsymbol{b}_1 = 2\boldsymbol{B}_1 \cos \omega t$ is also a "spin" condition that can vary over the sample. We start with the remark that the question is not so important here as, for example, in r.f. spectroscopy, with lumped circuits, since with microwaves one can use geometrical configurations of sample and field with a very good homogeneity. Keeping this in mind, let us first consider the inhomogeneity in orientation of $\boldsymbol{B}_1$. The problem will essentially be solved in the third chapter, where it is made clear that the available resonance signal is proportional to $\sin^2 \theta$, θ being the angle between $\boldsymbol{B}_s$ and $\boldsymbol{B}_1$. Hence an integration

$$\frac{1}{V} \int_V \sin^2\theta \, dv \tag{63}$$

over the sample is needed. Eventually however this integration has to be combined with the former integration over the $\boldsymbol{B}_s$ inhomogeneity and even with the inhomogeneity in magnitude of $\boldsymbol{B}_1$. Observe that θ is the angle between $\boldsymbol{B}_1$ and $\boldsymbol{B}_s$ at each point, and hence includes the effect of inhomogeneity in the orientation of $\boldsymbol{B}_s$. Consider now an inhomogeneity in the magnitude B_1 of $\boldsymbol{B}_1$, neglecting other effects. This inhomogeneity only effects the line if there is any saturation, since otherwise χ is dependent on B_1. And since it is in general difficult to saturate broad e.s.r. lines we can again restrict ourselves to the Lorentzian line shape, eq. (41). We write it as

$$\chi(B_d) = \frac{D(B_d - i\delta)}{B_d^2 + S^2\delta^2}$$

$$= \frac{D(B_d - i\delta)}{B_d^2 + \delta^2 + \gamma^2\tau_1\tau_2 B_1^2\delta^2}$$

$$= D\frac{(B_d - i\delta)}{(B_d^2 + \delta^2)\left(1 + \dfrac{\gamma^2\tau_1\tau_2 B_1^2}{1 + (B_d/\delta)^2}\right)}$$

$$= \frac{D}{B_d + i\delta}\left[1 - \frac{\beta^2}{1 + (B_d/\delta)^2} + \left\{\frac{\beta^2}{1 + (B_d/\delta)^2}\right\}^2 - \left\{\frac{\beta^2}{1 + (B_d/\delta)^2}\right\}^3 + \ldots\right]. \tag{64}$$

In the last equation we have introduced the abbreviation

$$\beta^2 = \gamma^2\tau_1\tau_2 B_1^2 \tag{65}$$

and we assume $\beta^2 < 1$ so that the expansion of eq. (51) may be used. Observe that only β^2 is space dependent. As in eq. (50) we now have for $\chi_{\text{exp}}(= \chi'_{\text{exp}} - i\chi''_{\text{exp}}$ and not $\chi'_{\text{exp}} - iS\chi''_{\text{exp}})$:

$$\chi_{\text{exp}} = \langle\chi\rangle = \frac{D}{B_d + i\delta}\left[1 - \frac{\langle\beta^2\rangle}{1 + (B_d/\delta)^2} + \frac{\langle\beta^4\rangle}{[1 + (B_d/\delta)^2]^2} - \ldots\right] \tag{66}$$

Of course B_1 has no influence on the g-factor, and hence neither has β^2. As for the *shape*, in first-order perturbation one has [compare eqs. (64) and (66)]:

$$\chi_{\text{exp}} = \chi_{B_1{}^2 = \langle B_1{}^2\rangle}, \tag{67}$$

i.e. the experimental line has the shape of the elementary line if B_1^2 is taken as the mean value over the sample. With the same assumption, we may write to second order

$$\chi_{\text{exp}} = \frac{D}{B_d + i\delta}\left[1 - \frac{\langle\beta^2\rangle}{1 + (B_d/\delta)^2} + \frac{\langle\beta^4\rangle}{[1 + (B_d/\delta)^2]^2}\right]. \tag{68}$$

χ_{exp} still has the elementary line shape, apart from a correction factor in the second-order term which amounts to $\langle\beta^4\rangle/\langle\beta^2\rangle^2 = \langle B_1^4\rangle/\langle B_1^2\rangle^2$. As an illustration we take a rectangular cavity in the lowest TE mode, as discussed below in Chapter 3, entirely filled with a homogeneous dielectric. In this case B_1^2 changes in space as

$$B_1^2 = (k_z^2 \sin^2 k_x x \cos^2 k_z z + k_x^2 \cos^2 k_x x \sin^2 k_z z) \text{ . constant} \quad (69)$$

and hence

$$\langle B_1^4\rangle/\langle B_1^2\rangle^2 = 1{\cdot}25 \quad \text{for} \quad k_x = k_z. \quad (70)$$

The calculation is straightforward. One supposes the cavity to be so oriented that the static field $\boldsymbol{B}_s$ is parallel to the HF electric field, so that everywhere $\boldsymbol{B}_1 \perp \boldsymbol{B}_s$.

The line width suffers no first-order correction if we use $\langle B_1^2\rangle$ for B_1^2. Finding the second-order correction is an exercise in differentiation.

5.5. Anisotropy broadening

(a) *General case*

Finally we discuss the shape of a line due to a powder of many microcrystals, each of which has an arbitrary orientation in the static and HF fields. In fact, it will become clear that the theory is also useful for some types of amorphous samples, for example free radicals in glass. But for clarity, let us consider microcrystals and powder. The question is, of course, trivial unless the line due to a single monocrystal of the powder is anisotropic, i.e. depends on the orientation of the crystal in the field. We first analyse how a line due to such a powder is composed. We start on a very general basis, in order to make it clear where simplifications are introduced and what particular cases can be dealt with.

Let us consider various "spin" packets in one microcrystal, corresponding to various situations. The nth packet corresponds to the nth situation, e.g. "the lowest level of the fluorine hyperfine structure". Each packet has a certain eigenfrequency $\omega_{(n)}$, or a certain resonance field $B_{0(n)}$, and also a certain relaxation $\alpha_{0(n)}$ or line shape $\chi_{(n)}$. Let there be $N_{(n)}$

"spins" in the nth packet. The line $\chi_{(n)}(B_{0(n)} + B_d)$ of these "spins" contributes to the line of the whole monocrystal:

$$\chi(\mu) = \frac{1}{\sum_n N_{(n)}} \sum_n N_{(n)} \chi_{(n)}(B_{0(n)} + B_d). \tag{71}$$

We have already covered the ground up to this point. Of course, the $\sum$ could be an $\int$. But now each packet belongs to a given microcrystal with orientation $\mu(\theta, \psi)$ with respect to the static field. The definition of the angles θ and ψ is illustrated in Fig. 5.2. $\omega_{(n)}$ or $B_{0(n)}$ as well as $\alpha_{0(n)}$ or $\chi_{(n)}$ may depend on this orientation—for any n. We therefore write $\omega_{(n,\mu)}$, $B_{0(n,\mu)}$, $\alpha_{0(n,\mu)}$, $\chi_{(n,\mu)}$. In order to get the total resonance line, we must sum over all the monocrystals. Let a fraction

$$dN_\mu / \int_{\text{all } \mu} dN_\mu$$

have crystal orientations between θ, ψ and $\theta + d\theta$, $\psi + d\psi$. Then

$$\chi_{\text{total}} = \frac{1}{\int_{\text{all } \mu} dN} \int_{\text{all } \mu} \chi_{(\mu)}\, dN_\mu$$

$$= \frac{1}{\int_{\text{all } \mu} dN} \int_{\text{all } \mu} \frac{1}{\sum_n N_{(n)}} \sum_n N_{(n)} \chi_{(n,\mu)} (B_{0(n,\mu)} + B_d). \tag{72}$$

There is one more complication, but we shall not mention it now. Those who are interested may look some pages ahead, after eq. (94). It concerns transition probabilities. It will be easier to deal with it when discussing an example. What is more in order now is *to simplify* the scheme, so that it may be used for practical applications.

A first rather obvious assumption is about the angular distribution of microcrystals, dN_μ. We assume any direction equally probable for a microcrystal, and therefore say the angular distribution is isotropic. This gives a definite expression for dN_μ:

$$dN_\mu = d\theta \,.\, \sin\theta\, d\psi; \quad \int_{\text{all } \mu} dN_\mu = 4\pi. \tag{73}$$

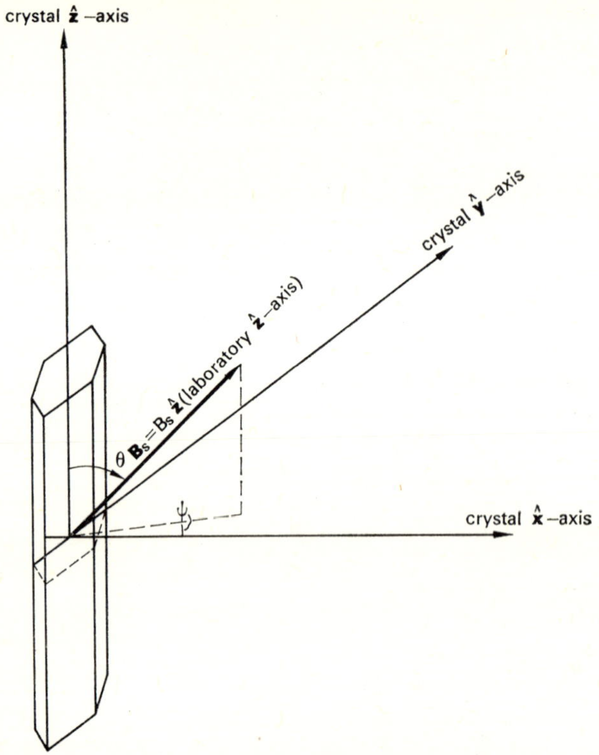

FIG. 5.2. The orientation of the μth microcrystal with respect to the static field $B_s = B_s\hat{z}$ is given by the angles θ and ψ. All directions of the laboratory $(\hat{x}, \hat{y})$ plane are equivalent with respect to the crystal orientation, at least if only one circularly polarized component of the HF is effective ($\omega_0\tau \gg 1$ for linearly polarized field).

If the crystals have axial symmetry, all crystals with the same θ behave in the same manner and, further, the crystals with angle θ behave in the same manner as crystals with angle $\pi - 0$. The line χ_μ is independent of ψ. In an isotropic distribution, a fraction dN_θ of monocrystals has an orientation between θ and $\theta + d\theta$ or between $\pi - \theta$ and $\pi - \theta - d\theta$ with respect to the static field.

$$dN_\theta = 2(d\theta \,.\, 2\pi \sin\theta)/4\pi = \sin\theta\, d\theta; \int_{\text{all } \theta} dN_\theta = 1. \qquad (74)$$

And the total line is

$$\chi_{\text{total}} = \int_0^{\pi/2} \frac{1}{\sum_n N_{(n)}} \sum_n N_{(n)} \chi_{(n,\theta)}(B_{0(n,\theta)} + B_d) \sin\theta \, d\theta . \qquad (75)$$

A more fundamental restriction, always made however, is to assume *a unique relaxation behaviour for all spins.* We already assumed α independent of the situation n of the "spin" packet in the monocrystals, when discussing the structure of a line. Now the shape of the "spin" packet line is also assumed to be isotropic. The reason for making this assumption is that it seems to give good results and principally that without it the problem would be hopelessly complicated. Indeed, relaxation involves time-dependent interaction with neighbours and with the HF field. For examples dipole–dipole interaction by no means has to be isotropic, and even exchange interaction may be anisotropic (Low, 1960, p. 156). There are still more possibilities of anisotropic relaxation. Cross relaxation, due to the overlap of the line of interest with another isotropic line, may be important for some orientations (where the line of interest overlaps the isotropic line) and less important for other orientations (where the line of interest is shifted away from the isotropic line). Finally, "spins" with some orientation may saturate more easily than "spins" with another orientation because they *see* a stronger effective HF field, due to the sine in eq. (3.30) of Chapter 3. However, we do not consider such effects for our discussion here and we assume the relaxation isotropic.†

Moreover, one generally assumes the relaxation to be of the form

$$e^{-t/\tau} \quad \text{or} \quad e^{-(\pi/4)(t/\tau)^2} \qquad (76)$$

which gives respectively a Lorentzian or a Gaussian line shape. Of course, this is also rather a drastic simplification. It will be useful to remember this, because it will make high precision, at a later stage, meaningless!

† The fact that one assumes a single relaxation behaviour does not mean that the lines due to each monocrystal all have the same shape or width. There may be an asymmetry in the monocrystal line due to the anisotropy in an unresolved hyperfine structure, as is the case for the well-known DPPH crystal.

The total composite line is now

$$\chi_{\text{total}} = \frac{1}{4\pi} \int\limits_{\text{sphere}} \frac{1}{\sum\limits_{g} N_n} \sum_{n} N_n \, \chi(B_{0(n,\theta,\psi)} + B_d) \sin\theta \, d\theta \, d\psi, \qquad (77)$$

with χ of Lorentzian or Gaussian shape. This expression contains the eigenfrequency spectrum of the monocrystal and its dependence on orientation. If this spectrum is known, it should, in principle, be possible to determine χ_{total}, although the mathematical difficulties may be such that a computer is needed. But in practice, one has an experimental line and wants to know something about the eigenfrequencies of the monocrystal. The only thing one can do is propose a theory about the crystal (based on some other data, such as the symmetry of its external shape) and to find out the eigenfrequency spectrum corresponding to this theory. Then one computes χ_{total} and checks if the postulated theory is valid, eventually adjusting some parameters.

Actually, once the angular dependence of each $\omega_{(n)}$ in the eigenfrequency spectrum, or rather of each resonance field $B_{0(n)}$ in the spectrum, is postulated, one first determines how many "spins" of the whole sample have a resonance field between B_0 and $B_0 + dB_0$, and then transforms the angular distribution into a field distribution. Then one only has to fold this distribution with the shape $\chi(B_0 + B_d)$ to get the total line. So one takes advantage of the fact that χ is the same for all "spin" packets. If the fraction $dN/N = f(B_0)\, dB_0$ of the spins has the resonance field B_0, the total line is

$$\chi_{\text{total}} = \int_0^\infty \chi(B_0 + B_d)\, f(B_0)\, dB_0 . \qquad (78)$$

As to the theory which must give the eigenfrequency spectrum, Abragam and Pryce (1951) have given important contributions. They defined an effective electron spin S, by setting the multiplicity of the electronic energy levels equal to $2S + 1$. Then the behaviour of the energy levels in the ionic paramagnetic crystal could be represented by the following Hamiltonian:

$$H = \beta_e \boldsymbol{S}\{g\} \cdot \boldsymbol{B}_s + \boldsymbol{S} \cdot \{D\}\, \boldsymbol{S} + \boldsymbol{S} \cdot \{A\}\, \boldsymbol{I} + \boldsymbol{I}\, \{P\}\, \boldsymbol{I} - \gamma\beta_m \boldsymbol{I} \cdot \boldsymbol{B}_s . \qquad (79)$$

The first term gives the well-known Zeeman interaction between our effective spin $\boldsymbol{S}$ and the external static field $\boldsymbol{B}_s$. The "spin" $\boldsymbol{S}$ may precess around a direction different from that of $\boldsymbol{B}_s$, depending on the orientation of the crystal with respect to $\boldsymbol{B}_s$. Therefore $\{g\}$ is a tensor. In the same way $\{D\}$, $\{A\}$ and $\{P\}$ are tensors, and all these together will result in an anisotropic line for a single monocrystal. It is beyond the scope of this book to discuss this Hamiltonian and the theory of Abragam and Pryce. We quoted eq. (79) only for reference purpose. The theory can be found in the original paper and in the books by Pake (1962) and Low (1960). See also, for example, Bleaney and Stevens (1953).

Given this Hamiltonian, one must solve the Schrödinger equations in order to obtain the energy levels, i.e. the eigenfrequencies. General formulae can be given for these, only in restricted cases. We refer again to the quoted books by Pake and Low.

The remaining problem is now:

(a) Given an eigenfrequency spectrum as a function of the orientation for the monocrystal, what is the distribution function $f(B_0)$?

(b) What is the total line, the folding of $f(B_0)$ with a Lorentzian or with a Gaussian shape?

This is a *mathematical* problem. That it can be stated in such a way is due to the following assumptions:

(a) isotropic distribution of monocrystals,

(b) unique relaxation behaviour for all spins,

(c) Lorentzian or Gaussian relaxation.

Let us demonstrate the procedure by considering the simplest example. Even so, we shall still meet considerable mathematical problems.

(b) *An example*

We consider a powder of microcrystals with axial symmetry and anisotropic g-factor. We assume that no fine or hyperfine structures are present, nor zero field splitting. The effective spin is $S = \frac{1}{2}$. The Hamiltonian is

$$H = \beta \boldsymbol{S}\, \{g\}\, \boldsymbol{B}_s. \tag{80}$$

Solving the Schrödinger equation, one finds that the unique eigenfrequency is given by

$$\hbar\omega = g\beta B_0 \tag{81}$$

with

$$g^2(\theta) = g_{\parallel}^2 \cos^2\theta + g_{\perp}^2 \sin^2\theta. \tag{82}$$

θ is the angle between the crystal axis and the static field $\boldsymbol{B}_s$. Since experimentally ω is held constant, the important fact is that the field of maximum χ'' or maximum $d\chi'/dB_s$ is given by

$$B_{0(\theta)} = \hbar\omega/\beta\, g(\theta) \tag{83}$$

for the "spins" of the microcrystals that make an angle θ with $\boldsymbol{B}_s$. This is the same field as for the spins making an angle $\pi - \theta$ with B_s:

$$B_{0(\theta)} = B_{0(\pi-\theta)}. \tag{84}$$

The "spins" of the $dN_{(\theta)}$ microcrystals, which are situated at an angle between θ and $\theta + d\theta$ or between $\pi - \theta$ and $\pi - \theta - d\theta$, belong to "spin" packets with same parameters (n, μ). The structure parameter n is unique (only one eigenfrequency) and for the orientation, only θ is important. All these spins give the elementary line characterized by the eigenfrequency or resonance field $B_{0(\theta)}$ and the unique spin-packet line shape. Because the monocrystals are isotropically distributed in space, the fraction of "spins" between θ and $\theta + d\theta$ *and* between $\pi - \theta$ and $\pi - \theta - d\theta$ is given by eq. (74):

$$dN_{(\theta)} = \sin\theta\, d\theta = -d\cos\theta.$$

With the aid of eq. (82) and eq. (83), we must now find the distribution of the eigenfrequencies of all the spins over the field axis. There are $dN(B_0)$ spins with eigenfrequency between B_0 and $B_0 + dB_0$. What is $dN(B_0)$? Or better, what is

$$f(B_0) = \frac{1}{N}\, dN(B_0)/dB_0? \tag{85}$$

This is a simple matter of calculus. Equation (82) gives us

$$\cos^2\theta = (g_{\perp}^2 - g_{\parallel}^2)/(g_{\parallel}^2 - g_{\perp}^2) \tag{86}$$

and eq. (83), now

$$\cos^2\theta = (B_0^{-2} - B_{0\perp}^{-2})/(B_{0\parallel}^{-2} - B_{0\perp}^{-2}). \tag{87}$$

Hence, first of all

$$B_\parallel \leqq B_0 \leqq B_\perp \quad \text{or} \quad B_\parallel \geqq B_0 \geqq B_\perp \tag{88}$$

and further

$$dN = -N d\cos\theta = -N \frac{B_{0\parallel}B_{0\perp}^2}{\sqrt{B_{0\perp}^2 - B_{0\parallel}^2}} \frac{1}{B_0^2\sqrt{B_{0\perp}^2 - B_0^2}} dB_0$$

$$= N \,.\, f(B_0)\, dB_0. \tag{89}$$

The experimental line is thus the folding of the elementary line

$$\chi = \chi(B_0 + B_d) \tag{90}$$

with the "spin" distribution over the field

$$f(B_0) = \frac{1}{N}\frac{dN}{dB_0} = \frac{B_{0\parallel}B_{0\perp}^2}{\sqrt{B_{0\perp}^2 - B_{0\parallel}^2}} \frac{1}{B_0^2\sqrt{B_{0\perp}^2 - B_0^2}} \tag{91}$$

giving

$$\chi_{\text{exp}} = \pm \int_{B_\parallel}^{B_\perp} f(B_0)\,\chi(B_0 + B_d)\, dB_0. \tag{92}$$

The $\pm$ sign means + for $B_\perp > B_\parallel$ and − for $B_\parallel > B_\perp$.
Of course

$$\pm \int_{B_\parallel}^{B_\perp} f(B_0)\, dB_0 = 1 \tag{93}$$

(and not 2π). If $\chi(B_0 + B_d)$ is much narrower than $|B_{0\perp} - B_{0\parallel}|$ the experimental line χ_{exp} has the shape of $f(B_0)$. This fact is sometimes quoted as "the delta-function approximation". When one has calculated $f(B_0)$, one has at once χ_{total} if a delta function is assumed as an approximation to the actual shape of an absorption line. If $|B_{0\perp} - B_{0\parallel}|$ is much less than the width of the elementary line, χ_{exp} gives the elementary line. If the elementary line width is comparable to $|B_{0\parallel} - B_{0\perp}|$, we must assume some convenient function for the elementary line shape, and integrate eq. (92). The situation is similar to that concerned with inhomogeneous static fields, but here we know the shape of $f(B_0)$. We can, for instance, fold this $f(B_0)$ with the two usually considered line shapes for χ, i.e. Lorentzian and Gaussian. For the Lorentzian shape we get an integral of the form

$$\int_a^b \frac{dx}{(x+y)\,x^2\sqrt{b^2-x^2}} \tag{94}$$

with $y \equiv B_d + i\delta$ and $a \equiv B_{\parallel}$ and $b \equiv B_{\perp}$. This integral is not so simple. The Gaussian line is still more complicated. We do not calculate the integrals because in fact, even for our simple case of axial symmetry and only g-anisotropy, the function $f(B_0)$ as given is not correct. We overlooked an important feature. It is the complication referred to at the beginning of this section and which has now to be explained.

We shall see later that the signal intensity, which measures the paramagnetic resonance susceptibility, depends on the angle between the static field and the HF field, and g-anisotropy means a distortion of the effective direction of the static field. The effect has been calculated by Bleaney (1960) for axial symmetry. It comes out that the signal is proportional to

$$\frac{g_{\parallel}^2 + g_{(\theta)}^2}{g_{(\theta)}^2} \tag{95}$$

and hence the total signal is proportional to

$$\int \chi(B_{0(\theta)} + B_d)\,\frac{g_{\parallel}^2 + g_{(\theta)}^2}{g_{(\theta)}^2}\sin\theta\, d\theta \tag{96}$$

rather than to

$$\int \chi(B_{0(\theta)} + B_d)\sin\theta\, d\theta\,. \tag{97}$$

This results in a different distribution function. For example, for $B_{\parallel} > B_{\perp}$,

$$f'(B_0) = A\,\frac{1 + B_{0\parallel}^{-2}B_0^2}{\sqrt{B_0^2 - B_{0\perp}^2}}\,. \tag{98}$$

A is a constant which could be fixed, for example, by normalizing $f'(B_0)$. This, however, is meaningless. Remember that now the folding of $f'(B_0)$ with $\chi(B_0 + B_d)$ no longer gives the total χ but the signal corresponding to it. The relation between signal and χ is no longer the same for all "spins".

The mathematical problem of folding $f'(B_0)$ with χ is the same as for $f(B_0)$. As an illustration, you may study the folding of $f'(B_0)$ with a Lorentzian absorption line as given by Ibers and Swalen (1962). The second term of the equation is half a page. We may consider it a "solution". But for a computer programmer it is, of course, easier to look directly for the first term, as observed by Searl *et al.* (1961). No closed algebraic expression is necessary. For comparison with experiment one must still take the derivative of that equation since the derivative of the line is generally plotted. A numerical example with graphs may be found in the quoted article of Searl *et al.* (1961).

(c) *Some final notes*

In view of the complications of these composition formulae, one may ask if it is not much simpler and more interesting to take measurements on single crystals, as a function of the orientation. Of course it is. And one gets much more information from such monocrystal measurements. But first of all, even for a crystalline product, it is sometimes impossible to obtain sufficiently large monocrystals in order to get enough sensitivity or even to be able to orient them properly. On the other hand, it may happen that the monocrystal itself is already a complex of a small number of similar elements with certain positions relative to each other. In this case the parameter n of each "spin" packet is double, $n(m, p)$, m giving the element of the complex and p the packet inside an element. If the relative position of the elements is unknown, it is sometimes easier to deal with an isotropic mixture of elements rather than with an unknown complex of elements. Such an isotropic mixture is obtained using a powder sample. A rather trivial reason for using a powder sample is that one likes having an isotropic reference sample. In this case, however, one is no longer interested in the interpretation of the spectrum, but one must take care of the fact that the saturation is determined by the width of the elementary line and not by the width of the total line.

Now when a structure has to be determined from the experimental line of a powder sample, we may still hope that the mathematical work has already been done for the case of interest, i.e. for the situation one supposes to exist and would like to test.

For the spin Hamiltonian given by Abragam and Pryce, the eigenfrequency spectrum has been deduced in various cases. We refer to the already quoted books by Low (1960) and Pake (1962). For these eigenfrequency spectra, the distribution function has been calculated in many cases, and these distribution functions have been folded with Lorentzian and with Gaussian absorption lines in some cases. A very good 1961 review of all the work concerning this distribution function and folding with Lorentzian and Gaussian lines is given by Drăgicescu (1963), who also introduces the problem very systematically. This review has apparently been overlooked in much of the more recent literature, probably because the text is in Romanian. An abundant 1963 list of references can be found in an article by Weil and Hecht (1963). In earlier studies, an effort was sometimes made to get closed algebraic expressions, eventually in an approximated form. However, to fit a calculated line to an experimental one requires in general an iteration procedure. Therefore, one has to use a computer in any case, and then there is no reason to prefer closed algebraic expressions.

References

ABRAGAM, A. (1961), *The Principles of Nuclear Magnetism*. Clarendon Press, Oxford.
ABRAGAM, A. and PRYCE, M. H. L. (1951), *Proc. Roy Soc.* A**205**, 135.
ANGOT, A. (1961), *Compléments de Mathématiques*. Ed. de la Revue d'Optique, Paris.
BLEANEY, B. (1960), *Proc. Phys. Soc.* **75**, 621.
BLEANEY, B. and STEVENS, K. W. H. (1953), *Rep. Progr. in Phys.* **66**, 107.
BLOEMBERGEN, N., SHAPIRO, S., PERSHAN, P. S., and ARTMAN, J. G. (1959), *Phys. Rev.* **114**, 445.
DRĂGICESCU, P. (1963), *Stud. Cercetari Fiz.* (*Rumania*) **14**, 201.
FAGOT, J. and MAGNE, P. (1961), *Frequency Modulation Theory*. Pergamon, Oxford.

GABILLARD, R. and PONCHEL, B. (1963), Observation of lateral frequency-modulation bands in E.S.R. at medium fields. Application to a new measurement procedure for relaxation time T_2. (In French). In: J. SCHMIDT (Ed.) *Magnetic and Electric Resonance and Relaxation*. North Holland, Amsterdam.

GRANT, W. J. C. (1964), *Physica* **30**, 1433.

HAMBURGER, H. (1920), *Mathematische Annalen* **81**, 235; **82**, 120.

HERVÉ, J. (1957), *C.R. Acad. Sci.* **244**, 1182.

HERVÉ, J. (1960), La forme des raies en résonance paramagnetique et la mesure directe des moments. (Thesis) Masson (Ann. Phys.), Paris.

HILGEVOORD, J. (1962), *Dispersion Relations and Causal Description*. North Holland, Amsterdam.

HUGHES, D. G. and MCDONNALD, D. K. C. (1961), *Proc. Phys. Soc.* **78**, 75.

IBERS, J. A. and SWALEN, J. D. (1962), *Phys. Rev.* **127**, 1914.

KAPLAN, T. I. (1965), *J. Chem. Phys.* **42**, 3789.

KARPLUS, R. (1948), *Phys. Rev.* **73**, 1027.

KRONIG, R. DE L. (1926), *J. of the Opt. Soc. Am. and Rev. Sc. Instr.* **12**, 547.

KRAMERS, H. A. (1927), *Atti Congr. Fiz. Como*, p. 545.

KUBO, R. and TOMITA, K. (1954), *J. Phys. Soc. Jap.* **9**, 888.

LACROIX, R. (1954), *Helvet. Phys. Acta* **27**, 283,

LEBEDEV, YA. S., CHERNIKOVA, D. M., TIKHOMIROVA, N. N., and VOEVODSKII, V. V. (1963), *Atlas of Electron Spin Resonance Spectra*. Consultants Bureau, New York.

LHÔTE, G., MOTCHANE, J. L., and THEOBALD, J. G. (1963, 1964), *C.R. Acad. Sci.* **257**, 630; **258**, 2771.

LOW, W. (1960), *Paramagnetic Resonance in Solids*. Academic Press, New York.

MACOMBER, J. D. and WAUGH, J. S. (1965), *Phys. Rev.* **140**, A 1494.

MANUS, C., BÉNÉ, G., DENIS, P., EXTERMANN, R., and MERCIER, R. (1954), *C.R. Acad. Sci.* **239**, 414.

MESSIAH, A. (1960), *Mécanique Quantique*. Dunod, Paris.

MOORE, L. (1968), *Brit. J. Appl. Phys.* (*J. Phys. D.*) **1**, 237.

MOTCHANE, J. L., THEOBALD, J. G., and UEBERSFELD, J. (1963), Study of the structure of electron spin resonance lines. In: W. LOW (Ed.) *Paramagnetic Resonance*, p. 490. Academic Press, New York.

PAKE, G. E. (1962), *Paramagnetic Resonance*. Benjamin, New York.

POINCARÉ, H. (1886), *Acta Math.* **8**, 295.

POOLE, C. P. (1967), *Electron Spin Resonance*. Interscience, New York.

PORTIS, A. M. (1953), *Phys. Rev.* **91**, 1071.

ROSCHDESTWENSKY, D. S. (1912), *Ann. d. Phys.* **39**, 307.

ROTARU, M., VALERIU, A., and WEINER, M. (1964), *Revue Roumaine de Physique* **9**, 269.

SEARL, J. W., SMITH, R. C., and WYARD, S. J. (1961), *Proc. Phys. Soc.* **78**, 1174.

SOLOMON, I. and EZRATTY, J. (1962), *Phys. Rev.* **127**, 78.

STIELTJES, T. J. (1894, 1895), *Ann. de la Fac. des Sci. de Toulouse*, **8**, J. 1; **9**, A. 1.

STOKES, A. R. (1948), *Proc. Phys. Soc.* **61**, 382.

SVARE, I. (1965), *Phys. Rev.* **138**, A 1718.

TALPE, J. (1967a), *Physica* **35**, 157.

TALPE, J. (1967b), *Am. J. Phys.* **35**, 114.

TALPE, J. and VAN GERVEN, L. (1966), *Phys. Rev.* **145**, 718.
VAN GERVEN, L. (1963), *Lijnvormen in Paramagnetische Resonantie.* Interuniversitair Instituut voor Kernwetenschappen, Brussels.
VAN GERVEN, L. and TALPE, J. (1967), Two modifications and generalizations of Bloch's magnetodynamic equations. In: R. BLINC (Ed.), *Magnetic Resonance and Relaxation*, p. 845. North Holland, Amsterdam.
VAN TIGGELEN, P. J. (1964), *Can. J. Chem.* **42**, 246.
VAN VLECK, J. H. (1957), *Nuovo Cim.* (*Suppl.*) **6** (S. **10**), 993.
VON DOLEGA, U. (1955), *Ann. Physik*, **16**, 153.
WEIL, J. A. and HECHT, H. G. (1963), *J. Chem. Phys.* **38**, 281.

CHAPTER 3

The Paramagnetic Resonance Signal

1. Introduction

After having analysed in the second chapter what should be measured, a paramagnetic resonance line with various interesting parameters, we are in this chapter concerned with the problem of how to measure this line. More precisely, we should like to study how to get a signal related to the HF susceptibility at a given frequency and static field. The next chapter will deal with the further problem of how to enhance the signal above noise.

The frequency used in e.s.r. studies is generally in the microwave region. Indeed line widths in e.s.r. range typically from 0·1 mT to 10 mT and the condition $\delta \ll B_0$ or $\omega_0\tau \gg 1$ (§ 2.4 of Chapter 2) thus requires a field above 0·1 T. With the typical magnetomechanical ratio of $\gamma/2\pi = 3 \times 10^{10}$ Hz/T this means a frequency $\omega/2\pi \gtrsim 3$ GHz. E.s.r. experiments have been done in fields as low as 0·1 mT, corresponding to $\omega/2\pi \approx 3$ MHz (Van Gerven, 1963). In the very first experiments on e.s.r. a radiofrequency was used by Zavoisky. But Zavoisky himself soon used microwave techniques for improving the static field to line width ratio. We shall restrict ourselves to microwave frequencies although part of our consideration are equally well applicable to the techniques used at lower frequencies.

The paramagnetic resonance signal is usually obtained by electromagnetic detection, i.e. by analysing the changes in electromagnetic observables, which are due to the HF susceptibility. Although some other techniques may be actually more sensitive in some cases (Gorter, 1936; Schmidt and Solomon, 1966; Alzetta *et al.*, 1967) we shall limit ourselves to electromagnetic detection. Microwave technology has been developed extensively because of its application in radar technology and the Radiation Laboratory has published a famous collection of books on the subject. But the microwave techniques for radar are not the same as the microwave techniques for paramagnetic resonance spectroscopy. In radar applications, one uses high powers as sources and detects weak signals. In paramagnetic resonance experiments one uses comparatively low-power sources and detects small variations of a strong signal. From this spectroscopic point of view, an important compilation of data has been published by Poole (1967). We shall make frequent reference to this book, which contains a very extensive bibliography.

We first give an introduction on microwaves in cavities and in wave guides using from the beginning the electromagnetic field quantities of interest. Then the HF susceptibility is related to cavity parameters. Finally we analyse how to measure these parameters.

2. Electromagnetic Fields in a Microwave Structure

2.1. Introduction

A straightforward technique for producing a magnetic field is to construct a solenoid and pass a current through it. An alternating current will produce an alternating field. If one does not want to lose the magnetic energy after each cycle, one stores this energy in a capacitor of appropriate dimensions so as to use it again in the next cycle. In other words, a HF magnetic field may be produced in the coil of a LC circuit. The energy contained in the magnetic field is transformed into energy of the electric field in the capacitor and transferred back in the next cycle. The only power to be supplied corresponds to the losses accompanying this transfer. The frequency, the number of such cycles per second, is determined by the rate at which magnetic energy, which disappears from the coil, induces an e.m.f., storing electric energy in the capacitor, or by the rate at which decreasing electric energy in the capacitor produces a current, storing magnetic energy in the coil. This rate depends on the geometry of the systems that store the energy. For example, the rate at which a current has to change in order to store a certain amount of energy in a coil is given by the inductance L of the coil ($\phi \equiv L\, dj/dt$), a geometrical property.

At low frequencies one can easily store the magnetic energy in one place (for example in a coil) and the electric energy in another (in a capacitor), some centimetres away. But at high frequencies the time for transporting the energy from one place to another becomes too short. One would need transport velocities comparable to the velocity of light. Therefore it is easier, at high frequencies, to store magnetic and electric energy in the same place. This is exactly what happens in microwave structures.

In a microwave cavity, a closed metallic box, we may consider electric and magnetic fields vibrating at a certain frequency. At some moment there is only an electric field in the cavity. Then this field disappears, while in the same cavity, at a somewhat different place perhaps, a magnetic field is set up, taking over the energy of the electric field. At maximum magnetic field, the electric field vanishes, but when the magnetic field decreases, the electric field sets up again, and so on. Of course, these oscillations will be damped, and in order to maintain them, we have to supply energy, just as for a LC circuit.

The two important parameters of our circuit (the cavity) will be its *eigenfrequency* and its *damping*. These are the parameters that will be altered by the effect of a paramagnetic sample. We could envisage the following method for measuring these parameters: we apply some convenient d.c. fields; we switch then off suddenly and we look for the frequency and attenuation of the oscillations in the cavity. Such a method is feasible in studying, for example, the eigenfrequency and damping of a 1 metre pendulum. Even much faster events can be displayed on a scope. But with microwaves we can only imagine, not apply, this procedure. A much better way is to sustain the oscillations, to discover at what frequency they are most likely to be sustained, and to look for the power needed to sustain them.

Hence we shall analyse the electromagnetic energy in a cavity and how to feed in energy in order to compensate the losses. The energy in the cavity will behave like a standing electromagnetic wave, and energy will be transported by travelling waves that are reflected by the cavity and are partially absorbed. The *energy lost* and the *phase* of the reflected travelling wave are important factors which will tell us something about the eigenfrequency and damping of the cavity.

Let us start with some general remarks on the electromagnetic field and then deal with standing waves, with travelling waves and finally with the fields in a cavity.

2.2. Equations of the electromagnetic field

(a) *Maxwell's equations*

The electric and magnetic fields $\boldsymbol{e}$ and $\boldsymbol{b}$ satisfy everywhere and at any time Maxwell's equations:

$$\begin{aligned} \text{curl}\,\boldsymbol{e} + \frac{\partial c\boldsymbol{b}}{\partial ct} &= 0 \qquad & \text{div}\, c\boldsymbol{b} &= 0 \\ \text{div}\,\boldsymbol{e} &= \frac{1}{\varepsilon_0}\varrho \qquad & \text{curl}\, c\boldsymbol{b} &= \frac{\partial \boldsymbol{e}}{\partial ct} + \frac{1}{\varepsilon_0}\boldsymbol{j}/c. \end{aligned} \tag{1}$$

c is the velocity of light in a vacuum,† a constant, and ε_0 is defined by $4\pi\varepsilon_0 c^2 = 10^{-7}$ (m/s) per ohm.

In the presence of matter we may take into account the part of the charge density ϱ and of the current density $\boldsymbol{j}$ which is *structural.* The structural *charge* ϱ_s defines a polarization $\boldsymbol{p}$:

$$\text{div}\,\boldsymbol{p} = -\varrho_s \tag{2}$$

and a displacement current $\boldsymbol{j}_d$

$$\text{div}\,\boldsymbol{j}_d/c + \frac{\partial \varrho_s}{\partial ct} = 0 \tag{3}$$

† For symmetry, c will mostly multiply $\boldsymbol{b}$ and t in this section, so $\boldsymbol{e}$ and $c\boldsymbol{b}$ have the same dimensions, just as r and ct or ϱ and j/c. Our purpose is to aid those who still use the c.g.s. system. In this system $\boldsymbol{b}$ is found where we write $c\boldsymbol{b}$.

whence

$$\operatorname{div} \boldsymbol{j}_d/c = \frac{\partial(\operatorname{div} \boldsymbol{p})}{\partial ct} \quad \text{or} \quad \boldsymbol{j}_d/c = \frac{\partial \boldsymbol{p}}{\partial ct}. \tag{4}$$

The structural *current* density $\boldsymbol{j}_s$ defines a magnetization $\boldsymbol{m}$:

$$\operatorname{curl} \boldsymbol{m}/c = \boldsymbol{j}_s/c. \tag{5}$$

If the free charge and current densities are designated by

$$\varrho_f = \varrho - \varrho_s \quad \text{and} \quad \boldsymbol{j}_f = \boldsymbol{j} - \boldsymbol{j}_s - \boldsymbol{j}_d \tag{6}$$

we get more precise expressions for the inhomogeneous equations:

$$\operatorname{div}(\varepsilon_0 \boldsymbol{e} + \boldsymbol{p}) = \varrho_f \quad \text{and} \quad \operatorname{curl}(\varepsilon_0 c\boldsymbol{b} - \boldsymbol{m}/c) = \frac{\partial(\varepsilon_0 \boldsymbol{e} + \boldsymbol{p})}{\partial ct} + \boldsymbol{j}_f/c. \tag{7, 8}$$

Therefore we define

$$\boldsymbol{d} = \varepsilon_0 \boldsymbol{e} + \boldsymbol{p} \quad \text{and} \quad \boldsymbol{h}/c = \varepsilon_0 c\boldsymbol{b} - \boldsymbol{m}/c. \tag{9}$$

Now Maxwell's equations reduce to the phenomenological equations:

$$\begin{aligned} &\operatorname{curl} \boldsymbol{e} + \frac{\partial c\boldsymbol{b}}{\partial ct} = 0 \qquad \operatorname{div} c\boldsymbol{b} = 0 \\ &\operatorname{div} \boldsymbol{d} = \varrho_f \quad \operatorname{curl} \boldsymbol{h}/c = \frac{\partial \boldsymbol{d}}{\partial ct} + \boldsymbol{j}_f/c. \end{aligned} \tag{10}$$

In vacuo $\varrho = j/c = 0$ and Maxwell's equations can be combined to give:

$$\begin{aligned} &\operatorname{curl}\operatorname{curl} c\boldsymbol{b} + \frac{\partial^2 c\boldsymbol{b}}{\partial(ct)^2} - \frac{1}{\varepsilon_0} \operatorname{curl} \boldsymbol{j}/c = 0, \\ &\operatorname{curl}\operatorname{curl} \boldsymbol{e} + \frac{\partial^2 \boldsymbol{e}}{\partial(ct)^2} - \frac{1}{\varepsilon_0} \frac{\partial \boldsymbol{j}/c}{\partial ct} = 0 \end{aligned} \tag{11}$$

and since

$$\operatorname{curl}\operatorname{curl} \boldsymbol{g} = \operatorname{grad}\operatorname{div} \boldsymbol{g} - \nabla^2 \boldsymbol{g} \tag{12}$$

this yields†

$$\nabla^2 c\boldsymbol{b} = \frac{\partial^2 c\boldsymbol{b}}{\partial(ct)^2},$$
$$\nabla^2 \boldsymbol{e} = \frac{\partial^2 \boldsymbol{e}}{\partial(ct)^2}. \tag{13}$$

In a region where $\boldsymbol{p}$ and $\boldsymbol{m}$ are homogeneous and proportional to $\boldsymbol{e}$ and $\boldsymbol{b}$ respectively we may write

$$\boldsymbol{p} = \chi_{\text{electric}}\, \varepsilon_0 \boldsymbol{e}; \quad \boldsymbol{m}/c = \chi_{\text{magnetic}}\, \varepsilon_0 c\boldsymbol{b} \tag{14}$$

and hence

$$\boldsymbol{d} = \varkappa_e \varepsilon_0 \boldsymbol{e}; \quad \boldsymbol{h}/c = \varkappa_m \varepsilon_0 c\boldsymbol{b}. \tag{15}$$

If then no free charges or currents are present ($\boldsymbol{j}_f = \varrho_f = 0$) the phenomenological equations can be combined to

$$\nabla^2 c'\boldsymbol{b} = \frac{\partial^2 c'\boldsymbol{b}}{\partial(c't)^2},$$
$$\nabla^2 \boldsymbol{e} = \frac{\partial^2 \boldsymbol{e}}{\partial(c't)^2}. \tag{16}$$

We have the same equations as above [eq. (13)] but with reduced light speed:

$$c' = c\sqrt{\varkappa_m/\varkappa_e}. \tag{17}$$

We shall not usually make any distinction between c and c'. We shall write c, and this has to be read as c' if the medium is homogeneous, not a vacuum.

In a homogeneous region of space enclosed by material walls eq. (13) or eq. (16) will be valid and subject to certain boundary conditions, appropriate to the walls. A component of $\boldsymbol{e}$ parallel to a good conducting

† The notation ∇^2 stands for

$$\nabla^2 \boldsymbol{g} = \left(\frac{\partial^2}{\partial x^2} + \frac{\partial^2}{\partial y^2} + \frac{\partial^2}{\partial z^2}\right)(g_x \hat{\boldsymbol{x}} + g_y \hat{\boldsymbol{y}} + g_z \hat{\boldsymbol{z}})$$

which is equal to

$$\sum_i (\text{div grad } g_i)\, \hat{\boldsymbol{x}}_i$$

only in *Cartesian* coordinates.

wall, as well as a component of $\partial c\boldsymbol{b}/\partial ct$ normal to such a wall, will induce a current in this wall. Hence these components will rapidly disappear if the fields $\boldsymbol{e}$ and $\boldsymbol{b}$ are varying at high frequency. Therefore we define a *perfectly conducting wall* S'' by

$$\begin{aligned} \boldsymbol{e} &\perp S'', \\ c\boldsymbol{b} &\parallel S'' \end{aligned} \tag{18a}$$

at this wall. We call the wall S'' a *metallic* wall. Later [eq. (148)] we shall also use the *complementary* boundary condition, a wall S' on which

$$\begin{aligned} \boldsymbol{e} &\parallel S', \\ c\boldsymbol{b} &\perp S' \end{aligned} \tag{18b}$$

called a *dielectric* wall.

(b) *Energy flow and energy density*

After this summary of the electromagnetic theory, we must look in more detail at two quantities that will be fundamental for us: the energy density and the energy flow. Let us start with the Poynting vector

$$\boldsymbol{s} = \boldsymbol{e} \wedge \boldsymbol{h}. \tag{19}$$

We may expand its outward flux per volume, or more precisely its divergence, by using a general vector theorem

$$\operatorname{div} \boldsymbol{e} \wedge \boldsymbol{h} = \boldsymbol{h} \operatorname{curl} \boldsymbol{e} - \boldsymbol{e} \operatorname{curl} \boldsymbol{h}$$

and from Maxwell's equations, eq. (10), we get

$$\operatorname{div}(\boldsymbol{e} \wedge \boldsymbol{h}) + \boldsymbol{e} \,.\, \boldsymbol{j} = -\left(\boldsymbol{h}\frac{\partial c\boldsymbol{b}}{\partial ct} + \boldsymbol{e}\frac{\partial \boldsymbol{d}}{\partial ct}\right). \tag{20}$$

We read: "the decrease in the electromagnetic free energy density (R.H.S. term) equals the Joule losses ($\boldsymbol{e} \,.\, \boldsymbol{j}$) plus the flux of energy leaving the point of interest." Hence $\boldsymbol{e} \wedge \boldsymbol{h}$ is the energy flow per unit area of the electromagnetic field. In many cases of interest for us, $\boldsymbol{j}$ will be zero. For example, we may integrate eq. (20) over a volume V

with surface, S_{inner}, entirely *inside* a cavity, but just along the wall, using Gauss's theorem:

$$\int_{S_{\text{inner}}} \boldsymbol{s} \cdot d\boldsymbol{a} = -\int_V \left(\boldsymbol{h}\frac{c\boldsymbol{b}}{ct} + \boldsymbol{e}\frac{c\partial \boldsymbol{d}}{\partial ct}\right) dv + 0. \tag{21}$$

On the other hand, the fields *outside* the cavity are zero and hence the surface integral over S_{outer}, entirely involving the cavity, is zero. But now $\boldsymbol{j}$ inside V is not zero:

$$\int_{S_{\text{outer}}} \boldsymbol{s} \cdot d\boldsymbol{a} = 0 = -\int_V \left(\boldsymbol{h}\frac{\partial c\boldsymbol{b}}{\partial ct} + \boldsymbol{e}\frac{c\partial \boldsymbol{d}}{\partial ct}\right) dv - \int_V \boldsymbol{e} \cdot \boldsymbol{j}\, dv. \tag{22}$$

An ideal cavity will be characterized as a volume enclosed by walls and from which no energy is lost. Then the energy inside is constant and

$$\int_V \boldsymbol{e} \cdot \boldsymbol{j}\, dv = 0 \tag{23}$$

or

$$\int_{S_{\text{inner}}} \boldsymbol{s} \cdot d\boldsymbol{a} = \int_{S_{\text{outer}}} \boldsymbol{s} \cdot d\boldsymbol{a} = 0. \tag{24}$$

Instead of S_{inner} or S_{outer}, we may even consider a surface $S_{\Delta\boldsymbol{\alpha}}$ which is just inside at $\Delta\boldsymbol{\alpha}$ and outside elsewhere. Since elsewhere $\boldsymbol{s} = 0$, one has in any case

$$\int_{S_{\Delta\boldsymbol{\alpha}}} \boldsymbol{s} \cdot d\boldsymbol{a} = 0 \tag{25}$$

or, on the whole surface, $(\boldsymbol{e} \wedge \boldsymbol{h}) \cdot d\boldsymbol{\alpha} = 0$, i.e.

$$\boldsymbol{e} \perp S \quad \text{or} \quad \boldsymbol{b} \perp S \tag{26}$$

(since $\boldsymbol{b} \sim \boldsymbol{h}$).

Let us now consider more particular fields, with harmonic time-dependence, of frequency $\omega'/2\pi$ and damping ω''. With $\omega = \omega' + i\omega''$, we get

$$\begin{aligned}
\boldsymbol{e} &= \mathscr{R}\, \boldsymbol{E}(\boldsymbol{r}) \exp(i\omega t) = \tfrac{1}{2}\,[\boldsymbol{E}(\boldsymbol{r}) \exp(i\omega t) + \boldsymbol{E}^*(\boldsymbol{r}) \exp(-i\omega^* t)], \\
\boldsymbol{h} &= \mathscr{R}\, \boldsymbol{H}(\boldsymbol{r}) \exp(i\omega t) = \tfrac{1}{2}\,[\boldsymbol{H}(\boldsymbol{r}) \exp(i\omega t) + \boldsymbol{H}^*(\boldsymbol{r}) \exp(-i\omega^* t)], \\
\boldsymbol{E} &= \boldsymbol{E}' + i\boldsymbol{E}'', \\
\boldsymbol{H} &= \boldsymbol{H}' + i\boldsymbol{H}''.
\end{aligned} \tag{27}$$

We consider only a weak damping, i.e. $\omega'' \ll \omega'$. Then we can consider a time mean defined by

$$\langle \ldots \rangle = \frac{1}{T} \int_{t-(T/2)}^{t+(T/2)} \ldots \, dt \tag{28}$$

with $1/\omega' \ll T \ll 1/\omega''$.

In practice, it is sufficient to take T equal to small number of exact periods. Now

$$\langle \boldsymbol{s} \rangle = \langle \boldsymbol{e} \wedge \boldsymbol{h} \rangle = \mathscr{R}\, \tfrac{1}{2}\, \boldsymbol{E}(\boldsymbol{r}) \wedge \boldsymbol{H}^*(\boldsymbol{r}) \exp(-2\omega'' t). \tag{29}$$

If we take the origin of time so that $\boldsymbol{E}(\boldsymbol{r})$ is real, we find

$$\langle \boldsymbol{s} \rangle = \tfrac{1}{2}\, \boldsymbol{E} \wedge \boldsymbol{H}' \exp(-2\omega'' t). \tag{30}$$

The mean density of the energy flow is obtained by taking the in phase component of $\boldsymbol{H}$ with respect to $\boldsymbol{E}$ in the Poynting vector.

As an important example, consider a hollow pipe of constant cross-section, a waveguide, through which energy can be fed to a system. The energy flows along the pipe so that $\boldsymbol{e} \wedge \boldsymbol{h}$ is parallel to the pipe axis, taken as the z-axis. Such a waveguide of rectangular cross-section is drawn in Fig. 2.1. Two cross surfaces S_1' and S_2' may be considered, each with its normal unit vector $\hat{\boldsymbol{n}}_1'$ and $\hat{\boldsymbol{n}}_2'$ respectively, $\hat{\boldsymbol{n}}_2' = -\hat{\boldsymbol{n}}_1'$. There may be some losses in the guide, e.g. energy may flow into the

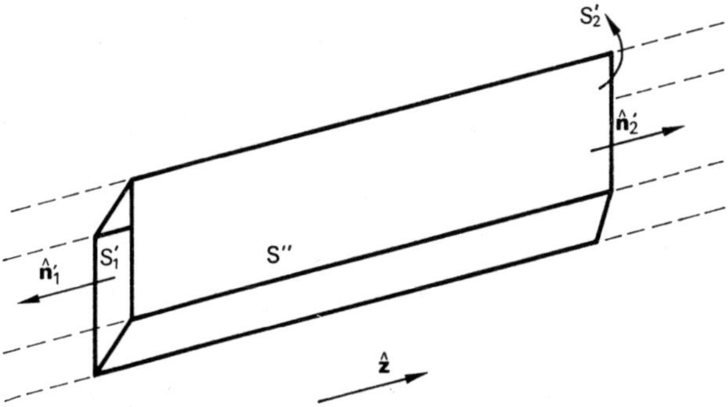

FIG. 2.1. A section of a rectangular waveguide. The losses are equal to the flux of the Poynting vector through S'', S_1' and S_2 (if the guide is evacuated).

side wall, but in any case the losses in the guide are equal to

$$\text{Losses} = \left\langle \int_{S_1'} \boldsymbol{s} \cdot \hat{\boldsymbol{n}}_1' \, da + \int_{S_2'} \boldsymbol{s} \cdot \hat{\boldsymbol{n}}_2' \cdot da + \int_{S''} \boldsymbol{s} \cdot \hat{\boldsymbol{n}}'' \, da \right\rangle. \qquad (31)$$

The surface S'' is chosen in order to close the volume between S_1' and S_2' and $\hat{\boldsymbol{n}}''$ is the normal to it, pointing outwards. We may take for S'', for example, the outside wall of the guide or any surface outside the guide. On any outside wall the fields are zero and this term vanishes. Losses inside are, for example, Joule losses in the wall of the guide. If one takes for S'' the inner surface of the wall there are no losses inside the guide (if the guide is evacuated) but the third term of eq. (31) does not vanish now and represents Joule losses. In any case, using eq. (27) and the fact that $\hat{\boldsymbol{n}}_1' = -\hat{\boldsymbol{n}}_2'$, we find, apart from a common factor $e^{-2\omega'' t}$:

$$\mathscr{R} \tfrac{1}{2} \int_{S_1'} \boldsymbol{E} \wedge \boldsymbol{H}^* \cdot \hat{\boldsymbol{n}}_1' da = \mathscr{R} \tfrac{1}{2} \int_{S_2'} \boldsymbol{E} \wedge \boldsymbol{H}^* \cdot \hat{\boldsymbol{n}}_1' da$$
$$+ \text{ losses between } S_1' \text{ and } S_2' \qquad (32)$$

and $\mathscr{R} \frac{1}{2} \int_{S'} \boldsymbol{E} \wedge \boldsymbol{H}^* \cdot \boldsymbol{da}$ is the energy flow through a section S' of a guide, in the direction of $\boldsymbol{da}$.

We may now ask if

$$\mathscr{I} \tfrac{1}{2} \int_{S} \boldsymbol{E} \wedge \boldsymbol{H}^* \boldsymbol{da} \qquad (33)$$

also has any meaning. Let us therefore return to eq. (21). Instead of defining $\boldsymbol{e}$ and $\boldsymbol{h}$ as in eq. (27) we consider the complex quantities:

$$\begin{aligned} \boldsymbol{e}_c &= \boldsymbol{e}' + i\boldsymbol{e}'' = E(\boldsymbol{r})\, e^{i\omega t}, \\ \boldsymbol{h}_c &= \boldsymbol{h}' + i\boldsymbol{h}'' = H(\boldsymbol{r})\, e^{i\omega t} \end{aligned} \qquad (34)$$

and similarly, for $\boldsymbol{b}_c$ and $\boldsymbol{d}_c$.

The actual fields are $\boldsymbol{e}'$ and $\boldsymbol{h}'$. However, the field (e'', h'') is the same as (e_1', h_1'), only transformed in time over $(-\pi/2\omega')$ and damped a little:

$$\begin{aligned} \mathscr{I}\, E\, e^{i\omega t} &= \mathscr{R}\, [-iE\, e^{i\omega t}] \\ &= \mathscr{R}\, [E\, e^{i\omega t - i(\pi/2)(\omega/\omega' - i\omega''/\omega')}] \\ &= \mathscr{R}\, [E\, e^{i\omega(t-\pi/2\omega')}\, e^{-\omega''\pi/2\omega'}]. \end{aligned} \qquad (35)$$

We shall neglect this damping $\exp(-\omega''\pi/2\omega')$. Let us define

$$s_c = e_c \wedge h_c. \tag{36}$$

We have

$$\langle s_c \rangle = \langle e' \wedge h' \rangle - \langle e'' \wedge h'' \rangle - i\langle e' \wedge h'' \rangle + i\langle e'' \wedge h' \rangle \tag{37}$$

and by direct calculation, or from eq. (35), one finds that

$$\begin{aligned} \langle e' \wedge h' \rangle &= -\langle e'' \wedge h'' \rangle, \\ \langle e' \wedge h'' \rangle &= -\langle e'' \wedge h' \rangle. \end{aligned} \tag{38}$$

Hence

$$\mathcal{R}\,\langle s_c \rangle = 2\langle e' \wedge h' \rangle = \mathcal{R}\, E \wedge H^* \exp(-2\omega'' t). \tag{39}$$

Now what about $\mathcal{I}\; E \wedge H^*$? Of course, the theorem of eq. (20) also holds for e_c and h_c, as do Maxwell's equations, which are linear.

Hence we have

$$\int_S s_c \,.\, da = \int_S e_c \wedge h_c^* da = -\int_V \left(h_c^* \frac{\partial b_c}{\partial t} + e_c \frac{\partial d_c^*}{\partial t} \right) dv \tag{40}$$

as in eq. (21), or

$$\int_S s_c\, da = \int_S E \wedge H^*\, da\, e^{-2\omega'' t}$$

$$= -\int_V (i\omega H^* \,.\, B - i\omega^* ED^*)\, dv\, e^{-2\omega'' t}. \tag{41}$$

We have already seen [eq. (39)] that

$$\mathcal{R} \int_S E \wedge H^* da\, e^{-2\omega'' t} \tag{42}$$

is twice the losses through the wall S of the volume. If, on the one hand, H and B and on the other, E and D are *in phase* with each other, then H^*B and ED^* are real, and twice the losses gives [eq. (41)]

$$\omega'' \int (H^*B + ED^*)\, dv\, e^{-2\omega'' t}. \tag{43}$$

But we know that the total energy stored at resonance in the cavity is

$$W = \mathcal{R}\left[\int \frac{h \,.\, b + e \,.\, d}{2}\, dv \right] = \frac{1}{2} \int_V \frac{H^*B + ED^*}{2}\, dv\, e^{-2\omega'' t} \tag{44}$$

and the damping was already characterized by ω''. We see now that

$$\left\langle \int_S \boldsymbol{s} \, . \, d\boldsymbol{a} \right\rangle = \mathcal{R} \tfrac{1}{2} \int_S \boldsymbol{s}_c d\boldsymbol{a} = \mathcal{R} \tfrac{1}{2} \int_S \boldsymbol{E} \wedge \boldsymbol{H}^* \, d\boldsymbol{a} \, e^{-2\omega'' t}$$

$$= (2\omega''/\omega') \, \omega' W. \tag{45}$$

At resonance, the energy lost by damping during one radian ($1/2\pi$ of a period or $1/\omega'$) is $(2\omega''/\omega')$ times the energy stored in the volume. The factor $2\omega''/\omega'$ is called the eigendamping and its inverse, the Q-factor,

$$\frac{2\omega''}{\omega'} = 1/Q_0 . \tag{46}$$

The imaginary part of eq. (41) may be written as

$$I \int_S \boldsymbol{E} \wedge \boldsymbol{H}^* \, d\boldsymbol{a} = \omega' \int_V (\boldsymbol{H}^* \boldsymbol{B} - \boldsymbol{E}\boldsymbol{D}^*) \, d\boldsymbol{a} \tag{47}$$

if $\boldsymbol{H}^*\boldsymbol{B}$ and $\boldsymbol{E}\boldsymbol{D}^*$ are again real. We define

$$\alpha = \frac{\int_V \boldsymbol{H}^* . \boldsymbol{B} \, dv}{\int_V \boldsymbol{E} . \boldsymbol{D}^* \, dv} \tag{48}$$

and now of course

$$\mathcal{I} \frac{1}{2} \int \boldsymbol{s}_c \, d\boldsymbol{a} = \mathcal{I} \frac{1}{2} \int \boldsymbol{E} \wedge \boldsymbol{H}^* \, d\boldsymbol{a} = 2\left(\frac{\alpha - 1}{\alpha + 1}\right) \omega' W. \tag{49}$$

We call $2\left(\frac{\alpha - 1}{\alpha + 1}\right)$ the energy imbalance. Hence the imaginary part of the complex Poynting vector gives the energy imbalance in a volume.

It may be interesting to calculate α for a simple LC circuit, with eigenfrequency $\omega_a = (\mathrm{LC})^{-\frac{1}{2}}$, driven by a generator at frequency ω. In any case

$$\alpha = \frac{\frac{1}{2} L I I^*}{\frac{1}{2} C V V^*} \tag{50}$$

and for a parallel circuit (Fig. 2.2) the voltage over the capacitor is the voltage over the inductor, given by $(iL\omega I)$, so that

$$\alpha_{\text{parallel}} = \frac{L I I^*}{C(iL\omega I)(-iL\omega^* I^*)} = \frac{\omega_a^2}{\omega . \omega^*} . \tag{51}$$

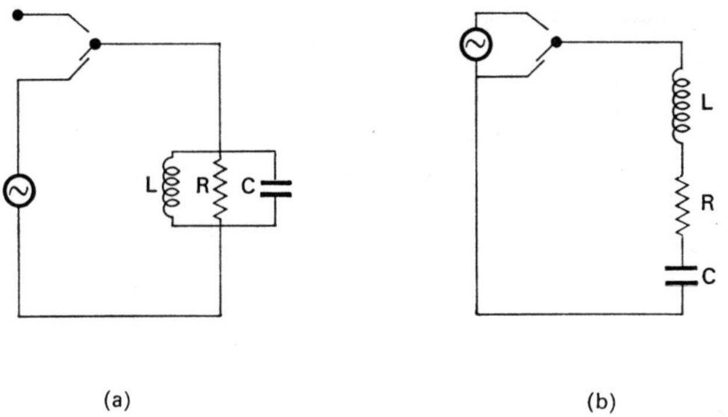

FIG. 2.2. (a) A parallel or "common voltage" circuit. (b) A series or "common current" circuit.

For a series circuit, one finds easily

$$\alpha_{\text{series}} = \frac{|\omega|^2}{\omega_a^2} = \alpha(_{\text{parallel}})^{-1}. \tag{52a}$$

We shall show later [eq. (3.35), see also eq. (82)] that for a metallic boundary cavity

$$\alpha = \omega\omega^*/\omega^2. \tag{52b}$$

From this equation, we now obtain

$$2\,\frac{\alpha - 1}{\alpha + 1} = 2\,\frac{\omega\omega^* - \omega^2}{\omega\omega^* + \omega^2} \cong 2\,\frac{|\omega| - \omega_a}{\omega_a}. \tag{53}$$

Summarizing:

$$\begin{aligned}
\frac{1}{2}\int_S \boldsymbol{s} \, . \, d\boldsymbol{a} = \frac{1}{2}\int_S \boldsymbol{E} \wedge \boldsymbol{H}^* \, d\boldsymbol{a} &= \left(\frac{2\omega''}{\omega} + i2\,\frac{\alpha - 1}{\alpha + 1}\right)\omega' W \\
&= \left(1/Q_0 + i2\,\frac{\omega\omega^* - \omega^2}{\omega\omega^* + \omega^2}\right)\omega' W \\
&\approx \left(1/Q_0 + i2\,\frac{|\omega| - \omega_a}{\omega_a}\right)\omega' W \\
&\approx |2\omega'' + 2i\,(|\omega| - \omega_a)|\, W
\end{aligned} \tag{54}$$

the last approximation $\approx$ holds for $|(|\omega| - \omega_a)| \ll \omega_a$. We may also write eq. (41) directly as

$$\int_S \boldsymbol{E} \wedge \boldsymbol{H}^* \, d\boldsymbol{a} = -i(\omega - \omega^*/\alpha) \int_V \boldsymbol{H} . \boldsymbol{B} \, dv$$

$$= -i(\alpha\omega - \omega^*) \int_V \boldsymbol{E} . \boldsymbol{D}^* \, dv. \qquad (55)$$

2.3. Standing waves

(a) *The modes of vibration of fields in a cavity*

Inside a cavity, a box enclosed by conducting walls, we shall now analyse the configurations of the magnetic field which do not move away, i.e. the configurations only appear or disappear, but do not enter the cavity or leave it through a hole or a wall. A completely static configuration is modulated in time, simultaneously at every point. We can also find a similar configuration for the electric field and it represents, by definition, a standing wave, a wave that does not move its pattern from one place to another. One may think of a vibrating string with a "standing" pattern. One knows that such a configuration can be described by the product of a factor which depends only on time and a factor which depends only on position.

In this cavity, eq. (13) [or eventually eq. (16)] holds and, for a standing wave, $\boldsymbol{b}(r, t)$ can be written as the product of a space-dependent factor and a time-dependent factor

$$\boldsymbol{b}(\boldsymbol{r}, t) = \boldsymbol{B}(\boldsymbol{r}) . \theta(t). \qquad (56)$$

We put this in eq. (13):

$$(\nabla^2 B_x)\, \theta(t) = B_x \frac{\partial^2 \theta(t)}{\partial (ct)^2} \quad \text{or} \quad \frac{\nabla^2 B_x}{B_x} = \frac{\partial^2 \theta(t)/(\partial ct)^2}{\theta(t)}. \qquad (57)$$

Since $\Delta^2 B_x/B_x$ is independent of time and $[(\partial^2 \theta(t)/(\partial\, ct)^2]/\theta(t)$ is independent of space coordinates, both members have to be constant The same holds for the other components and we find

$$\frac{\partial^2 \theta(t)/(\partial ct)^2}{\theta(t)} = \frac{\nabla^2 B_x}{B_x} = \frac{\nabla^2 B_y}{B_y} = \frac{\nabla^2 B_z}{B_z} = \text{constant}. \qquad (58)$$

We first look for $\theta(t)$

$$\frac{\partial^2\theta(t)}{\partial(\partial ct)^2} - (\text{constant}) \,.\, \theta(t) = 0 \,. \tag{59}$$

We write $(-\omega^2/c^2)$ for the constant, so that

$$\theta(t) = A_+ e^{i\omega t} + A_- e^{-i\omega t}; \tag{60}$$

of course $(-\omega^2/c^2)$ could *a priori* be positive. We write, even more generally, for ω:

$$\omega = \omega' + i\omega'' \,. \tag{61}$$

ω is a complex frequency. ω' gives the number of events per 2π units of time and $e^{-\omega'' t}$ gives the decrease in amplitude, i.e. the damping. If $\theta(t)$ has to be finite for $t \to \infty$, A_- has to be zero if $\omega'' > 0$ and A_+ has to be zero if $\omega'' < 0$. If $\theta(t)$ has also to be real, the only possibilities are

$$\begin{array}{lll} A_+ = A_- = 0 & \text{if} \;\; \omega'' \neq 0, & \omega' \neq 0 \\ A_- = 0; \;\; A_+ = A_+^* & \text{if} \;\; \omega'' > 0, & \omega' = 0 \\ A_+ = 0; \;\; A_- = A_-^* & \text{if} \;\; \omega'' < 0, & \omega' = 0 \\ A_- = A_+^* & \text{if} \;\; \omega'' = 0 \,. & \end{array} \tag{62}$$

For example, the function $\mathscr{R}(A_+ e^{i\omega t})$ is not a solution of eq. (59) if $\omega'' \neq 0$. This means that damped oscillations with time dependence

$$e^{-\omega'' t} \cos(\omega' t + \varphi) \tag{63}$$

are not possible as standing waves. This is because eq. (59) contains no damping term of the form $\partial\theta/\partial t$. We shall see below that damped oscillations are indeed accompanied by energy flow, which means that the wave is no longer standing. Only when an energy flow entering the cavity balances out the losses shall we again have an undamped oscillation. It will be a standing wave with ω'', due to damping, accompanied by a $(-\omega'')$ term, due to the energy fed in to sustain oscillations. Hence for standing waves $\omega'' = 0$ and

$$\theta(t) = \mathscr{R}\, 2A\, e^{i\omega' t} = |2A| \cos(\omega' t + \varphi_A) \,. \tag{64}$$

The space configuration $\boldsymbol{B}(\boldsymbol{r})$ now obeys the equation

$$\begin{aligned} \nabla^2 B_x &= -(\omega'/c)^2\, B_x, \\ \nabla^2 B_y &= -(\omega'/c)^2\, B_y, \\ \nabla^2 B_z &= -(\omega'/c)^2\, B_z. \end{aligned} \tag{65}$$

But the fields also have to obey some boundary conditions. The consequence will be that solutions only exist for certain values of ω'. For instance, for the rectangular box represented in Fig. 2.3 we may try a solution for $B_x(r)$ of the type

$$B_x(r) = f(x)\, g(y)\, h(z). \tag{66}$$

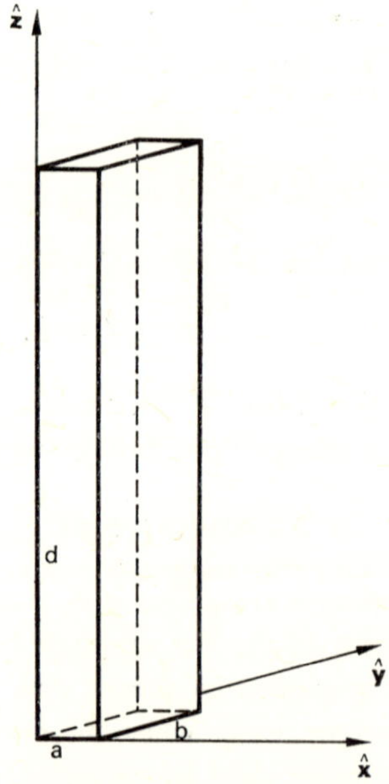

FIG. 2.3. A rectangular cavity.

Then

$$\frac{1}{f}\frac{\partial^2 f}{\partial x^2} + \frac{1}{g}\frac{\partial^2 g}{\partial y^2} + \frac{1}{h}\frac{\partial^2 h}{\partial z^2} = -(\omega'/c)^2. \tag{67}$$

The term $\dfrac{1}{f}\dfrac{\partial^2 f}{\partial x^2}$ is independent of y and z and equals something independent of x.

Hence $\dfrac{1}{f}\dfrac{\partial f}{\partial x^2}$ equals something independent of any coordinate, say $(-k_x^2)$, a constant. The same holds for the other terms:

$$\frac{\partial^2 f}{\partial x^2} = -k_x^2 f; \quad \frac{\partial^2 g}{\partial y^2} = -k_y^2 g; \quad \frac{\partial^2 h}{\partial z^2} = -k_z^2 h; \tag{68}$$

with

$$k_x^2 + k_y^2 + k_z^2 = (\omega'/c)^2. \tag{69}$$

The solution

$$f = F \mathscr{R}\, e^{i(k_x x + \varphi_x)} \tag{70}$$

has to satisfy the boundary condition, eq. (18a), and thus $B_x = 0$ for $x = 0, a$. Hence $\varphi_x = \pi/2$ and $k_x = m\pi/a$ with $m = 0, 1, 2, 3, \ldots$ Similar conditions will appear for k_y and k_z and so we see why only certain discrete values of ω' are possible. In our example

$$(\omega'/c)^2 = \left(\frac{m\pi}{a}\right)^2 + \left(\frac{n\pi}{b}\right)^2 + \left(\frac{p\pi}{c}\right)^2 \tag{71}$$

with m, n and p integers. In this way the whole field pattern for $\boldsymbol{B}$ and for $\boldsymbol{E}$ may be established. The patterns for $\boldsymbol{B}$ and $\boldsymbol{E}$ are, of course, related by Maxwell's equations, eqs. (1).

We shall not deduce the whole field pattern. The solution of this mathematical problem for a rectangular cavity and for other shapes may be found in various books (e.g. Montgomery *et al.*, 1948; Slater, 1950). Here we should only like to stress the existence of such modes of vibration in any cavity, each with its own eigenfrequency. Any cavity admits an infinite series of such modes. We shall represent them by

$$\begin{aligned} &\boldsymbol{B}_a\, e^{i\omega_a t}, \\ &\boldsymbol{E}_a\, e^{i\omega_a t}. \end{aligned} \tag{72}$$

ω_a are always real numbers, so we dropped the prime of ω'. The importance of these modes is that any field configuration in a cavity may be expressed as a linear combination of such modes. This looks like a Fourier expansion. A curve $y(x)$ may be represented by a sum of sines and cosines:

$$y(x) = \sum_n a_n \cos nkx + \sum_m b_m \sin mbx.$$

Consider a vibrating string: any configuration $y(x)$ of the string may be described by a linear combination of the standing wave patterns of the string, sines and cosines. Of course it is not interesting to write, for example, $y = \ln x$ as a sum of sines and cosines, but a distorted wave may be written as a series of harmonics, and for an actual vibrating string, the configuration will be at any time approximately a sine. Hence the sine expansion will have a good convergence. In the same way, we shall express actual fields in a cavity by a series of modes. The actual magnetic field will be given by a series of $\boldsymbol{B}_a$-modes and the electric field by a series of $\boldsymbol{E}_a$-modes. But, for example, curl $\boldsymbol{e}$ is better represented by a series of $\boldsymbol{B}_a$-modes, since it is a $\boldsymbol{b}$-like field. There is one restriction: since div $\boldsymbol{E}_a$ = div $\boldsymbol{B}_a = 0$, we cannot get a field whose divergence is not zero. We still need a different collection of fields, say $\boldsymbol{F}_a$, with div $\boldsymbol{F}_a \neq 0$. Incidentally, curl $\boldsymbol{F}_a$ may be zero.

(b) *The field pattern in a rectangular cavity*

We did not derive the complete field pattern for a cavity because it is a pure question of mathematics, not because it is unimportant to know the field pattern. One needs the pattern of a certain mode, in order to choose an appropriate shape for the cavity, to determine the best sample location, to calculate the filling factor, i.e. the importance of the field at the sample compared to the main field in the cavity, and finally, to determine the intensity of the field. On the other hand, from the field pattern, one may form an estimate of the eigenfrequency and damping of a cavity that has to be designed, although these parameters are much more accurately measured directly.

As an example, which will be useful later in order to represent things more concretely, we shall give the field pattern of a rectangular cavity. The actual fields in a cavity made of copper or silver and machined to a certain precision will, of course, be different. They will be a linear combination of the modes of the ideal rectangular cavity. But for a good cavity, with low losses, the lowest mode by itself will be a very good approximation to the actual fields.

The normal-mode fields for the shape illustrated in Fig. 2.3 can be expressed in terms of sines and cosines. These modes are conveniently divided into two sets, the transverse-electric (TE) and transverse-magnetic (TM) modes. Transverse means that the electric or magnetic field is orthogonal to a certain axis, generally labelled as the z-axis. TE modes have no E_z component, TM modes have no B_z component. The next specification is in terms of the integers already met in eq. (71), by TE_{mnp} and TM_{mnp}:

$$\begin{aligned} m &= \text{number of half-period variations of } \boldsymbol{E} \text{ and } \boldsymbol{B} \text{ along } x, \\ n &= \text{number of half-period variations of } \boldsymbol{E} \text{ and } \boldsymbol{B} \text{ along } y, \\ p &= \text{number of half-period variations of } \boldsymbol{E} \text{ and } \boldsymbol{B} \text{ along } z. \end{aligned} \tag{73}$$

The field patterns are given by

$$\begin{aligned} E_x &\sim \cos k_x x \sin k_y y \sin k_z z, \\ E_y &\sim \sin k_x x \cos k_y y \sin k_z z, \\ E_z &\sim \sin k_x x \sin k_y y \cos k_z z, \\ B_x &\sim \sin k_x x \cos k_y y \cos k_z z, \\ B_y &\sim \cos k_x x \sin k_y y \cos k_z z, \\ B_z &\sim \cos k_x x \cos k_y y \sin k_z z. \end{aligned} \tag{74}$$

The coefficients of proportionality are different for TE and for TM modes (e.g. $E_z = 0$ for TE and $B_z = 0$ for TM). They are given, for example, by Poole (1967). One can easily calculate them by applying Maxwell's equations, eq. (1), together with $E_z = 0$ or $B_z = 0$.

The resonant frequencies are given by

$$(\omega/c)^2 = k_x^2 + k_y^2 + k_z^2 \tag{75}$$

and

$$k_x = \frac{m}{2a} 2\pi; \quad k_y = \frac{n}{2b} 2\pi; \quad k_z = \frac{p}{2d} 2\pi. \tag{76}$$

a, b and d are the dimensions of the cavity, as given in Fig. 2.3. It is clear that we have a whole set of eigenfrequencies. A rectangular cavity used in paramagnetic resonance is usually a piece of waveguide, closed at its ends. The z-axis is along the guide and the dominant mode, the lowest possible, is the TE_{10p} mode. The dimensions of the waveguide are a and b; let the length of the cavity be d. We call d' the length of one-half wavelength along the z-axis:

$$d' = d/p. \tag{77}$$

For such a cavity, the fields of the TE_{10p} mode ($k_x = \pi/a$; $k_y = 0$, $k_z = \pi/d'$) are given by:

$$\begin{aligned}
e_x(\boldsymbol{r}, t) &= 0, \\
e_y(\boldsymbol{r}, t) &= +2c'B_1 \sin(\pi x/a) \sin(\pi z/d') \sin \omega t, \\
e_z(\boldsymbol{r}, t) &= 0, \\
b_x(\boldsymbol{r}, t) &= +(\lambda/2d')\, 2B_1 \sin(\pi x/a) \cos(\pi z/d') \cos \omega t, \\
b_y(\boldsymbol{r}, t) &= 0, \\
b_z(r, t) &= -(\lambda/2a)\, 2B_1 \cos(\pi x/a) \sin(\pi z/d') \cos \omega t.
\end{aligned} \tag{78}$$

We assume the medium in the cavity (i.e. $\varkappa_e$ and $\varkappa_m$) to be homogeneous. *In vacuo* $c' = c$ (compare eq. (13) with eq. (16)). We have abbreviated $\omega/2\pi c'$ by $1/\lambda$. λ is the wavelength a *non-guided* wave of frequency $\omega/2\pi$ would have in the same homogeneous medium. B_1^2 is the mean value of $\boldsymbol{B}^2(\boldsymbol{r})$ over the whole cavity

$$\left(\frac{1}{V}\right) \int (\boldsymbol{b} \,.\, \boldsymbol{b}\, dv) = B_1^2 \cos^2 \omega t \tag{79}$$

since $\lambda^{-2} = (2d')^{-2} + (2a)^{-2}$ from eq. (75). The field pattern is given by Poole (1967, p. 264).

The energy of the electric field is

$$\int \boldsymbol{e} \,.\, \boldsymbol{d}\, dv = \varkappa_e \varepsilon_0 \,.\left[4c'^2 B_1^2 \int_0^a \int_0^b \int_0^d \sin^2(\pi x/a) \sin^2(\pi z/d')\, dx\, dy\, dz\right] \sin^2 \omega t$$

$$= V \varkappa_e \varepsilon_0 c'^2 B_1^2 \sin^2 \omega t \tag{80}$$

and of the magnetic field:

$$\int \boldsymbol{b} \,.\, \boldsymbol{h}\, dv = V \varkappa_m \varepsilon_0 c^2 B_1^2 \cos^2 \omega t \left[\frac{(2d')^{-2} + (2a)^{-2}}{\lambda^{-2}}\right]. \tag{81}$$

One can easily verify that α, defined in eq. (48), is given by:

$$\alpha = \frac{(2d')^{-2} + (2a)^{-2}}{\lambda^{-2}} = \frac{\omega^2}{\omega_0^2} \tag{82}$$

consistent with eq. (52). [We have used eq. (17).] The total energy at resonance, i.e. when $\lambda^{-2} = (\omega/2\pi c')^2 = (2d')^{-2} + (2a)^{-2}$, is always

$$\varkappa_m \varepsilon_0 c^2 B_1^2 V \tag{83}$$

but this energy oscillates to and fro between magnetic and electric fields.

For such a field pattern, one can now calculate the damping that would occur in an actual cavity in which this mode oscillates. The losses are due to an energy flow into the walls, given by the Poynting vector. Let us only quote here the results for our rectangular cavity:

$$\frac{1}{Q} = \delta\left(b^{-1} + \frac{2}{1+u^2}a^{-1} + \frac{2}{1+u^2}d^{-1}\right) \tag{84}$$

where $u = a/d'$ and δ is the skin depth. For a normal cavity $u \approx 1$ and

$$\frac{1}{Q} = \approx \frac{\delta}{a} + \frac{\delta}{b} + \frac{\delta}{d}. \tag{85}$$

The skin depth is proportional to $\omega^{-1/2}$ and hence, since the dimensions are proportional to ω^{-1}, for a given geometry, $1/Q$ will be proportional to $\omega^{1/2}$.

2.4. Travelling waves

In a former section, we considered fields with a standing pattern. Now we must consider the moving pattern of a field that will be able to transport energy. We shall only consider field patterns moving along a waveguide, a metallic tube of constant section. We choose the z-axis along the guide. Hence the field pattern must be of the type $F(x, y) \times f(kz - \omega t)$. We shall limit ourselves to waves with harmonic time dependence:

$$\begin{aligned} \boldsymbol{e} &= \mathscr{R}\, \boldsymbol{E}(x, y) \exp[i(\omega t - kz)], \\ \boldsymbol{b} &= \mathscr{R}\, \boldsymbol{B}(x, y) \exp[i(\omega t - kz)] \end{aligned} \tag{86}$$

and we shall call them travelling waves.

A priori, $k \equiv k' + ik''$, being complex. The wave may be attenuated along the z-axis ($k'' < 0$):

$$e^{i(\omega t - kz)} = e^{i(\omega t - k'z)}\, e^{+k''z}. \qquad (87)$$

However, $|k''| \ll |k'|$ for our applications and since all the waveguides used in a spectrometer are only a few number of wavelengths in length, $k'z$ will not exceed a few units and $k''z \ll 1$. Thus we may neglect k'' and drop the prime on k'. From now on, k is real. Incidentally, k will be positive for a wave travelling along the z-axis and negative for a wave travelling in the opposite direction. Observe that the relations

$$\frac{\partial}{\partial t} = i\omega \quad \text{and} \quad \frac{\partial}{\partial z} = -ik \qquad (88)$$

will be very helpful in finding the field equations.

The coefficients $\boldsymbol{E}(x, y)$ and $\boldsymbol{B}(x, y)$ are not independent of each other, of course. They must satisfy Maxwell's equations and some boundary conditions. A solution with only longitudinal components, i.e. with $e_x = e_y = b_x = b_y = 0$, is impossible. Indeed,

$$-\frac{\partial c b_z}{\partial c t} = \text{curl}_z\, \boldsymbol{e} = 0 \quad \text{and} \quad \frac{\partial e_z}{\partial c t} = \text{curl}_z\, c\boldsymbol{b} = 0 \qquad (89)$$

so that b_z and e_z would only be a constant field. By arguments of this kind (Montgomery *et al.*, 1948, p. 20), although slightly more complicated, one can prove that in a waveguide the only solutions are waves with $e_z = 0$ and $b_z \neq 0$, called TE or transverse electric waves and $b_z = 0$ and $e_z \neq 0$, called TM or transverse magnetic waves. We shall only use TE waves because, on one hand they are almost exclusively used in e.s.r. techniques and, on the other hand, the discussion about TM waves is completely parallel and can easily be carried out. Hence

$$\boxed{e_z = 0 \quad \text{(TE waves) from now on.}} \qquad (90)$$

We also used c instead of c'. We shall consider evacuated guides. The influence of a homogeneous $\varkappa_m$ or $\varkappa_e$ may easily be introduced, as in

§ 2.3. From eqs. (1) we now have $\partial cb_z/\partial ct = -\text{curl}_z\, \boldsymbol{e}$ or

$$B_z(x, y) = (i/\omega)\,(\partial E_y/\partial x - \partial E_x/\partial_y) \tag{91}$$

and for the other components

$$-i\omega \boldsymbol{B}_{\text{tr}} = -ik(E_x\hat{y} - E_y\hat{x}) = -ik(\hat{z} \wedge \boldsymbol{E}) \quad \text{or} \quad \boldsymbol{B}_{\text{tr}} = (\boldsymbol{k}/\omega) \wedge \boldsymbol{E}_{\text{tr}}. \tag{92}$$

$\boldsymbol{E}_{\text{tr}}$ and $\boldsymbol{B}_{\text{tr}}$ refer to the transverse component of the field:

$$\boldsymbol{A}_{\text{tr}} = A_x\hat{\boldsymbol{x}} + A_y\hat{\boldsymbol{y}}, \tag{93}$$

and we define $\boldsymbol{k}$ along the direction of propagation. Observe that if $\boldsymbol{E}_{\text{tr}}$ is real, then so is $\boldsymbol{B}_{\text{tr}}$, while B_z is purely imaginary.

It is important to know that a travelling wave in a given guide and mode is completely specified by $\boldsymbol{e}$ only, i.e. by $\boldsymbol{E}_{\text{tr}}$ and $\boldsymbol{k}$, since $\boldsymbol{b}$ is then given by eqs. (91) and (92).

The actual field pattern of $\boldsymbol{E}(x, y)$ and $\boldsymbol{B}(x, y)$ may be deduced from the boundary conditions, just as for the cavity. We shall not solve this mathematical problem for different cross-sections. But let us only indicate the procedure. We shall also find different modes, just as for a cavity. We take the various TE modes in a rectangular guide as our example. This mode has by far the widest application in e.s.r. spectroscopy. If we introduce eqs. (88) together with $e_z = 0$ in Maxwell's equations, eqs. (1), we get a set of relations between the components $E_x, E_y, E_z, B_x, B_y, B_z$. For instance,

$$\left[\left(\frac{\omega}{c}\right)^2 - k^2\right] B_z = -\left(\frac{\partial^2 B_z}{\partial x^2} + \frac{\partial^2 B_z}{\partial y^2}\right), \tag{94}$$

$$\left[\left(\frac{\omega}{c}\right)^2 - k^2\right] B_y = -ik\, \partial B_z/\partial y, \tag{95}$$

$$\left[\left(\frac{\omega}{c}\right)^2 - k^2\right] B_x = -ik\, \partial B_z/\partial x. \tag{96}$$

Equation (94) is similar to eq. (65). The boundary conditions are also the same and one gets

$$B_z \sim \cos k_x x \cos k_y y \tag{97}$$

with

$$k_x^2 + k_y^2 = \left(\frac{\omega}{c}\right)^2 - k^2 = \left(\frac{2\pi}{\lambda}\right)^2 - k^2 \tag{98}$$

and

$$k_x = m\pi/a; \quad k_y = n\pi/b. \tag{99}$$

Equations (95) and (96) then give B_x and B_y. One has similar equations for E_x and E_y. For more details we refer to a textbook on microwaves, e.g. Montgomery *et al.* (1948), p. 30. The modes are labelled TE_{mn} and TM_{mn} as for the cavity.

Let us only write down the field pattern of the TE_{10} mode, i.e. with $m = 1$ and $n = 0$. The travelling wave is given by

$$\begin{aligned} e_y &= \mathscr{R}\, cB_1 \sin(\pi x/a)\, e^{i(\omega t - kz)}, \\ b_x &= \mathscr{R}\, (-k/\omega)\, cB_1 \sin(\pi x/a)\, e^{i(\omega t - kz)}, \\ b_z &= \mathscr{R}\, (i\pi/a\omega)\, cB_1 \cos(\pi x/a)\, e^{i(\omega t - kz)}. \end{aligned} \tag{100}$$

The field lines for this and various other patterns are drawn by Poole (1967, p. 100).

Observe that $k_y = 0$ and

$$(\omega/c)^2 = k^2 + k_x^2 = k^2 + (\pi/a)^2 \tag{101}$$

[eqs. (76) and (98)]. Hence $|\omega/c|$ has to be greater than (π/a) since k is assumed real. The wavelength $\lambda = 2\pi c/\omega$, which would correspond to a *non-guided* wave of frequency $\omega/2\pi$ in the same medium as that of the guide, has to be less than $2a$:

$$\frac{2\pi c}{\omega} = \lambda < 2a. \tag{102}$$

The guide can only transmit power at a frequency above a certain cut-off frequency $\omega_{\text{cut-off}}$ given by

$$\frac{2\pi c}{\omega_{\text{cut-off}}} = \lambda_{\text{cut-off}} = 2a. \tag{103}$$

$2\pi c/\omega_{\text{cut-off}}$ is called the cut-off wavelength. The "wavelengths" λ and $\lambda_{\text{cut-off}}$ are parameters, not really wavelengths. For example, λ gives essentially the frequency and $\lambda_{\text{cut-off}}$ is a geometrical parameter of the guide. The real wavelength of the travelling wave is

$$\lambda_{\text{guide}} = 2\pi/k. \tag{104}$$

Of course

$$\lambda^{-2} = \lambda_{\text{guide}}^{-2} + \lambda_{\text{cut-off}}^{-2} \tag{105}$$

or

$$\omega^2 = \omega_{\text{guide}}^2 + \omega_{\text{cut-off}}^2 \tag{106}$$

if we define a parameter ω_{guide} by

$$\frac{\omega_{\text{guide}}}{c} = k. \tag{107}$$

At that point in the waveguide defined by $x = \frac{1}{4}a$ or $x = \frac{3}{4}a$, we have $\sin \pi x/a = \cos \pi x/a$. If we choose the origin of the z-axis so that $kz/2\pi$ is an integer, we get for the fields at this point

$$\begin{aligned} b_x &= -k/\omega \frac{cB_1}{\sqrt{2}} \cos \omega t, \\ b_z &= -\pi/a\omega \frac{cB_1}{\sqrt{2}} \sin \omega t, \end{aligned} \tag{108}$$

and one has an elliptically polarized HF field. For $k = k_x = \pi/a$ or $\omega = \sqrt{2}\omega_{\text{cut-off}}$ one has a *rotating HF field of amplitude* $B_1/\sqrt{2}$.

The Poynting vector may be integrated for a travelling wave over the cross-section of the guide:

$$\int_S \mathbf{s}\, d\mathbf{a} = \varepsilon_0 c^2 \int_{0,0}^{a,b} (\mathbf{e} \wedge \mathbf{b})_z \, dx\, dy = \varepsilon_0 c^2 (kc/\omega)\, B_1^2 \frac{ab}{2} \cos^2 (\omega t - kz). \tag{109}$$

For the mean energy flow, one then obtains

$$\int_S \mathbf{s}\, d\mathbf{a} = \mathcal{R} \int_S \mathbf{s}_c\, d\mathbf{a} = \mathcal{R} \frac{1}{2} \varepsilon_0 c^2 \int_{S_1} (\mathbf{e}_c \wedge \mathbf{b}_c^*)\, dx\, dy = \varepsilon_0 c^2 (kc/\omega)\, B_1^2 \frac{ab}{4}. \tag{110}$$

2.5. Reflection coefficient and admittance

(a) *Reflection coefficient*

Let us now analyse how a travelling wave feeds energy into a microwave cavity, where energy is stored in standing waves.

A given guide may carry along electromagnetic energy by travelling waves in various modes and in both directions. We write such a wave as

$$\boldsymbol{e} = \mathscr{R}\, \boldsymbol{E}_{\mathrm{tr}}\, e^{i(\omega_a t - k_a z)}. \tag{111}$$

The sign of k_a gives the direction. Equation (111) completely defines the wave, since $\boldsymbol{b}$ may be deduced from it by eqs. (91) and (92) [remember eq. (90)]. We shall now limit ourselves to the dominant mode. The main reason for this is that only this mode is influenced by e.s.r. unless the line is so broad that $\omega\tau \simeq \frac{1}{2}$. We measure at a Larmor frequency in the neighbourhood of the dominant mode frequency only. (The dominant mode has the lowest frequency. The next mode frequency is in general twice as high. We do not consider here mixtures of TE and TM modes.) Secondly, only this mode is sustained by the microwave oscillator, since second and higher harmonics are in general negligible. The higher modes in the guide may also be generated by some nonlinear element in the circuit, e.g. the sample or a detector crystal, but these effects are also small and the higher modes in the guide are damped out more heavily. There remain two types of waves in a given guide, corresponding to the two directions of propagation. For $k > 0$, the wave specified by

$$\vec{\boldsymbol{e}} = \mathscr{R}\, \vec{\boldsymbol{E}}_{\mathrm{tr}}\, e^{i(\omega t - kz)} \tag{112a}$$

travels along $\hat{z}$ and the wave

$$\overleftarrow{\boldsymbol{e}} = \mathscr{R}\, \overleftarrow{\boldsymbol{E}}_{\mathrm{tr}}\, e^{i[\omega t - (-k)z]} \tag{112b}$$

travels in the reverse direction (along $-\hat{z}$).

We wrote $-(-k)$ instead of $+k$ because it is important here to use $(-k)$ in eq. (92) for finding $\boldsymbol{b}$. Now let a source feed energy into some termination of a guide. This termination may be, for example, a conducting wall closing the guide, or an open end together with objects in the laboratory that may reflect energy back just into the open end of the guide. It may also be a cavity, a transverse plate with a hole in it, a pin introduced into the guide or a combination of all these things. In any case, some wavelengths away from the termination, say at a section S_0, we observe a dominant mode wave travelling towards the termination and another travelling back from the termination. (Too close to the termination, the field pattern is heavily disturbed and one does not have a clear dominant mode pattern.) Let $z = 0$ at S_0. The forward wave is given by eq. (112a):

$$\vec{e} = \mathscr{R}\,\vec{E}_{tr}\,e^{i(\omega t-kz)}$$

and we may now write the reverse wave as

$$\overleftarrow{e} = \mathscr{R}\,r\vec{E}_{tr}\,e^{i(\omega t+kz)}. \qquad (112c)$$

In this way we define a *reflexion coefficient* r, which gives the complex amplitude of the reflected wave per unit amplitude of the incident wave. Observe that r is complex, since the phase of the reflected wave may be different.

$$r = \mathscr{R}^{i\varphi} = x + iy \qquad (113)$$

r also depends on the position of S_0. This dependence is rather simple. $\vec{e}$ may be written as

$$\vec{e} = \mathscr{R}\,\vec{E}_{tr}\,e^{-ikz_0}\,e^{i[\omega t-k(z-z_0)]} \qquad (114a)$$

so that the amplitude with reference to $z = z_0$ instead $z = 0$ is $\vec{E}_{tr}\,e^{-ikz_0}$. And

$$\overleftarrow{e} = \mathscr{R}\,[r\,\vec{E}_{tr}\,e^{ikz_0}\,e^{i[\omega t+k(z-z_0)]}] = \mathscr{R}\,[r\,e^{2ikz_0}\,\vec{E}_{tr}\,e^{-ikz_0}\,e^{i[\omega t-k(z-z_0)]}] \qquad (114b)$$

so that

$$r_{z_0} = e^{2ikz_0}\,r_0. \qquad (115)$$

The phase changes by $2kz_0$. One must be aware of the fact that the phase is *relative*. We may, for example, choose the time origin so that $\vec{E}_{tr}$ is real and choose z_0 so as to make r real. The phase enters when multiple reflections are considered.

A rather simple termination is a perfectly conducting wall, across the guide. At this wall $\boldsymbol{e}_{tr}$ has to be zero or $\overrightarrow{\boldsymbol{e}} = -\overleftarrow{\boldsymbol{e}}$. If $z = 0$ at this wall then $\overrightarrow{\boldsymbol{E}}_{tr} = -\overleftarrow{\boldsymbol{E}}_{tr}$ or $r = -1$. We find then from eq. (91) that $B_z = -B_z$ i.e. the total normal component of $\boldsymbol{b}$ at the wall is also zero, as it ought to be.† From eq. (92) $\overrightarrow{\boldsymbol{B}}_{tr} = \overleftarrow{\boldsymbol{B}}_{tr}$ since k also changes. Hence the Poynting vector reverses, but remains of constant amplitude, $\overleftarrow{\boldsymbol{s}} = -\overrightarrow{\boldsymbol{s}}$, i.e. all the energy is reflected and returns back along the guide. Let us for clarity write down the fields in this case. Note the signs. The forward wave is

$$\overrightarrow{\boldsymbol{e}} = \mathscr{R}\, \overrightarrow{\boldsymbol{E}}_{tr}\, e^{i(\omega t - kz)},$$

$$\overrightarrow{\boldsymbol{b}} = \mathscr{R}\, [(\boldsymbol{k}/\omega) \wedge \overrightarrow{\boldsymbol{E}}_{tr} + (i/\omega)\, (\partial \overrightarrow{E}_y/\partial x - \partial \overrightarrow{E}_x/\partial y)\, \hat{z}]\, e^{i(\omega t - kz)} \tag{116a}$$

and the reverse wave

$$\overleftarrow{\boldsymbol{e}} = \mathscr{R}\, [-\, \overrightarrow{\boldsymbol{E}}_{tr}\, e^{i(\omega t - kz)}],$$

$$\overleftarrow{\boldsymbol{b}} = \mathscr{R}\, [(\boldsymbol{k}/\omega) \wedge \overrightarrow{\boldsymbol{E}}_{tr} - (i/\omega)\, (\partial \overrightarrow{E}_y/\partial x - \partial \overrightarrow{E}_x/\partial y)\, \hat{z}]\, e^{i(\omega t + kz)}. \tag{116b}$$

The total complex Poynting vector is

$$s_c = \varepsilon_0 c^2\, \overrightarrow{\boldsymbol{E}}_{tr}\, [e^{i(\omega t - kz)} - e^{i(\omega t + kz)}] \wedge \overrightarrow{\boldsymbol{B}}_{tr}\, [e^{-i(\omega t + kz)} + e^{-i(\omega t - kz)}]$$

$$= -\varepsilon_0 c^2\, (\overrightarrow{\boldsymbol{E}}_{tr} \wedge \overrightarrow{\boldsymbol{B}}^*_{tr})\, 2i \sin 2kz \tag{117}$$

which is indeed imaginary for a real incident wave.

If the wave is not entirely reflected, i.e., $r \neq 1$, then the Poynting vector is

$$s_c = \varepsilon_0 c^2\, \overrightarrow{\boldsymbol{E}}_{tr} \wedge \overrightarrow{\boldsymbol{B}}^*_{tr}\, (e^{ikz} + re^{-ikz})\, (e^{ikz} - r^* e^{ikz})$$

$$= \varepsilon_0 c^2\, (\overrightarrow{\boldsymbol{E}}_{tr} \wedge \overrightarrow{\boldsymbol{B}}_{tr})\, [(1 - rr^*) + 2i\, \mathscr{I} re^{-2ikz}]. \tag{118}$$

This reduces to eq. (113) for $r = -1$. For a perfectly reflecting wall, indeed $r = -1$. The forward energy flux was given by

$$\varepsilon_0 c^2\, \overrightarrow{\boldsymbol{E}}_{tr} \wedge \overrightarrow{\boldsymbol{B}}^*_{tr} \tag{119}$$

† We proceed as if the operator $\mathscr{R}$ were absent in eq. (111). In fact we must consider the case, e.g. for $t = 0$ and then again for $t = \pi/2\omega$. See eq. (34).

and we see that a fraction rr^* of this flux is reflected, since $(-rr^*)$ times the incident flux goes through S'. Therefore

$$rr^* \leqq 1 \tag{120}$$

if the termination is passive.

(b) *Admittance*

Observe that the total field in a guide is

$$\begin{aligned} \boldsymbol{e} &= \overrightarrow{\boldsymbol{e}} + \overleftarrow{\boldsymbol{e}} = \mathscr{R}\, \overrightarrow{\boldsymbol{E}}_{\text{tr}}\, (e^{-ikz} + re^{ikz})\, e^{i\omega t}, \\ \boldsymbol{b} &= \overrightarrow{\boldsymbol{b}} + \overleftarrow{\boldsymbol{b}} = \mathscr{R}\, (\overrightarrow{\boldsymbol{k}}/\omega) \wedge \overrightarrow{\boldsymbol{E}}_{\text{tr}}\, (e^{-ikz} - re^{ikz})\, e^{i\omega t} \\ &\quad + \mathscr{R}\, (i/\omega)\, (\partial E_y/\partial x - \partial E_x/\partial y)\, \hat{z}\, (e^{-ikz} + re^{ikz})\, e^{i\omega t}. \end{aligned} \tag{121}$$

We consider the wave as coming from $z = +\infty$ to $z = 0$ and going back along $\hat{z}$. Hence $k < 0$ here. For a metallic wall at $z = 0$ we have $r = -1$. Let us adjust the time origin for $\overrightarrow{\boldsymbol{E}}_{\text{tr}}$ to be real. Then

$$\begin{aligned} \boldsymbol{e} &= 2\overrightarrow{\boldsymbol{E}}_{\text{tr}} \sin kz \sin \omega t \\ \boldsymbol{b} &= 2\overrightarrow{\boldsymbol{k}}/\omega \wedge \overrightarrow{\boldsymbol{E}}_{\text{tr}} \cos kz \cos \omega t + (2/\omega)\, (\partial E_y/\partial x - \partial E_x/\partial y)\, \hat{z} \sin kz \cos \omega t \\ &\quad \text{with } (r = -1). \end{aligned} \tag{122}$$

This is a standing wave. If we put an infinitely thin metallic wall at $z = -n\pi/k$ ($n = 1, 2, 3 \ldots$) across the guide, the boundary conditions for $\boldsymbol{e}$ and $\boldsymbol{b}$ are still fulfilled. Indeed, eqs. (122) give the fields in a rectangular cavity of length $d = pd' = -p\pi/k$. This may be seen by comparison with eq. (78) and eq. (100). Take

$$\overrightarrow{\boldsymbol{E}}_{\text{tr}} = cB_1 \sin \pi x/a$$

and remember that $\lambda = 2\pi c/\omega$ (forget the prime on c'). However, the fields in this cavity will decrease, because of the losses. In order to sustain the oscillations, we may feed in some energy from the travelling wave. We make a little hole in the wall, located at $z = -n\pi/k$. At this hole the fields are now strongly disturbed and, for example, we no longer have $\overrightarrow{\boldsymbol{e}} = -\overleftarrow{\boldsymbol{e}}$. But at some wavelengths ahead of the hole, say at $z = z_2$, the fields are not so strongly disturbed. At $z = z_2$, we again distinguish a forward and a reverse wave. If no hole is present, then $r = -1$ with reference to $z = 0$ as well as to $z = -n\pi/k$ or to $z = z_2$, and $[\vec{e} = -\overleftarrow{e}]_{z=z_2}$. With $r \neq -1$ a significant parameter would be

$$Z = \left[\frac{\vec{e} - (-\overleftarrow{e})}{\vec{e} + (-\overleftarrow{e})}\right] = \frac{1+r}{1-r}. \tag{123}$$

If we take $z = z_2 + \frac{1}{2}\pi/k$ as a reference for r, then $r = +1$ for total reflection (i.e. no hole in the wall at $z = z_2$). Then $[\vec{e} = \overleftarrow{e}]_{z=z_2+\pi/2k}$, and a significant parameter giving the influence of the hole would be

$$Y = \frac{\vec{e} - \overleftarrow{e}}{\vec{e} + \overleftarrow{e}} = \frac{1-r}{1+r}. \tag{124}$$

We may consider Z and Y for any termination, and we define them by

$$Y = \frac{1-r}{1+r} = 1/Z. \tag{125a}$$

The inverse relation is:

$$r = \frac{1-Y}{1+Y} = \frac{Z-1}{Z+1}. \tag{125b}$$

We call Y the admittance and Z the impedance of the termination of the guide. We shall in fact only use the admittance.† We write the real and imaginary part‡ of Y as

$$Y = Y' + iY''. \tag{126}$$

The energy that enters the cavity in order to compensate the losses may now be considered at $z = z_2$.

† Y is dimensionless. In textbooks on microwaves, a characteristic admittance of a transmission line is often introduced. Our Y is then the reduced admittance, the admittance divided by this characteristic admittance. This is simply a question of taste, since lumped circuit currents and voltages cannot be uniquely defined.

‡ We do not use $G + iB$ in order to avoid confusion with the B of magnetic field.

We write the time mean of the incident flux of $\boldsymbol{s}_c$ [see eq. (36)] as

$$\varepsilon_0 c^2 \langle(\vec{\boldsymbol{e}}_c + \overleftarrow{\boldsymbol{e}}_c) \wedge (\vec{\boldsymbol{b}}_c^* + \overleftarrow{\boldsymbol{b}}_c^*)\rangle = (1 + r)(1 - r^*)\,\varepsilon_0 c^2 (\vec{\boldsymbol{e}}_c \wedge \vec{\boldsymbol{b}}_c^*) \tag{127a}$$

or

$$\langle \vec{\boldsymbol{s}}_c + \overleftarrow{\boldsymbol{s}}_c\rangle = (1 + r)(1 - r^*)\langle \vec{\boldsymbol{s}}_c\rangle \tag{127b}$$

and the real part of this flux, integrated over the guide section, is the net flux that enters the cavity, and equals the losses. These losses have been described by means of a damping ($1/Q_0$) and the stored energy. See eqs. (45) and (46). The complete expression is

$$\left\langle \frac{1}{2}\int_S (\vec{\boldsymbol{s}}_c + \overleftarrow{\boldsymbol{s}}_c)\, d\boldsymbol{a}\right\rangle = (1 + r)(1 - r^*)\left\langle \frac{1}{2}\int \vec{\boldsymbol{s}}_c\, d\boldsymbol{a}\right\rangle$$
$$= \left(\frac{1}{Q_0} + 2i\frac{\alpha - 1}{\alpha + 1}\right)\omega' W. \tag{128}$$

Suppose now that the fields in the guide suddenly disappear, and that instant $\boldsymbol{b} = 0$ at $z = z_2$, and only the fields in the cavity remain, i.e. we shall consider the attenuation of the fields in a cavity when free. The fields will be damped out by two effects. On the one hand, we have the losses in the walls, represented by $1/Q_0$, and on the other hand, energy will flow away through the guide. This last part will be called the external damping and will be represented by $1/Q_e$, i.e. the external losses are also proportional to the stored energy and are given by

$$\text{external losses} = \frac{1}{2}\left\langle \int_S \overleftarrow{\boldsymbol{s}}_e\, d\boldsymbol{a}\right\rangle = \frac{1}{Q_e}\omega' W. \tag{129}$$

Let us now investigate the flux $\overleftarrow{\boldsymbol{s}}_e$. At the instant of removing the fields in the guide, the electric field at $z = z_2$ is

$$\boldsymbol{e}(z_2) = \vec{\boldsymbol{e}}(z_2) + \overleftarrow{\boldsymbol{e}}(z_2) = (1 + r)\,\vec{\boldsymbol{e}}(z_2). \tag{130}$$

This will produce a travelling wave in the guide:

$$\overleftarrow{\boldsymbol{e}}_e = (1 + r)\vec{\boldsymbol{E}}_{\text{tr}}\, e^{i(\omega t - kz)} \tag{131}$$

and hence

$$\overleftarrow{\boldsymbol{b}}_e = (1 + r)(\overrightarrow{\boldsymbol{k}}/\omega) \wedge \overrightarrow{\boldsymbol{E}}_{\mathrm{tr}}\, e^{i(\omega t - kz)} + \overleftarrow{\boldsymbol{b}}_{ez}. \tag{132}$$

And the flux will be

$$\overleftarrow{\boldsymbol{s}}_e = (1 + r)(1 + r^*)\, \overrightarrow{\boldsymbol{s}}_c \tag{133}$$

or

$$\frac{1}{2}\left\langle \int \boldsymbol{s}_e\, da \right\rangle = (1 + r)(1 + r^*)\frac{1}{2}\left\langle \int \overrightarrow{\boldsymbol{s}}_c\, \overrightarrow{d\boldsymbol{a}} \right\rangle = \frac{1}{Q_e}\omega' W. \tag{134}$$

The factor $\left\langle \int \boldsymbol{s}_e\, da \right\rangle$ is of course real.

The total damping will be:

$$\frac{1}{Q_L} = \frac{1}{Q_0} + \frac{1}{Q_e} \tag{135}$$

and the attenuation of the free cavity will be $e^{-\omega_L'' t}$ with $\omega_L''/\omega' = 1/Q_L$. We may now divide eq. (128) by eq. (134) and find for the admittance

$$Y^* = \frac{1 - r^*}{1 + r^*} = \frac{\left(\dfrac{1}{Q_0} + 2i\dfrac{a - 1}{a + 1}\right)}{1/Q_e} \simeq \frac{1/Q_0}{1/Q_e} + 2i\frac{|\omega| - \omega_a}{\omega_a} Q_e$$

$$\simeq \frac{1/Q_0}{1/Q_e} + 2i\frac{\omega' - \omega_a}{\omega_a} Q_e, \tag{136a}$$

or

$$\boxed{Y = \frac{1 - r}{1 + r} = \frac{1/Q_0}{1/Q_e} - 2i\,.\,\frac{(\omega' - \omega_a)/\omega_a}{1/Q_e}.} \tag{136b}$$

Observe that eq. (136) may also be written as

$$Y = \frac{\left\langle \dfrac{1}{2}\displaystyle\int (\overrightarrow{\boldsymbol{s}}_c + \overleftarrow{\boldsymbol{s}}_c)\, da \right\rangle}{(1/Q_e)\omega' W} = \frac{\dfrac{1}{2}\displaystyle\int_{\substack{\text{guide}\\ \text{cross-section}}} \boldsymbol{E} \wedge \boldsymbol{H}^*\, da}{\dfrac{1}{Q_e}\dfrac{\omega'}{4}\left(1 + \dfrac{1}{\alpha}\right)\displaystyle\int_{\substack{\text{cavity}\\ \text{volume}}} \boldsymbol{B}\,.\,\boldsymbol{H}^*\, dv}. \tag{137}$$

In discussing paramagnetic resonance effects on a cavity, as well as in dealing with spectrometer schemes, we shall make ample use of eq. (137).

In fact, the quantities Y and r are accessible to measurement and, on the other hand, the properties of a paramagnetic sample in the cavity may be considered as a variation in $1/Q_0$ and in ω_0. The term $1/Q_e$ will also be an important factor and gives the coupling of the cavity to the guide. If $1/Q_e$ is small, little energy flows away but also little energy enters. The most sensitive situation will be:

$$1/Q_e \approx 1/Q_0. \tag{138}$$

This coupling is called "matching".

We now make one final remark. We considered only one mode in the cavity and one mode in the guide. In fact, we have an admittance Y for each mode of the cavity as couplet to each mode of the guide. The fields in a cavity are a superposition of all possible modes, each with its amplitude and complex eigenfrequency and any mode is coupled to a guide by a certain admittance. The question is still more involved if one considers different modes in the guide. Fortunately this is not necessary for paramagnetic resonance studies.

2.6. Field in the Cavity as a Function of the Orthonormal Modes

We now have to describe the electromagnetic field in an actual cavity. Even if the cavity is of a regular shape, the field pattern may be different from the field of the normal mode of vibration of the ideal cavity. There will be losses, and, in order to compensate them, an incoming net flux of energy will be necessary. However, the field pattern may be described *approximately* by one of the normal modes of vibration of the lossless cavity, even if the cavity is of irregular shape.

If we have to describe a distorted sine curve we may do it advantageously by a Fourier series. For example, the pattern of a vibrating string fixed at $x = 0$ and at $x = a$ may be described by $f(x) \,.\, \cos \omega t$ with

$$f(x) = \sum_0^\infty a_n \sin n(\pi x/a). \tag{139}$$

The coefficients are found by computing:

$$\frac{2}{a}\int_0^a f(x)\cdot a_n \sin n(\pi x/a)\,dx = \sum_{n=0}^{\infty}\frac{2}{a}\int_0^a a_m a_n$$
$$\times \sin m(\pi x/a)\sin n(\pi x/d)\,dx = a_n^2 \tag{140}$$

because the functions $\sin m(\pi x/a)$ are orthogonal:

$$\int_0^a \sin m(\pi x/a)\sin n(\pi x/a)\,dx = (\tfrac{1}{2}\,a)\,\delta_{nm}. \tag{141}$$

It is clear that, for a precise excitation frequency, one of the sines in eq. (139) by itself will be a very good approximation to the actual pattern. Each sine in eq. (139) is a mode of vibration (a solution of the differential equation plus boundary conditions) and will be a good approximation to the real pattern corresponding to a certain frequency of excitation, the eigenfrequency of this mode.

We shall describe the fields in a cavity also as a series of ideal modes of vibration. We have already mentioned these modes in the former section, when dealing with "ideal fields"

$$\begin{aligned} \boldsymbol{e}_a &= \mathscr{R}\,\boldsymbol{E}_a(x, y, z)\,e^{i\omega_a t}, \\ \boldsymbol{b}_a &= \mathscr{R}\,\boldsymbol{B}_a(x, y, z)\,e^{i\omega_a t}. \end{aligned} \tag{142}$$

The field patterns $\boldsymbol{E}_a$ and $\boldsymbol{B}_a$ (one for each eigenfrequency ω_a) will serve as the sine in eq. (139), to express any field. We shall describe a $\boldsymbol{b}$-like field (as $\boldsymbol{b}$ or curl $\boldsymbol{e}$) by the set $\boldsymbol{B}_a$ and an $\boldsymbol{e}$-like field by the set $\boldsymbol{E}_a$, in order to get better convergence.

Of course $\text{div}\,\boldsymbol{e}_a = \text{div}\,\boldsymbol{b}_a = 0$ and hence $\text{div}\,\boldsymbol{E}_a = \text{div}\,\boldsymbol{B}_a = 0$. But we shall not only describe fields with zero divergence. Hence we shall still need another collection of fields, say $\boldsymbol{F}_a$, with curl $\boldsymbol{F}_a = 0$ but with $\text{div}\,\boldsymbol{F}_a \neq 0$. But let us first establish some properties of our collections $\boldsymbol{E}_a$ and $\boldsymbol{B}_a$.

We have already seen that

$$\text{div}\,\boldsymbol{E}_a = \text{div}\,\boldsymbol{B}_a = 0. \tag{143}$$

Applying the other Maxwell equations to $\boldsymbol{e}_a$ and $\boldsymbol{b}_a$ one easily shows that

$$\begin{aligned} \text{curl } i\boldsymbol{E}_a &= (\omega_a/c)\, c\boldsymbol{B}_a, \\ \text{curl } c\boldsymbol{B}_a &= (\omega_a/c)\, i\boldsymbol{E}_a. \end{aligned} \tag{144}$$

We write "$i\boldsymbol{E}_a$" in order to emphasize that $\boldsymbol{e}_a$ is out of phase with $\boldsymbol{b}_a$ or that $i\boldsymbol{E}_a$ is real when $\boldsymbol{B}_a$ is.

We said that these ideal modes, by definition, are lossless. We assume that no energy flows out of the cavity. This is a more severe restriction than the statement that the outgoing flux in one part of the surface is compensated by an incoming flux through another part of the surface. We say that the normal component of $\boldsymbol{e}_a \wedge \boldsymbol{b}_a$ is zero on S at any time, or

$$(i\boldsymbol{E}_a \wedge \boldsymbol{B}_a) \,.\, \hat{\boldsymbol{n}} = 0 \quad \text{on} \quad S. \tag{145}$$

We may write this as

$$i\boldsymbol{E}_a \,.\, (\boldsymbol{B}_a \wedge \hat{\boldsymbol{n}}) = 0 \tag{146}$$

or

$$\boldsymbol{B}_a \,.\, (i\boldsymbol{E}_a \wedge \hat{\boldsymbol{n}}) = 0. \tag{147}$$

Hence either $i\boldsymbol{E}_a \wedge \hat{\boldsymbol{n}} = 0$ or $\boldsymbol{B}_a \wedge \hat{\boldsymbol{n}} = 0$ (or both are zero, of course). We may distinguish a surface S' where $\boldsymbol{B}_a$ is normal to the surface, $\boldsymbol{B}_a \wedge \boldsymbol{n} = \boldsymbol{0}$, and a surface S'' where $i\boldsymbol{E}_a$ is normal to the surface, $i\boldsymbol{E}_a \wedge \boldsymbol{n} = 0$. From $\boldsymbol{B}_a \wedge \boldsymbol{n} = \boldsymbol{0}$ on S' it follows that $\boldsymbol{E}_a$ is parallel to S', $\boldsymbol{E}_a \cdot \hat{\boldsymbol{n}} = 0$. Indeed, the line integral of $\boldsymbol{B}_a$ along any path lying in the surface S' is zero, since the tangential component of $\boldsymbol{B}_a$ is zero. Thus, by Stocke's theorem, $(\text{curl } \boldsymbol{B}_a)_{\text{normal}}$ to S' is zero. Hence by eq. (144b), $\boldsymbol{E}_a \,.\, \boldsymbol{n} = 0$. From $\boldsymbol{E}_a \wedge \boldsymbol{n} = \boldsymbol{0}$ on S'', it follows in the same way that $\boldsymbol{B}_a \,.\, \boldsymbol{n} = 0$ on S''. So we have two kinds of surfaces, with the following boundary conditions:

$$\left.\begin{aligned} \boldsymbol{B}_a \perp S' \quad &\text{or} \quad \boldsymbol{B}_a \wedge \boldsymbol{n} = \boldsymbol{0} \\ i\boldsymbol{E}_a \parallel S' \quad &\text{or} \quad i\boldsymbol{E}_a \,.\, \boldsymbol{n} = 0 \end{aligned}\right\} \text{on} \quad S', \tag{148a}$$

$$\left.\begin{aligned} i\boldsymbol{E}_a \perp S'' \quad &\text{or} \quad i\boldsymbol{E}_a \wedge \boldsymbol{n} = \boldsymbol{0} \\ \boldsymbol{B}_a \parallel S'' \quad &\text{or} \quad \boldsymbol{B}_a \,.\, \boldsymbol{n} = 0 \end{aligned}\right\} \text{on} \quad S''. \tag{148b}$$

We shall call S' a perfectly insulating wall and S'' a perfectly conducting wall. The boundary condition $i\boldsymbol{E}_a \perp S''$ is well known for static fields: since curl $i\boldsymbol{E}_a = \boldsymbol{0}$, one cannot have a discontinuity in the tangential component of $i\boldsymbol{E}_a$. Apply Stokes's theorem to a loop formed by two parallel paths, close to each other and to S'', but one inside and one outside the cavity. The tangential component has to be zero in the conductor and hence also inside the cavity near S''. In the same way one can show that $\boldsymbol{B}_a \perp S'$ for static fields if $\boldsymbol{B}_a$ is zero outside the cavity. Indeed, curl $c\boldsymbol{B} = \varepsilon_0^{-1}\boldsymbol{j}/c$ and since the wall S' is an insulator, there is no current $\boldsymbol{j}$.

In order to show why we call S' an insulator and S'' a conductor, for time-dependent fields also, let us consider a travelling wave incident on the wall. We consider a similar loop to which to apply Stokes's theorem, but now, using eq. (144),

$$\int_{\substack{1\\ \text{inside}}}^{2} i\boldsymbol{E}_a \cdot d\boldsymbol{s} - \int_{\substack{1\\ \text{outside}}}^{2} i\boldsymbol{E}_a \cdot d\boldsymbol{s} = \int_{\text{area}} \text{curl}\; i\boldsymbol{E}_a\, d\boldsymbol{a} = \int_{\text{area}} \omega_a \boldsymbol{B}_{a,\,\text{tr}}\, d\boldsymbol{a} \tag{149}$$

and $\boldsymbol{B}_{a,\text{tr}} = (\boldsymbol{k}/\omega) \wedge (i\boldsymbol{E}_{a,\text{tr}})$ with $\boldsymbol{k}$ normal to the wall [(eq. 92)]. Hence if the wall is a conductor then

$$\int_{\substack{1\\ \text{inside}\\ \text{cavity}}}^{2} i\boldsymbol{E}_a \cdot d\boldsymbol{s} = \int_{\substack{1\\ \text{conductor}}}^{2} i\boldsymbol{E}_a \cdot d\boldsymbol{s} - i \int_{\text{area}} \boldsymbol{k} \wedge (i\boldsymbol{E}_{a,\text{tr}})\, d\boldsymbol{a} \tag{150}$$

and both terms on the R.H.S. are zero, since $i\boldsymbol{E}_{a,\text{tr}}$ is zero in the conductor. (We choose the "area" so that the part "inside" is infinitesimal, i.e. the contribution to the surface integral is zero for the area "inside" the cavity.) Hence $(i\boldsymbol{E}_a)_{\text{tr}}$ is zero at the surface since eq. (150) holds for any path.

For a wall S', we can use a similar approach with $\boldsymbol{B}_a$, assuming $\boldsymbol{j}$ = zero everywhere since there is no conductor. The boundary condition on S'' is what we observe by reflection of light from a metal mirror. The boundary condition on S' is what we observe by reflection of light from a prism (Fig. 2.4).

It is now necessary to prove an orthogonality relation as in eq. (141).

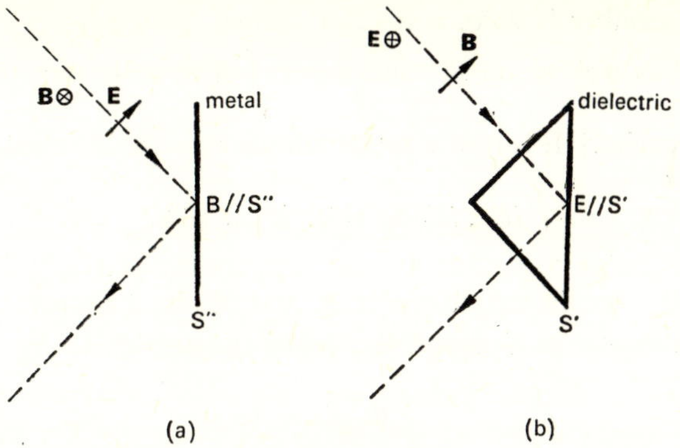

FIG. 2.4. (a) A perfectly conducting wall S'' with $\boldsymbol{B}//S''$. (b) A perfectly insulating wall S' with $\boldsymbol{E}//S'$.

We shall prove that

$$\int_V \boldsymbol{B}_a \,.\, \boldsymbol{B}_b \, dv = 0 \quad \text{if} \quad a \neq b. \tag{151}$$

We apply the vector identity div $(\boldsymbol{x} \wedge \boldsymbol{y}) = \boldsymbol{y} \operatorname{curl} \boldsymbol{x} - \boldsymbol{x} \operatorname{curl} \boldsymbol{y}$:

$$\begin{aligned} \operatorname{div}(\boldsymbol{B}_a \wedge \operatorname{curl} \boldsymbol{B}_b) - \operatorname{div}(\boldsymbol{B}_b \wedge \operatorname{curl} \boldsymbol{B}_a) &= \operatorname{curl} \boldsymbol{B}_b \operatorname{curl} \boldsymbol{B}_a \\ - \boldsymbol{B}_a \operatorname{curl} \operatorname{curl} \boldsymbol{B}_b - \operatorname{curl} \boldsymbol{B}_a \operatorname{curl} \boldsymbol{B}_b &+ \boldsymbol{B}_b \operatorname{curl} \operatorname{curl} \boldsymbol{B}_a \end{aligned} \tag{152}$$

and use now eq. (144) for all the curls:

$$\frac{\omega_b}{c^2} \operatorname{div}(\boldsymbol{B}_a \wedge i\boldsymbol{E}_b) - \frac{\omega_a}{c^2} \operatorname{div}(\boldsymbol{B}_b \wedge i\boldsymbol{E}_a) = - \boldsymbol{B}_a \frac{\omega_b^2}{c^2} \boldsymbol{B}_b + \boldsymbol{B}_b \frac{\omega_a^2}{c^2} \boldsymbol{B}_a; \tag{153}$$

and with Gauss's theorem

$$\begin{aligned} &\omega_b \int_V \operatorname{div}(\boldsymbol{B}_a \wedge i\boldsymbol{E}_b)\, dv - \omega_a \int_V \operatorname{div}(\boldsymbol{B}_b \wedge i\boldsymbol{E}_a)\, dv \\ &= \omega_b \int_S \boldsymbol{B}_a \wedge i\boldsymbol{E}_b \,.\, d\boldsymbol{a} - \omega_a \int_S \boldsymbol{B}_b \wedge i\boldsymbol{E}_a \, d\boldsymbol{a} \\ &= (\omega_a^2 - \omega_b^2) \int_V \boldsymbol{B}_a \boldsymbol{B}_b \, dv. \end{aligned} \tag{154}$$

The first member is zero, since the normal component of $E_a \wedge B_b$ is zero on S' as well as on S'', and hence $\int_V B_a B_b \, dv$ is zero for different eigenfrequencies.† It is now a rather simple exercise of calculus to prove also that

$$\int_V iE_a \, . \, iE_b \, dv = 0 \quad \text{if} \quad a \neq b. \tag{155}$$

We shall also fix the amplitude of B_a and iE_a by a normalization. This is simply a matter of elegance. We define the amplitudes by

$$\int_V B_a^2 \, dv = 1. \tag{156}$$

Now, again using the theorem div $(x \wedge y) = (\text{curl } x) \, . \, y - x \, . \, \text{curl } y$, we get

$$\begin{aligned} \text{div}\,(iE_a \wedge \text{curl } iE_a) &= (\text{curl } iE_a)^2 - iE_a \text{ curl curl } iE_a \\ &= +\,\omega_a^2 \, B_a^2 - iE_a \, [(\omega_a^2/c^2) \, iE_a] \\ &= +\omega_a^2 \, [B_a^2 - (iE_a)^2/c^2] \end{aligned} \tag{157}$$

and again by Stokes's theorem, just as before, one easily finds that

$$\int_V [B_a^2 - (iE_a)^2/c^2] \, dv = 0 \tag{158}$$

or

$$\int_V (iE_a)^2 \, dv = c^2 \int_V B_a^2 \, dv = c^2. \tag{159}$$

Since B_a and iE_a are also orthogonal, we may summarize the results using the Kronecker delta δ_{ab}, equal to one for $a = b$ and zero for $a \neq b$:

$$\int_V B_a B_b \, dv = \delta_{ab} \tag{160}$$

$$\int_V iE_a \, . \, iE_a \, dv = c^2 \delta_{ab}.$$

† The case of degeneration, i.e. different modes with the same eigenfrequency, may be resolved by the usual orthogonalization techniques that can be found in any standard text on vector spaces.

The fields $\boldsymbol{E}_a$ and $\boldsymbol{B}_a$ are the space-dependent parts of fields that satisfy Maxwell's equations in the absence of sources ϱ and $\boldsymbol{j}$, and satisfy the boundary condition $(\boldsymbol{E}_a \wedge \boldsymbol{B}_a) \wedge \boldsymbol{n} = 0$.

We have seen that for a certain ideal type of source, a perfect conductor or perfect dieletric, the given boundary conditions fully take account of the sources. In this ideal cavity the actual fields are given by $\boldsymbol{e}_a, \boldsymbol{b}_a$. However, in non-ideal conditions, such boundary conditions do not completely represent the effect of the sources. The fields $\boldsymbol{e}_a$ and $\boldsymbol{b}_a$ have zero divergence in the whole space, since they are defined by Maxwell's differential equations for $\varrho = 0$ and some boundary conditions. (In fact, the fields are zero outside the cavity.) The actual fields may for example be of the type "electrostatic field". The divergence is zero only in certain regions of space. We leave it to the mathematicians to prove that any field in the cavity with zero divergence may be represented by the collection $i\boldsymbol{E}_a$ or by the collection $\boldsymbol{B}_a$ (with time-dependent but not space-dependent coefficients) and also that any vector field may be represented by the sum of a field with zero divergence and a field with zero curl. We now have only to look for a field, say $\boldsymbol{F}_a$, with zero curl, to complement the description of an arbitrary field. In the static case we may observe that curl $\boldsymbol{E} = 0$ and choose $\boldsymbol{E}$ with div $\boldsymbol{E} = \varrho/\varepsilon_0$ for the field. But this $\boldsymbol{E}$ for the ideal cavity is $\boldsymbol{E}_a$ and does not have any divergence. If we define $\boldsymbol{a}_a$ by curl $\boldsymbol{a}_a = \boldsymbol{b}_a$, then another of Maxwell's equations gives

$$\operatorname{curl}\left(\boldsymbol{e}_a + \frac{\partial \boldsymbol{a}_a}{\partial t}\right) = 0. \tag{161}$$

The field

$$\boldsymbol{f}_a = \boldsymbol{e}_a + \frac{\partial \boldsymbol{a}_a}{\partial t} = \boldsymbol{F}_a e^{i\omega_a t}$$

will provide a good description of the fields. Its curl is zero, and hence we may define a scalar potential $\varphi_a = \phi_a e^{i\omega_a t}$ by

$$\boldsymbol{f}_a = -\operatorname{grad} \varphi_a. \tag{162}$$

We can define $\boldsymbol{a}_a$ even more completely. Since only curl $\boldsymbol{a}_a$ is defined, div $\boldsymbol{a}_a$ may still be arbitrarily defined. We choose

$$\operatorname{div} \boldsymbol{a}_a = -\frac{\partial \varphi_a}{\partial t}. \tag{163}$$

Now for any field

$$\varrho/\varepsilon_0 = \operatorname{div} \boldsymbol{e} = \left(\operatorname{div} \operatorname{grad} \varphi + \frac{\partial \operatorname{div} \boldsymbol{a}}{\partial t}\right) = -\left(\nabla^2 \varphi - \frac{\partial^2 \varphi}{\partial t^2}\right) \tag{164}$$

and therefore we assume this to hold for φ_a *inside* the cavity, where $\varrho = 0$:

$$\nabla^2 \varphi_a - \frac{\partial^2 \varphi_a}{c^2\, \partial t^2} = 0 \quad \text{or} \quad \nabla^2 \varphi_a = -\frac{\omega_a^2}{c^2} \varphi_a. \tag{165}$$

On the other hand, curl $\boldsymbol{f}_a = 0$ and, since we should like $(f_a)_{\text{tr}}$ to be zero outside, we shall have $(f_a)_{\text{tr}} = 0$ on the surface S or grad $\varphi_a \perp S$. Thus ϕ_a is constant on S, and we take this constant to be zero. Now it is a simple matter of calculus to prove some orthogonality relations. We also introduce a normalization condition:

$$\int_V \boldsymbol{F}_a \,.\, i\boldsymbol{E}_a \, dv = 0, \qquad \int_V \boldsymbol{F}_a \boldsymbol{F}_b \, dv = \delta_{ab}. \tag{166}$$

The proofs may be found in Slater (1950), and are similar to the calculations above. (They start with the vector equation for div $a\boldsymbol{x}$ instead of div $\boldsymbol{x} \wedge \boldsymbol{y}$.)

The fields $i\boldsymbol{E}_a$ and $\boldsymbol{B}_a$ are real vector fields, completely defined by

$$\begin{aligned} \operatorname{curl}(i\boldsymbol{E}_a) &= \omega_a(\boldsymbol{B}_a), \\ \operatorname{curl}(\boldsymbol{B}_a) &= \frac{\omega_a}{c^2}(i\boldsymbol{E}_a), \\ \operatorname{div} i\boldsymbol{E}_a &= \operatorname{div} \boldsymbol{B}_a = 0, \\ i\boldsymbol{E}_a \wedge \boldsymbol{B}_a \,.\, \hat{\boldsymbol{n}} &= 0 \text{ on the boundaries } S' \text{ and } S''. \end{aligned} \tag{167}$$

In fact $\mathscr{R}\, \boldsymbol{E}_a\, e^{i\omega_a t} = i\boldsymbol{E}_a \sin \omega_a t$ and $\mathscr{R}\, \boldsymbol{B}_a\, e^{i\omega_a t} = \boldsymbol{B}_a \cos \omega_a t$ are often good approximations to the actual fields of a certain mode of vibration of the cavity defined by the boundary S' and S''. But $i\boldsymbol{E}_a$ and $\boldsymbol{B}_a$ are to be regarded as a collection of real vector fields, furnishing a mathematical tool for the description of any actual field.

It is important to note that $\boldsymbol{iE_a}$ and $\boldsymbol{B_a}$ are real quantities; e.g.

$$\mathscr{R}(i\boldsymbol{E}_a \wedge \boldsymbol{h}) = i\boldsymbol{E}_a \wedge \mathscr{R}\,\boldsymbol{h}. \tag{168}$$

Therefore, we now write $i\boldsymbol{E}_a$ or $\mathscr{R}\, i(\boldsymbol{E}'_a + i\boldsymbol{E}''_a)$ as $(-\boldsymbol{E}''_a)$ and $\boldsymbol{B}_a$ as $\boldsymbol{B}'_a$. For reference

$$\begin{aligned} \operatorname{curl} \boldsymbol{E}''_a &= -\omega_a \boldsymbol{B}'_a, \\ \operatorname{curl} \boldsymbol{B}'_a &= -(\omega_a/c^2)\, \boldsymbol{E}''_a, \\ \operatorname{div} \boldsymbol{E}''_a &= \operatorname{div} \boldsymbol{B}'_a = 0, \\ \boldsymbol{E}''_a &\perp S'', \\ \boldsymbol{B}'_a &\perp S'. \end{aligned} \tag{169}$$

We now write all our actual fields $\boldsymbol{e}$, $\boldsymbol{d}$, $\boldsymbol{b}$, $\boldsymbol{h}$ and the current density $\boldsymbol{j}$, as functions of $\boldsymbol{E}''_a$, $\boldsymbol{F}_a$ and $\boldsymbol{B}'_a$. For $\boldsymbol{b}$ we choose $\boldsymbol{B}'_a$, ($\operatorname{div} \boldsymbol{b} = 0$), and for $\boldsymbol{e}$, $\boldsymbol{d}$ and $\boldsymbol{j}$ we choose $\boldsymbol{E}''_a$ and $\boldsymbol{F}_a$. This is necessary in order to get a good convergence, as already stressed above. However, for the same reason, it is convenient to write, for example, curl $\boldsymbol{h}$ as a function of $\boldsymbol{E}''_a$, since curl $\boldsymbol{h}$ is an $\boldsymbol{e}$-like field. For the same reason, we write curl $\boldsymbol{e}$ as a function of $\boldsymbol{B}'_a$. For instance,

$$\boldsymbol{e}(t) = \sum_a (\alpha_a \boldsymbol{E}''_a + \beta_a \boldsymbol{F}_a) \tag{170}$$

(α_a and β_a are time-dependent). But

$$\int_V \boldsymbol{e} \,.\, \boldsymbol{E}''_a \, dv = \sum_b \left(\alpha_b \int_V \boldsymbol{E}''_b \boldsymbol{E}''_a \, dv + \beta_b \int_V \boldsymbol{E}''_b \boldsymbol{F}_a \, dv \right) = +\alpha_a c^2 \tag{171}$$

because of the orthogonality and normalization conditions. Thus

$$\alpha_a = c^{-2} \int_V \boldsymbol{e} \,.\, \boldsymbol{E}''_a \, dv. \tag{172}$$

We find β_a in the same way and hence,

$$\boldsymbol{e} = \sum_a \left(c^{-2} \int_V \boldsymbol{e} \,.\, \boldsymbol{E}''_a \, dv \right) \boldsymbol{E}''_a + \left(\int_V \boldsymbol{e} \,.\, \boldsymbol{F}_a \, dv \right) \boldsymbol{F}_a. \tag{173}$$

For curl $\boldsymbol{e}$ we write

$$\operatorname{curl} \boldsymbol{e} = \sum_a \boldsymbol{B}'_a \int_V \operatorname{curl} \boldsymbol{e} \,.\, \boldsymbol{B}'_a \, dv \tag{174}$$

and again using

$$\operatorname{div}(\boldsymbol{x} \wedge \boldsymbol{y}) = \boldsymbol{y} \operatorname{curl} \boldsymbol{x} - \boldsymbol{x} \operatorname{curl} \boldsymbol{y} \tag{175}$$

and eqs. (144) we get

$$\int_V \boldsymbol{B}'_a \,.\, \operatorname{curl} \boldsymbol{e}\, dv = \int_V \boldsymbol{e} \,.\, \operatorname{curl} \boldsymbol{B}'_a\, dv + \int_V \operatorname{div}(\boldsymbol{e} \wedge \boldsymbol{B}'_a)\, dv$$

$$= -\frac{\omega_a}{c^2} \int_V \boldsymbol{e} \,.\, \boldsymbol{E}''_a\, dv + \int_{S'S''} \boldsymbol{e} \wedge \boldsymbol{B}'_a \,.\, d\boldsymbol{a}. \tag{176}$$

With $\boldsymbol{n} \,.\, \boldsymbol{e} \wedge \boldsymbol{B}'_a = \boldsymbol{e} \,.\, \boldsymbol{B}'_a \wedge \boldsymbol{n}$ and the boundary conditions, we obtain:

$$\operatorname{curl} \boldsymbol{e} = \sum_a \left(\frac{-\omega_a}{c^2} \boldsymbol{B}'_a \int_V \boldsymbol{e} \,.\, \boldsymbol{E}''_a\, dv + \boldsymbol{B}'_a \int_{S''} \boldsymbol{e} \wedge \boldsymbol{B}'_a\, d\boldsymbol{a} \right). \tag{177}$$

We can make a similar calculation for curl $\boldsymbol{h}$. Observe that it is not necessary that $\boldsymbol{h} \sim \boldsymbol{b}$ throughout the whole volume. For curl $\boldsymbol{h}$ we write

$$\operatorname{curl} \boldsymbol{h} = \sum_a \boldsymbol{E}''_a\, c^{-2} \int_V (\operatorname{curl} \boldsymbol{h} \,.\, \boldsymbol{E}''_a)\, dv \tag{178}$$

and again

$$\int_V \boldsymbol{E}''_a \,.\, \operatorname{curl} \boldsymbol{h}\, dv = -\omega_a \int_V \boldsymbol{h} \,.\, \boldsymbol{B}_a\, dv + \int_{S'S''} (\boldsymbol{h} \wedge \boldsymbol{E}''_a)\, d\boldsymbol{a} \tag{179}$$

or

$$\operatorname{curl} \boldsymbol{h} = \sum_a \boldsymbol{E}''_a\, c^{-2} \left\{ -\omega_a \boldsymbol{h} \,.\, \boldsymbol{B}_a\, dv - \int_{S'} \boldsymbol{E}''_a \wedge \boldsymbol{h}\, d\boldsymbol{a} \right\}. \tag{180}$$

Finally we get the following set of equations:

$$\boldsymbol{e} = \sum_a \left\{ \boldsymbol{E}''_a\, c^{-2} \int_V \boldsymbol{e} \,.\, \boldsymbol{E}''_a\, dv + \boldsymbol{F}_a \int_V \boldsymbol{e} \,.\, \boldsymbol{F}_a\, dv \right\}, \tag{181 a}$$

$$\boldsymbol{d} = \sum_a \left\{ \boldsymbol{E}''_a\, c^{-2} \int_V \boldsymbol{d} \,.\, \boldsymbol{E}''_a\, dv + \boldsymbol{F}_a \int_V \boldsymbol{d} \,.\, \boldsymbol{F}_a\, dv \right\}, \tag{181 b}$$

$$\boldsymbol{j} = \sum_a \left\{ \boldsymbol{E}''_a\, c^{-2} \int_V \boldsymbol{j} \,.\, \boldsymbol{E}''_a\, dv + \boldsymbol{F}_a \int_V \boldsymbol{j} \,.\, \boldsymbol{F}_a\, dv \right\}, \tag{181 c}$$

$$\boldsymbol{b} = \sum_a \left\{ \boldsymbol{B}'_a \int_V \boldsymbol{b} \,.\, \boldsymbol{B}'_a\, dv + 0 \right\}, \tag{181 d}$$

$$\operatorname{curl} \boldsymbol{e} = \sum_a \boldsymbol{B}'_a \left\{ -\omega_a c^{-2} \int_V \boldsymbol{e} \cdot \boldsymbol{E}''_a \, dv + \int_{S''} \boldsymbol{e} \wedge \boldsymbol{B}'_a \cdot \boldsymbol{da} \right\}, \qquad (181\text{e})$$

$$\operatorname{curl} \boldsymbol{h} = \sum_a \boldsymbol{E}''_a c^{-2} \left\{ -\omega_a \int_V \boldsymbol{h} . \boldsymbol{B}'_a \, dv - \int_S \boldsymbol{E}''_a \wedge \boldsymbol{h} \, \boldsymbol{da} \right\}. \qquad (181\text{f})$$

Introducing these expressions into Maxwell's equations we obtain equations for the coefficients. For example, $\operatorname{curl} \boldsymbol{e} + \partial \boldsymbol{b}/\partial t = 0$ becomes

$$\sum_a \boldsymbol{B}'_a \left\{ -\omega_a c^{-2} \int_V \boldsymbol{e} \cdot \boldsymbol{E}''_a \, dv + \int_{S''} \boldsymbol{e} \wedge \boldsymbol{B}'_a \, \boldsymbol{da} + \frac{\partial}{\partial t} \int_V \boldsymbol{b} . \boldsymbol{B}'_a \, dv \right\} = 0 \qquad (182)$$

and $\operatorname{curl} \boldsymbol{h} = \partial \boldsymbol{d}/\partial t + \boldsymbol{j}$ becomes

$$\sum_a c^{-2} \boldsymbol{E}''_a \left\{ -\omega_a \int_V \boldsymbol{h} \cdot \boldsymbol{B}'_a \, dv - \int_{S'} \boldsymbol{E}''_a \wedge \boldsymbol{h} \, \boldsymbol{da} - \frac{\partial}{\partial t} \int_V \boldsymbol{d} \cdot \boldsymbol{E}''_a \, dv - \int_V \boldsymbol{j} \cdot \boldsymbol{E}''_a \, dv \right\} + \sum_a \boldsymbol{F}_a \left\{ -\frac{\partial}{\partial t} \int_V \boldsymbol{d} \cdot \boldsymbol{F}_a \, dv - \int_V \boldsymbol{j} \cdot \boldsymbol{F}_a \, dv \right\} = 0. \qquad (183)$$

When $\sum_a K_a B_a = 0$, then each K_a is zero, because of the orthogonality. Indeed, then

$$\int_V B_b \left(\sum_a K_a B_a \right) dv = 0 = \sum_a K_a \int_V B_b B_a \, dv = \sum_a K_a \delta_{ab} = K_a. \qquad (184)$$

Hence for each mode (for each a):

$$-\omega_a \int_V \boldsymbol{e} \cdot \boldsymbol{E}''_a \, dv + c^2 \int_{S''} \boldsymbol{e} \wedge \boldsymbol{B}'_a \, \boldsymbol{da} + c^2 \frac{\partial}{\partial t} \int_V \boldsymbol{b} \cdot \boldsymbol{B}'_a \, dv = 0,$$

$$-\omega_a \int_V \boldsymbol{h} \cdot \boldsymbol{B}'_a \, dv - \int_{S'} \boldsymbol{E}''_a \wedge \boldsymbol{h} \, \boldsymbol{da} - \frac{\partial}{\partial t} \int_V \boldsymbol{d} \cdot \boldsymbol{E}''_a \, dv - \int_V \boldsymbol{j} \cdot \boldsymbol{E}''_a \, dv = 0, \qquad (185)$$

$$\frac{\partial}{\partial t}\int_V \boldsymbol{d}\,.\,\boldsymbol{F}_a\,dv + \int_V \boldsymbol{j}\,.\,\boldsymbol{F}_a\,dv = 0.$$

These equations give us information about the cavity. Their solutions will depend on the actual condition of the cavity and this will be discussed in the next section. Let us only consider here an evacuated cavity, without losses, and entirely closed. The surface integrals are zero and $\boldsymbol{h} = \varepsilon_0 c^2 \boldsymbol{b}$ while $\boldsymbol{d} = \varepsilon_0 \boldsymbol{e}$. Then the first two eqs. (185) may be combined to give:

$$\frac{\partial^2}{\partial t^2}\int_V \boldsymbol{b}\,.\,\boldsymbol{B}'_a\,dv + \omega_a^2\int_V \boldsymbol{b}\,.\,\boldsymbol{B}'_a\,dv = 0 \tag{186}$$

which is a differential equation for each of the coefficients of $\boldsymbol{b}$ in

$$\boldsymbol{b} = \sum_a \boldsymbol{B}'_a \int_V \boldsymbol{b}\,.\,\boldsymbol{B}'_a\,dv, \tag{187}$$

i.e.

$$\boldsymbol{b} = \sum_a \boldsymbol{B}'_a\,(K_a^+ e^{i\omega_a t} + K_a^- e^{-i\omega_a t}) = \sum_a \boldsymbol{B}'_a |K_a|\, e^{i\varphi_a}\, e^{i\omega_a t}. \tag{188}$$

The field is a superposition of the normal modes, each with a complex amplitude given by the initial conditions.

In an actual cavity, the "equation of motion" for the coefficients $\int_V \boldsymbol{b}\,.\,\boldsymbol{B}'_a\,dv$ will be more complicated. But at this point we are ready for the section about susceptibility and cavity parameters.

3. High-frequency Susceptibility and Cavity Parameters

3.1. Introduction

In the preceding section we obtained a method for describing the fields in a cavity. The fields are given by eqs. (2.181), and for the coefficients we have the differential equations, eqs. (2.185).

Fortunately, we shall not need to solve these equations rigorously. The fields $i\boldsymbol{E}''_a e^{i\omega' t}$ and $\boldsymbol{B}'_a\, e^{i\omega' t}$ are a first approximation to the actual fields in the cavity, if $\omega' \cong \omega_a$. The volume integrals

$$\int_V \boldsymbol{d} \,.\, i\boldsymbol{E}_a''\, dv \quad \text{and} \quad \int_V \boldsymbol{h} \,.\, \boldsymbol{B}_a'\, dv$$

may easily be recognized as expressions for the electric and magnetic energy in the cavity. The integrals

$$\int_V \boldsymbol{e} \,.\, i\boldsymbol{E}_a''\, dv \quad \text{and} \quad \int_V \boldsymbol{b} \,.\, \boldsymbol{B}_a'\, dv$$

may be related to the former ones by the paramagnetic and dielectric parameters of the material in the cavity. We shall assume that no currents are present inside the cavity, since the coupling to a cavity by a loop is rather rare in paramagnetic resonance experiments. The surface integrals may be recognized as an energy flux. The integral over S'' represents the losses inside the cavity walls and the integral over S' is essentially the wave that drives the cavity, the admittance Y of § 2.5. In the present section we shall express Y, the measurable quantity, as a function of the paramagnetic sample characteristics. We shall first do this for monochromatic fields. At the end of the section we shall discuss this apparent limitation.

Our starting-point is eqs. (2.185)

$$-\omega_a \varepsilon_0 \int_V \boldsymbol{e} \,.\, \boldsymbol{E}_a''\, dv + \varepsilon_0 c^2 \int_{S''} \boldsymbol{e} \wedge \boldsymbol{B}_a'\, da + \varepsilon_0 c^2 \frac{\partial}{\partial t} \int_V \boldsymbol{b} \,.\, \boldsymbol{B}_a'\, dv = 0, \tag{1a}$$

$$-\omega_a \int_V \boldsymbol{h} \,.\, \boldsymbol{B}_a'\, dv - \int_{S'} \boldsymbol{E}_a'' \wedge \boldsymbol{h}\, da - \frac{\partial}{\partial t} \int_V \boldsymbol{d} \,.\, \boldsymbol{E}_a''\, dv = 0. \tag{1b}$$

We have multiplied eq. (2.185a) by ε_0 and have put $\boldsymbol{j} = 0$ in eq. (2.185b). We shall not use eq. (2.185c). In eqs. (1) $\boldsymbol{e}$ and $\boldsymbol{b}$ have arbitrary time-dependence. For monochromatic fields without damping (we use ω for ω' since $\omega'' = 0$):

$$\boldsymbol{e} = \mathscr{R}\, \boldsymbol{E}\, e^{i\omega t} \quad (= \mathscr{I}\, \boldsymbol{E}\, e^{i(\omega t - \pi/2)}), \tag{2a}$$

$$\boldsymbol{b} = \mathscr{R}\, \boldsymbol{B}\, e^{i\omega t}, \tag{2b}$$

$$\boldsymbol{d} = \mathscr{R}\, \boldsymbol{D}\, e^{i\omega t}, \tag{2c}$$

$$\boldsymbol{h} = \mathscr{R}\, \boldsymbol{H}\, e^{i\omega t}. \tag{2d}$$

Introducing these expressions in eqs. (1) for $t = 0$ and for $t = \pi/2\omega$ we get the real and imaginary part of

$$-\omega_a \varepsilon_0 \int_V \boldsymbol{E} \cdot i\boldsymbol{E}_a'' \, dv + i\varepsilon_0 c^2 \int_{S''} \boldsymbol{E} \wedge \boldsymbol{B}_a' \, da - \varepsilon_0 c^2 \int_V \boldsymbol{B} \cdot \boldsymbol{B}_a' \, dv = 0 \tag{3a}$$

and

$$-\omega_a \int_V \boldsymbol{H} \cdot \boldsymbol{B}_a' \, dv + i \int_{S'} i\boldsymbol{E}_a'' \wedge \boldsymbol{H} \, da - \int_V \boldsymbol{D} \cdot i\boldsymbol{E}_a'' \, dv = 0. \tag{3b}$$

3.2. Paramagnetic filling function for monochromatic fields

(a) *Definition of* $\langle \chi \rangle$ *and* $\langle \varepsilon \rangle$

Our paramagnetic sample will, of course, disturb the $\boldsymbol{h}$ field or the $\boldsymbol{b}$ field in the cavity. This is precisely what we want to measure. At the moment, we shall not deal with the question of whether it is $\boldsymbol{h}$ or $\boldsymbol{b}$ which remains unperturbed. One would think that it is $\boldsymbol{h}$, since $\boldsymbol{h}$ represents the free current distribution, unperturbed by the sample. However, these free currents are due to $\boldsymbol{e}$, which is in turn due to $\boldsymbol{b}$. The "internal impedance" of the current source is not infinite. One could then think that $\boldsymbol{b}$ is unperturbed, since $\boldsymbol{b}$ is generated by $\boldsymbol{e}$ and $\boldsymbol{e}$ is independent of paramagnetism. However, $\boldsymbol{e}$ is not independent of the currents, which are proportional to $\boldsymbol{h}$. The "internal impedance" of the $\boldsymbol{e}$-source is not zero. In fact, neither $\boldsymbol{b}$ nor $\boldsymbol{h}$ remains unperturbed, but *in any situation* and *anywhere* in the cavity

$$\boldsymbol{h} = \varepsilon_0 c^2 \boldsymbol{b} - \boldsymbol{m} \tag{4}$$

where $\boldsymbol{m}$ is the magnetization. And hence

$$\int_V \boldsymbol{h} \cdot \boldsymbol{B}_a \, dv = \int_V \varepsilon_0 c^2 \boldsymbol{b} \cdot \boldsymbol{B}_a \, dv - \int_V \boldsymbol{m} \cdot \boldsymbol{B}_a \, dv. \tag{5}$$

We have already assumed that $\boldsymbol{b}$ and $\boldsymbol{e}$ are monochromatic. If the system is such that $\boldsymbol{m}$ is monochromatic also,

$$\boldsymbol{m} = \mathscr{R} \, \boldsymbol{M} \, e^{i\omega t}, \tag{6}$$

then we may define the complex susceptibility tensor $\chi = \chi' - i\chi''$ by

$$\boldsymbol{M} = \chi\varepsilon_0 c^2 \boldsymbol{B}. \tag{7}$$

Let us now define a certain *scalar* mean susceptibility†

$$\langle\chi\rangle = \langle\chi' - i\chi''\rangle = \langle\chi\rangle' - i\langle\chi\rangle'', \tag{8}$$

a susceptibility weighted *over the cavity*, by

$$\int_V \boldsymbol{M} \cdot \boldsymbol{B}_a \, dv = \langle\chi\rangle \int_V \varepsilon_0 c^2 \boldsymbol{B} \cdot \boldsymbol{B}_a \, dv. \tag{9}$$

(Here the meaning of $\langle\rangle$ is different from the time mean defined in eq. (2.28).) Now,

$$\int_V \boldsymbol{h} \cdot \boldsymbol{B}_a \, dv = \mathscr{R}\left(\int_V \boldsymbol{H} \cdot \boldsymbol{B}_a \, dv\right) e^{i\omega t} \tag{10}$$

$$= \mathscr{R}\left(\int_V \varepsilon_0 c^2 \boldsymbol{B} \cdot \boldsymbol{B}_a \, dv\right) e^{i\omega t} - \mathscr{R}\left(\int_V \boldsymbol{M} \cdot \boldsymbol{B}_a \, dv\right) e^{i\omega t}$$

or

$$\mathscr{R}\left(\int_V \boldsymbol{H} \cdot \boldsymbol{B}_a \, dv\right) e^{i\omega t} = \mathscr{R}\left[(1 - \langle\chi\rangle) \int_V \varepsilon_0 c^2 \boldsymbol{B} \cdot \boldsymbol{B}_a \, dv\right] e^{i\omega t}. \tag{11}$$

This holds at any time, i.e. also for $t' = t + \pi/2\omega$, and hence for the imaginary parts. Dropping the common factor $e^{i\omega t}$ we get

$$\int_V \boldsymbol{H} \cdot \boldsymbol{B}_a \, dv = (1 - \langle\chi\rangle) \int_V \varepsilon_0 c^2 \boldsymbol{B} \cdot \boldsymbol{B}_a \, dv. \tag{12a}$$

Incidentally,

$$\left(\int_V \boldsymbol{H} \cdot \boldsymbol{B}_a \, dv\right)_{\chi=0} = \left(\int_V \varepsilon_0 c^2 \boldsymbol{B} \cdot \boldsymbol{B}_a \, dv\right)_{\chi=0}$$

$$= (1 - \theta \langle\chi\rangle) \int_V \varepsilon_0 c^2 \boldsymbol{B} \cdot \boldsymbol{B}_a \, dv \tag{12b}$$

with $0 < \theta < 1$, since the integrals for $\chi = 0$ lie between the integrals of eq. (12a).

† Note the difference between $\langle\chi'\rangle$ and $\langle\chi\rangle'$. The operator $\langle\rangle$ is not always linear.

Similarly, for $\boldsymbol{d}$ and $\boldsymbol{e}$:

$$\boldsymbol{e} = \mathscr{R}\, \boldsymbol{E} e^{i\omega t}, \tag{13a}$$

$$\boldsymbol{d} = \mathscr{R}\, \boldsymbol{D} e^{i\omega t}. \tag{13b}$$

Instead of using $\boldsymbol{D} = \varepsilon \boldsymbol{E}$, we define a mean dielectric constant $\langle \varepsilon \rangle = \langle \varepsilon' - i\varepsilon'' \rangle$ by

$$\int_V \boldsymbol{D} \,.\, i\boldsymbol{E}_a \, dv = \langle \varepsilon \rangle \int_V \boldsymbol{E} \,.\, i\boldsymbol{E}_a \, dv. \tag{14}$$

The constant corresponding to $\langle \chi \rangle$ would be $(\langle \varepsilon \rangle - \varepsilon_0)/\varepsilon_0$ but we prefer to use ε and χ instead of, for example, χ_m and χ_e in order to avoid confusion arising from too many subscripts. In paramagnetic resonance experiments $\langle \varepsilon \rangle$ will in general be a constant, with no further importance, and $\langle \chi \rangle$ will be the quantity accessible to measurements, and from which χ may be deduced. $\langle \chi \rangle$ depends on how the cavity is filled with a sample of susceptibility χ. Therefore we call it the "filling function". In certain special cases $\langle \chi \rangle = \eta \,.\, \chi$ with η representing the filling factor, to be defined in eq. (20). Let us consider more accurately the relation between $\langle \chi \rangle$ and χ.

(b) *Meaning of* $\langle \chi \rangle$

The scalar quantity $\langle \chi \rangle$ is defined by

$$\int_V \boldsymbol{M} \,.\, \boldsymbol{B}'_a \, dv = \langle \chi \rangle \int_V \boldsymbol{B} \,.\, \boldsymbol{B}'_a \, dv = \frac{\langle \chi \rangle}{(1 - \langle \chi \rangle)} \int_V \boldsymbol{H} \,.\, \boldsymbol{B}'_a \, dv. \tag{15}$$

Let V_s be the volume occupied by the paramagnetic sample. $\boldsymbol{M} = 0$ outside V_s. We only may augment this definition, if we make some further assumptions. A first assumption will be that χ is homogeneous throughout the sample. Let $\boldsymbol{M}_{\|}$, $\boldsymbol{B}_{\|}$ and $\boldsymbol{H}_{\|}$ be the components of $\boldsymbol{M}$, $\boldsymbol{B}$ and $\boldsymbol{H}$ parallel to $\boldsymbol{B}_a$. Of course

$$\varepsilon_0 c^2 \boldsymbol{B}_{\|} = \boldsymbol{H}_{\|} + \boldsymbol{M}_{\|}. \tag{16}$$

We may thus define some scalar susceptibility χ_{sc} by

$$\boldsymbol{M}_{\|} = \chi_{sc} \varepsilon_0 c^2 \boldsymbol{B}_{\|} \tag{17}$$

or
$$H_{\parallel} = (1 - \chi_{sc})\, \varepsilon_0 c^2 B_{\parallel}$$
and hence
$$M_{\parallel} = \frac{\chi_{sc}}{1-\chi_{sc}} H_{\parallel}. \tag{18}$$

Consider first an infinitely flat sample, which is everywhere *normal* to $\boldsymbol{B}$. The field $\boldsymbol{B}$ is continuous inside and outside V_s, since div $\boldsymbol{B} = 0$ and so we assume $\boldsymbol{B} = \boldsymbol{B}_{\parallel}$. Then
$$\langle\chi\rangle = \chi_{sc} \frac{\int\limits_{V_s} \boldsymbol{B}_{\parallel} \,.\, \boldsymbol{B}'_a \, dv}{\int\limits_{V} \boldsymbol{B}_{\parallel} \,.\, \boldsymbol{B}'_a \, dv} = \chi_{sc} \frac{\int\limits_{V_s} \boldsymbol{B}(\chi = 0) \,.\, \boldsymbol{B}'_a \, dv}{\int\limits_{V} \boldsymbol{B}(\chi = 0) \,.\, \boldsymbol{B}'_a \, dv}. \tag{19}$$

We define a filling factor η as
$$\eta = \frac{\int\limits_{V_s} \boldsymbol{B}(\chi = 0)\, \boldsymbol{B}'_a \, dv}{\int\limits_{V} \boldsymbol{B}(\chi = 0)\, \boldsymbol{B}'_a \, dv} \tag{20}$$

and hence for this case $\langle\chi\rangle = \chi_{sc} \cdot \eta$.

If on the other hand the sample is infinitely flat but *parallel* to $\boldsymbol{H}$, then $\boldsymbol{H}$ remains unperturbed, since curl $\boldsymbol{H} = 0$, and from eq. (15):
$$\langle\chi\rangle (1 - \langle\chi\rangle)^{-1} = \frac{\int\limits_{V_s} \boldsymbol{M} \,.\, \boldsymbol{B}'_a \, dv}{\int\limits_{V} \boldsymbol{H} \,.\, \boldsymbol{B}'_a \, dv} = \frac{\chi_{sc}}{1-\chi_{sc}} \frac{\int\limits_{V_s} \boldsymbol{H}(\chi = 0)\, \boldsymbol{B}'_a \, dv}{\int\limits_{V} \boldsymbol{H}(\chi = 0)\, \boldsymbol{B}'_a \, dv}$$
$$= \frac{\chi_{sc}}{1-\chi_{sc}} \eta. \tag{21}$$

In the general case neither $\boldsymbol{B}$ nor $\boldsymbol{H}$ will remain unperturbed and we shall have something between these two limiting cases. Anyhow, from the definition of $\langle\chi\rangle$, eq. (15),
$$\langle\chi\rangle = \frac{\varepsilon_0 c^2 \int\limits_{V_s} \boldsymbol{M}_{\parallel} \boldsymbol{B}'_a \, dv}{\varepsilon_0 c^2 \int\limits_{V} \boldsymbol{B}_{\parallel} \boldsymbol{B}'_a \, dv}.$$

For the numerator one uses eq. (12b), and for the denominator one has $M_{\|} = \chi_{sc} B_{\|}$ and $B_{\|}(\chi = 0)$ lies between $B_{\|}$ and $H_{\|}/\varepsilon_0 c^2 = (1 - \chi_{sc})\, B_{\|}$ so that $B_{\|}(\chi = 0) = (1 - \theta_1 \chi_{sc})\, B_{\|}$. Hence

$$\frac{\langle\chi\rangle}{1 - \theta\langle\chi\rangle} = \frac{\chi_{sc}}{1 - \theta_1 \chi_{sc}}\, \eta. \tag{22}$$

with $0 < \theta < 1$ and now also $0 < \theta_1 < 1$. The correction θ is unimportant since always in practice $\langle\chi\rangle \ll 1$. However, χ_{sc} may not be negligible compared to unity. For example, $(\chi'_{max} - \chi'_{min}) \approx 0{\cdot}4$ for DPPH at 15°K and a static field of 0·3 T. (In such a case $\langle\chi\rangle$ remains small because $\eta \ll 1$.) So we must consider θ_1. This will be possible only if we make further assumptions about the sample.

If we assume an ellipsoidal sample, then we may define a constant N, the demagnetization factor,† by

$$\varepsilon_0 c^2 \boldsymbol{B}_{outside} = \varepsilon_0 c^2 \boldsymbol{B}_{inside} - N\boldsymbol{M}. \tag{25}$$

Since

$$\boldsymbol{M}_{\|} = \chi_{sc}\, \varepsilon_0 c^2 \boldsymbol{B}_{inside} \tag{26}$$

one has

$$\varepsilon_0 c^2 \boldsymbol{B}_{outside} = (1 - N\chi_{sc})\, \boldsymbol{B}_{inside}. \tag{27}$$

Thus

$$\theta_1 = N \tag{28}$$

if we assume

$$\boldsymbol{B}(\chi = 0) = \boldsymbol{B}_{outside}. \tag{29}$$

Remark. Both $\langle\chi\rangle$ and χ_{sc} are complex quantities. Hence, for example, $\langle\chi\rangle = \eta \cdot \chi_{sc}/(1 - N\chi_{sc})$ does not mean that $\langle\chi\rangle' = \eta\chi'_{sc}/(1 - N\chi'_{sc})$. We shall return to this question below.

† The coefficient N is one minus (4π) times the factor tabulated by Osborn (1945),

$$4\pi N_{tabulated} + N = 1, \tag{23}$$

since Osborn uses the definition

$$(\varepsilon_0 c^2 \boldsymbol{B}_{outside}) = \boldsymbol{H}_{outside} = \boldsymbol{H}_{inside} + 4\pi \boldsymbol{N}_{tabulated}\, \boldsymbol{M} \tag{24}$$

usual in the c.g.s. system of units.

A final question now is how to establish which quantity is given by χ_{sc}. We assume $\boldsymbol{B} \parallel \boldsymbol{H} \parallel \boldsymbol{B}_a$ in V_s. This is verified for the ellipsoidal sample and is a less rigid limitation than putting $\theta_1 = 0$ for an arbitrary sample. If the HF field is normal to the static field $\boldsymbol{B}_s = B_s\hat{z}$, then χ_{sc} is the component of χ usually designated by χ_{xx}. If the HF field is parallel to $\boldsymbol{B}_s$, then χ_{sc} is the HF drag χ_l for parallel fields. If the HF fields makes an angle ψ with $\boldsymbol{B}_s$ then

$$\chi_{sc} = \chi_{xx} \sin^2 \psi + \chi_l \cos^2 \psi. \tag{30}$$

This may be seen from Fig. 3.1. The component of $\boldsymbol{B}_{\parallel}$ normal to $\boldsymbol{B}_s$ is $\boldsymbol{B}_{\parallel} \sin \psi$ and produces a magnetization M_x, given by $M_x = \chi_{xx}(\boldsymbol{B}_{\parallel} \sin\psi)$

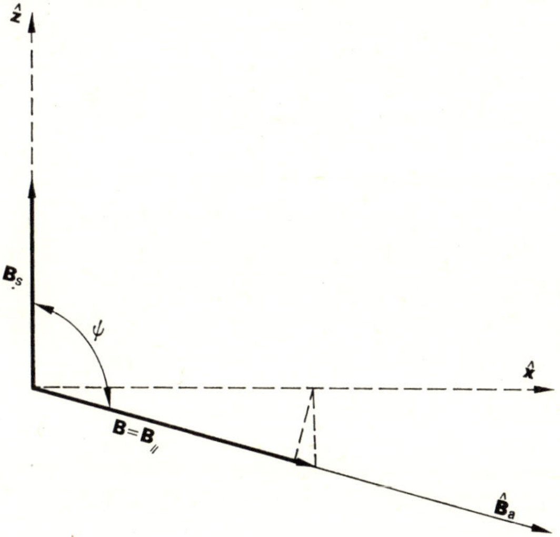

FIG. 3.1. The relation between χ_{sc} and χ_{xx} and χ_e is obtained by projecting twice each component of $\boldsymbol{B}_{\parallel}$. The result is $\chi_{sc} = \chi_{xx} \sin^2 \psi + \chi_e \cos^2 \psi$.

along this normal, the projection of which on $\boldsymbol{B}_{\parallel}$ is $\chi_{xx} \sin^2 \psi \boldsymbol{B}_{\parallel}$. The component of $\boldsymbol{B}_{\parallel}$ parallel to $\boldsymbol{B}_s$ produces a magnetization $\boldsymbol{M} = \boldsymbol{M}_{\parallel}$ along $\boldsymbol{B}_s$ and its projection on $\boldsymbol{B}_{\parallel}$ is $\chi_l \cos^2 \psi \boldsymbol{B}_{\parallel}$. $\boldsymbol{M}_{\parallel}$ is the sum of both, and eq. (30) follows from the definition $\boldsymbol{M}_{\parallel} = \chi_{sc}\boldsymbol{B}_{\parallel}$.

3.3. THE ADMITTANCE AS A FUNCTION OF $\langle\chi\rangle$

With the definition of $\langle\chi\rangle$ and $\langle\varepsilon\rangle$ we may now analyse eqs. (3):

$$-\omega_a \int_V \varepsilon_0 \boldsymbol{E} \, . \, i\boldsymbol{E}_a'' \, . \, dv + i\varepsilon_0 c^2 \int_{S''} \boldsymbol{E} \wedge \boldsymbol{B}_a' \, da - \varepsilon_0 c^2 \int_V \boldsymbol{B} \, . \, \boldsymbol{B}_a' \, dv = 0 \tag{31a}$$

$$-\omega_a (1 - \langle\chi\rangle) \, \varepsilon_0 c^2 \int_V \boldsymbol{B} \, . \, \boldsymbol{B}_a' \, dv + i \int_{S'} i\boldsymbol{E}_a'' \wedge \boldsymbol{H} \, da$$
$$-\omega \frac{\langle\varepsilon\rangle}{\varepsilon_0} \int_V \boldsymbol{E} \, . \, i\boldsymbol{E}_a'' \, dv = 0. \tag{31b}$$

We eliminate the integral over $\boldsymbol{E} \, . \, i\boldsymbol{E}_a''$ from both equations:

$$\left(\frac{1 - \langle\chi\rangle}{\langle\varepsilon\rangle/\varepsilon_0} \, \frac{\omega_a}{\omega} - \frac{\omega}{\omega_a} \right) \omega_a \int_V \varepsilon_0 c^2 \, \boldsymbol{B} \, . \, \boldsymbol{B}_a' \, dv + i\varepsilon_0 c^2 \int_{S''} \boldsymbol{E} \wedge \boldsymbol{B}_a' \, da$$
$$= i \frac{\omega_a}{\omega} \, \frac{1}{\langle\varepsilon\rangle/\varepsilon_0} \int_{S'} i\boldsymbol{E}_a'' \wedge \boldsymbol{H} \, da. \tag{31c}$$

Although not necessary, we shall now assume $\langle\varepsilon\rangle = \varepsilon_0$ because it facilitates writing the equations and it has no serious influence on the theory. Suppose for a while that there is a perfectly reflecting wall closing the hole S' of the cavity. Then we shall have a free oscillation with complex frequency $\omega = \omega' + i\omega''$. The integral over S' vanishes and eq. (31c) becomes

$$\frac{\varepsilon_0 c^2 \int_{S''} \boldsymbol{E} \wedge \boldsymbol{B}_a \, . \, da}{\omega_a \varepsilon_0 c^2 \int_V \boldsymbol{B} \, . \, \boldsymbol{B}_a \, dv} = i \left[(1 - \langle\chi\rangle) \frac{\omega_a}{\omega} - \frac{\omega}{\omega_a} \right]. \tag{32}$$

Let us write this again for $\chi = 0$, using a subscript "0". For example, ω_0 is the complex frequency to which ω would tend if χ were quenched. On S'' we assume $\chi = 0$ in any case:

$$\frac{\varepsilon_0 c^2 \int_{S''} \boldsymbol{E} \wedge \boldsymbol{B}_a \, da}{\omega_a \left(\varepsilon_0 c^2 \int_V \boldsymbol{B} \, . \, \boldsymbol{B}_a \, dv \right)_0} = -i \left(\frac{\omega_0}{\omega_a} - \frac{\omega_a}{\omega_0} \right). \tag{33}$$

Equation (33) gives us the free oscillation frequency ω_0 of the cavity for $\chi = 0$; or it gives a relation between

$$\int_{S''} \boldsymbol{E} \wedge \boldsymbol{B}_a \, da \quad \text{and} \quad \left(\int_V \boldsymbol{B} \, . \, \boldsymbol{B}_a \, dv \right)_0$$

if ω_0 is known. Recall now eqs. (2.41) and (2.48)

$$\frac{\int\limits_{S''+S'} \boldsymbol{E} \wedge \boldsymbol{H}^* \, da}{\int\limits_V \boldsymbol{B} \, . \, \boldsymbol{H}^* \, da} = i(\omega_0^*/\alpha - \omega_0) \tag{34}$$

for the actual fields. If we assume $\boldsymbol{H}^*$ proportional to $\boldsymbol{B}_a$ in our cavity (for $\chi = 0$) then it follows from eqs. (33) and (34) that

$$\alpha = \frac{\omega_0 \omega_0^*}{\omega_a^2} \, . \tag{35}$$

This equation was already mentioned in eq. (2.52b) and also holds if ω_0 is not the free oscillation frequency but an excitation through a very small hole, $S' \ll S''$. Here $S' = 0$ and since at free oscillation magnetic energy is converted into electrical and vice versa, $\alpha = 1$ or

$$\omega_0 \omega_0^* = \omega_0'^2 + \omega_0''^2 = \omega_a^2 \, . \tag{36}$$

Now eq. (33) becomes

$$\frac{\varepsilon_0 c^2 \int\limits_{S''} \boldsymbol{E} \wedge \boldsymbol{B}_a' \, da}{\varepsilon_0 c^2 \int\limits_V (\boldsymbol{B} \, . \, \boldsymbol{B}_a \, dv)_0} = 2\omega_0'' \, . \tag{37}$$

Note that

$$\frac{2\omega_0''}{\omega_0'} = 1/Q_0 \tag{38}$$

is the eigendamping of the cavity. The approximation $\boldsymbol{B}_a \sim \boldsymbol{H}^*$ on S' and inside V is reasonable for a metallic boundary cavity. Remember that $\boldsymbol{B}_a' \parallel S''$ and $\boldsymbol{E}_a'' \perp S''$. On S' one has $(\boldsymbol{B}_a')_{\text{tangent}} = 0$ so that $\boldsymbol{B}_a \sim \boldsymbol{H}^*$ would be an incorrect approximation for

$$\int_{S'} \boldsymbol{E} \wedge \boldsymbol{B}_a^* \, da \, .$$

Let us now consider the cavity coupled to the guide. The integral over S' will not vanish but will be substantially given by the admittance Y. Indeed, we write eq. (2.137) as

$$Y = \frac{1}{(1/Q_e)} \frac{\int_{S'} \boldsymbol{E} \wedge \boldsymbol{H}^* \, da}{\omega' \left(\frac{1+\alpha^{-1}}{2}\right) \int_V \boldsymbol{B} . \boldsymbol{H}^* \, dv}. \tag{39}$$

$1/Q_e$ is a parameter which gives the coupling between guide and cavity. Energy will be supplied through S' in order to compensate the losses and the oscillation will be stationary: $\omega'' = 0$ or $\omega = \omega'$.

Let us now consider $\boldsymbol{E}_{\parallel}$ on S' and $\boldsymbol{B}$ inside V, in the first approximation, equal to $i\boldsymbol{E}_a$ and $\boldsymbol{B}_a$ respectively, at least for $\chi = 0$. Remember that $iE_a \parallel S'$ while $B_a \perp S''$. Thus

$$Y = \frac{1}{(1/Q_e)} \frac{\int_{S'} i\boldsymbol{E}_a \wedge \boldsymbol{H}^* \, da}{\omega \left(\frac{1+\alpha^{-1}}{2}\right) \left(\int_V \boldsymbol{B}_a \boldsymbol{H}^* \, dv\right)_0} \frac{\left(\int_V \boldsymbol{B}\,\boldsymbol{H}^* \, dv\right)_0}{\int_V \boldsymbol{B} . \boldsymbol{H}^* \, dv}. \tag{40}$$

We again assume $\chi = 0$ at S'.

We may write eq. (31c) again, using eq. (37) for the integral over S'' and the complex conjugate of eq. (40) for the integral over S'. If we use eqs. (12), then a common term $\left(\int_V \varepsilon_0 c^2 \boldsymbol{B} . \boldsymbol{B}'_a \, da\right)$ may be dropped. The result of these manipulations is

$$\left[(1 - \langle\chi\rangle)\frac{\omega_a}{\omega} - \frac{\omega}{\omega_a}\right] + 2i\frac{\omega_0''}{\omega_a}(1 - \theta\langle\chi\rangle)$$

$$= iY^* \frac{1}{Q_e} \frac{(1+\alpha^{-1})}{2} \frac{\int_V \boldsymbol{B}^*\boldsymbol{H} \, dv}{\left(\int_V \boldsymbol{B}^*\boldsymbol{H} \, dv\right)_0} (1 - \theta\langle\chi\rangle). \tag{41}$$

We may write

$$\left(\int_V \boldsymbol{B}^*\boldsymbol{H} \, dv\right)_0 = (1 - \theta_2\langle\chi\rangle) \int_V \boldsymbol{B}^*\boldsymbol{H} \, dv \tag{42}$$

as in eq. (12b) but with $\theta_2 \neq \theta$. We still have $0 < \theta_2 < 1$, and $(1 - \theta\langle\chi\rangle)/(1 - \theta_2\langle\chi\rangle) = (1 - \theta_3\langle\chi\rangle)$, with $-1 < \theta < 1$, now.
Then

$$(1 - \theta_3 \langle\chi\rangle)\left(\frac{\alpha + 1}{2\alpha}\right) i(1/Q_e)\, Y^* = (1 - \langle\chi\rangle)\frac{\omega_a}{\omega} - \frac{\omega}{\omega_a}$$
$$+ (1 - \theta\langle\chi\rangle)(2i\omega_0''/\omega_a). \tag{43}$$

Let us first see what this means for $\chi = 0$. We know that ω and ω_a are real. For the real part we have:

$$\frac{\alpha + 1}{2\alpha}(1/Q_e)\, Y'' = \frac{\omega_a}{\omega} - \frac{\omega}{\omega_a}, \tag{44}$$

and for the imaginary part,

$$\frac{\alpha + 1}{2\alpha} 1/Q_e\, Y' = \frac{2\omega_0''}{\omega}\frac{\omega}{\omega_a} = \frac{1}{Q_0}\frac{\omega}{\omega_a}. \tag{45}$$

On the other hand, from eq. (2.136),

$$\frac{\alpha + 1}{2\alpha}\left(\frac{1}{Q_e} Y^*\right) = \left(\frac{\alpha + 1}{2\alpha}\right)\left(\frac{1}{Q_0} + 2i\frac{\alpha - 1}{\alpha + 1}\right)$$
$$= \frac{\alpha + 1}{2\alpha}\frac{1}{Q_0} + i\frac{\alpha - 1}{\alpha}. \tag{46}$$

Hence

$$\frac{\alpha + 1}{2\alpha} = \frac{\omega}{\omega_a} \quad \text{and} \quad -\frac{\alpha - 1}{\alpha} = \frac{\omega_a}{\omega} - \frac{\omega}{\omega_a}. \tag{47a}$$

Let us put $\alpha = \omega^2/\omega_a^2$ [from eq. (35)] in eq. (47a):

$$\frac{\omega^2 + \omega_a^2}{2\omega^*\omega_a} = \frac{\omega^2}{\omega_a^2} \quad \frac{\omega_a^2 - \omega^2}{\omega^2} = \frac{\omega_a^2 - \omega^2}{\omega_a}. \tag{47b}$$

This is indeed satisfied for $\omega = \omega_a$. Then $\alpha = 1$ and $Y'' = 0$. The approximations $\boldsymbol{E}_{\parallel} = i\boldsymbol{E}_a$ on S' and $\boldsymbol{B}_{\parallel} = \boldsymbol{B}_a'$ on S'' are indeed best for $\omega = \omega_a$. This is the case of the freely oscillating cavity but with no losses (the losses being compensated). One sees, however, from eqs. (47b), that the approximation is still good if only $\omega \approx \omega_a$. The

R.H.S. of eq. (43) may be written as

$$\left(\frac{\omega_a}{\omega} - \frac{\omega}{\omega_a}\right) + \frac{2i\omega_0''}{\omega_a} - \langle\chi\rangle\left[\frac{\omega_a}{\omega} - \theta\,\frac{2i\omega_0''}{\omega_a}\right]. \tag{48}$$

ω/ω_a is of the order of unity and $2\omega_0''/\omega_a$ is the cavity damping $1/Q_0$. Since

$$1/Q_0 \ll 1 \tag{49}$$

(e.g. $1/Q_0 < 10^{-3}$) in general, we may neglect θ. Incidentally, it would be rather difficult to calculate θ. Now

$$\frac{\omega_a^2 - \omega^2}{\omega_a} + \frac{2i\omega_0''}{\omega_a^2} - \langle\chi\rangle = i(1/Q_e)\,Y^*\,\frac{\omega^2 + \omega_0^2}{2\omega^2}(1 - \theta_3\,\langle\chi\rangle). \tag{50}$$

We have used $\alpha = (\omega/\omega_a)^2$. We may neglect θ_3 for $\omega \approx \omega_a$, if

$$[(1/Q_e)\,Y^*] \approx 1/Q_0 - i(1/Q_e)\,Y^* \ll 1. \tag{51}$$

This is generally achieved, because one chooses $1/Q_e \approx 1/Q_0$ and $Y'' \lesssim 1$, but it can be a reason for inaccurate measuring if the spectrometer is not well adjusted. We shall now neglect θ and θ_3 and assume $\omega \approx \omega_a$. Equation (43) becomes:

$$(1/Q_e)\,Y = \frac{2\omega_0''}{\omega_a} - 2i\,\frac{\omega - \omega_a}{\omega_a} - i\,\langle\chi\rangle^*. \tag{52}$$

The approximation used here ($\theta = \theta_3 = 0$) is better than one part in 10^3 for $\langle\chi\rangle$, for a well-constructed spectrometer. For higher precision one must even at this stage take into account the shape of the sample. [Another problem is θ_1 which also depends on the shape of the sample, eq. (22).] Observe that the approximation in eq. (52) is *not* based on $\langle\chi\rangle \ll 1$, but on $1/Q_0 \ll 1$. Let us still write eq. (52) as

$$(1/Q_e)\,Y = (1/Q_e)\,Y_0 - i\langle\chi\rangle^* \tag{53}$$

where the subscript "0" represents $\chi = 0$. We may also write it as

$$Y' = Y_0' + \frac{\langle\chi\rangle''}{1/Q_e}, \tag{54a}$$

$$Y'' = Y_0'' - \frac{\langle\chi\rangle'}{1/Q_e}, \tag{54b}$$

or

$$1/Q_m = 1/Q_0 + \langle\chi\rangle'', \tag{55}$$

$$\left(2\frac{\omega - \omega_a}{\omega_a}\right)_m = \left(2\frac{\omega - \omega_a}{\omega_a}\right)_0 + \langle\chi\rangle'. \tag{56}$$

The effect of $\langle\chi\rangle''$ is an additional damping and $\langle\chi\rangle'$ produces a shift in the eigenfrequency ω_a of the cavity:

$$\langle\chi\rangle'' = \Delta(1/Q_0) = \Delta(2\omega_0''/\omega_a), \tag{57a}$$

$$\langle\chi\rangle' = 2\omega\left(\frac{1}{(\omega_a)_m} - \frac{1}{(\omega_a)_0}\right) = -2\frac{\omega_{am} - \omega_{a0}}{\omega_{a0}} = -2\frac{\Delta\omega_a}{\omega_a}. \tag{57b}$$

If we write $\omega_0 = \omega_0' + i\omega_0''$ for the complex eigenfrequency of the driven cavity (i.e. $\omega_a = \omega_0'$ and not $\omega_a = |\omega_0|$ as for the free cavity) then

$$\langle\chi\rangle = -2\frac{\Delta\omega_0}{\omega_0'} \tag{58}$$

for $\omega \approx \omega_a$.

We indicated by $1/Q_m$ the eigendamping and by ω_m' the eigenfrequency of the cavity with the paramagnetic sample. (This is *not* what one calls a "loaded" cavity. "Loaded" here means connected to a guide, with $1/Q_e \neq 0$. The "loaded" damping $1/Q_L$ is $1/Q_e + 1/Q_0$ or eventually $1/Q_e + 1/Q_m$.)

3.4. Non-monochromatic fields

We may now finally discuss the limitation to monochromatic fields. What we measure, Y, is a quantity defined for monochromatic fields. Even if higher modes are generated in the cavity, we only measure at one frequency because of the limited bandwidth of the waveguide and detector. The higher modes are so rapidly damped that they do not influence the measurement of Y. One could write the fields e, h, b, d of eqs. (1), for example, as

$$e = \mathscr{R}(E_1\, e^{i\omega t} + E_2\, e^{i2\omega t} + \ldots + E_n\, e^{in\omega t} + \ldots). \tag{59}$$

This would give final equations for each $e^{in\omega t}$ but the only things we measure are the quantities of the equation for $e^{i\omega t}$. One distinction must be made about $\langle\chi\rangle$ (and about $\langle\varepsilon\rangle$, but we limit the discussion to $\langle\chi\rangle$). We defined $\langle\chi\rangle$ as

$$\int_V \boldsymbol{M} \cdot \boldsymbol{B}_a \, dv = \langle\chi\rangle \int_V \boldsymbol{B} \cdot \boldsymbol{B}_a \, dv. \tag{60}$$

But now each harmonic of $\boldsymbol{B}$ may generate a magnetization and this magnetization may have components at each multiple of the frequency of the $\boldsymbol{B}$-harmonic:

$$\boldsymbol{M}_i = \sum_j \chi^{ij} \boldsymbol{B}_j \tag{61}$$

and we may also define a *harmonic-space* tensor by

$$\int_V \boldsymbol{M}_i \boldsymbol{B}_a \, dv = \sum_j \langle\chi\rangle^{ij} \int \boldsymbol{B}_j \cdot \boldsymbol{B}_a \, dv. \tag{62}$$

$\langle\chi\rangle$ may be considered to be a tensor in the harmonic-space, transforming a harmonic-space "vector" with "components"

$$\int_V \boldsymbol{B}_n \cdot \boldsymbol{B}_a \, dv$$

in the space with unit vectors $e^{i\omega t}$, $e^{i2\omega t}$, ..., into a "vector" with "components"

$$\int_V \boldsymbol{M}_n \boldsymbol{B}_a \, dv.$$

Of course $\langle\chi\rangle^{ij} = 0$ for $i < j$.

In our arrangement, we only have multiples of the dominant frequency, i.e. ω, 2ω, 3ω, etc., and the only "component" of $\boldsymbol{M}$ at frequency ω is generated by $\boldsymbol{B}_1 e^{i\omega t}$. Hence the $\langle\chi\rangle$ that we measure is in fact $\langle\chi\rangle''$.

4. Measurement of Cavity Parameters

4.1. Introduction

In the former sections [eq. (3.53)] we have deduced that the admittance of the cavity is given by

$$Y = Y_0 - \frac{i\langle\chi\rangle^*}{1/Q_e}. \tag{1}$$

We have discussed how $\langle\chi\rangle$ may furnish us with the required information about the sample. Now the only remaining point about electromagnetic detection is how to measure Y, and in particular small variations in Y. At this point, one can already see that a high sensitivity will require a low value of

$$(1/Q_e)\, Y_0 = 1/Q_0 + i2\frac{\omega - \omega_a}{\omega_a} \tag{2}$$

of which $i\langle\chi\rangle^*$ represents a variation. Of course, one cannot choose the damping $1/Q_0$ to be arbitrarily low. The limits are imposed by technical problems and depend on what one wants to measure. For example, if we have to investigate a sample with a high content of water, the damping will be high because of the dielectric losses in the water. If there is not sufficient space in a dewar for a cylindrical cavity, we must use a rectangular one and this has a higher damping. Besides this, $\langle\chi\rangle$ cannot be chosen arbitrarily high; it is determined by the characteristics of the sample to be studied. For our discussion, we assume $1/Q_0$ and $\langle\chi\rangle$ already optimized. They are constants of the problem. Then, we have a cavity with a certain eigendamping and this cavity is filled with a certain paramagnetic material, in a certain way. The variables of our problem are Y_0, i.e. Y_0' and Y_0''. We may, in the absence of resonance, couple the cavity to a certain extent choosing Q_e^{-1} or $Y_0' = Q_0^{-1}/Q_e^{-1}$. And we may choose the exciting frequency and hence the deviation $2(\omega' - \omega_a)/\omega_a$ in frequency, or $Y_0'' = -[2(\omega' - \omega_a)/\omega_a]/Q_e^{-1}$. We therefore write eq. (1) as

$$Y = Y_0 - i(\langle\chi\rangle^*/Q_0^{-1})\, Y_0' \tag{3}$$

or

$$\frac{\Delta Y}{Y_0'} = -i\langle\chi\rangle^*/Q_0^{-1}. \tag{4}$$

Thus the problem is reduced to measuring a small deviation $\Delta Y/Y_0'$. Actually we cannot measure ΔY straightforwardly. We can only measure changes in the microwave power which are related to ΔY. This is done with the aid of a microwave spectrometer. A wave of constant amplitude A is reflected by the admittance. The reflected wave is of amplitude rA; it leads to the knowledge of the changes in the admittance, but what we measure are changes in rA or in $|rA|^2$. This microwave power is to be detected, i.e. to be transformed into a signal accessible to further non-microwave amplification and analysis. We begin with a very simple scheme. Afterwards, various refinements will be discussed in order to eliminate or reduce spurious effects and improve the performance.

A relation exists between Y and r or ΔY and Δr, since $r = (1 - Y)/(1 + Y)$. Remember, however, that Y and r are complex quantities. Therefore we first explain the Smith diagram.

4.2. Paramagnetic resonance in the Smith diagram

(a) *Smith diagram*

We have defined the reflection coefficient $r = R^{i\varphi}$, related to the admittance $Y = Y' + iY''$ by

$$r = \frac{1 - Y}{1 + Y} \quad \text{or} \quad Y = \frac{1 - r}{1 + r}. \tag{5}$$

The relation between R, φ and Y', Y'' is easily found, but yields rather complicated expressions compared to the simplicity of eqs. (5). These equations define what we call a bilinear transformation between r and Y. We may consider a complex plane with the points r and another complex plane with the points Y. The transformation equation eq. (5) establishes a correspondence between each point of the r-plane and each point of the Y-plane, and vice versa. It so happens that straight lines in the Y-plane (e.g. lines $Y' =$ constant or $Y'' =$ constant or $aY' + bY'' =$ constant) transform into circles in the r-plane. This is emphasized in Fig. 4.1.

This property is used in a Smith diagram. Such a diagram *is an r-plane* in which the circles corresponding to $Y' =$ constant and to $Y'' =$ constant are drawn for the various values of the constant. For each point of the r-plane one easily finds the r-coordinates, R and φ, the distance from the centre and the angle the radius vector makes with

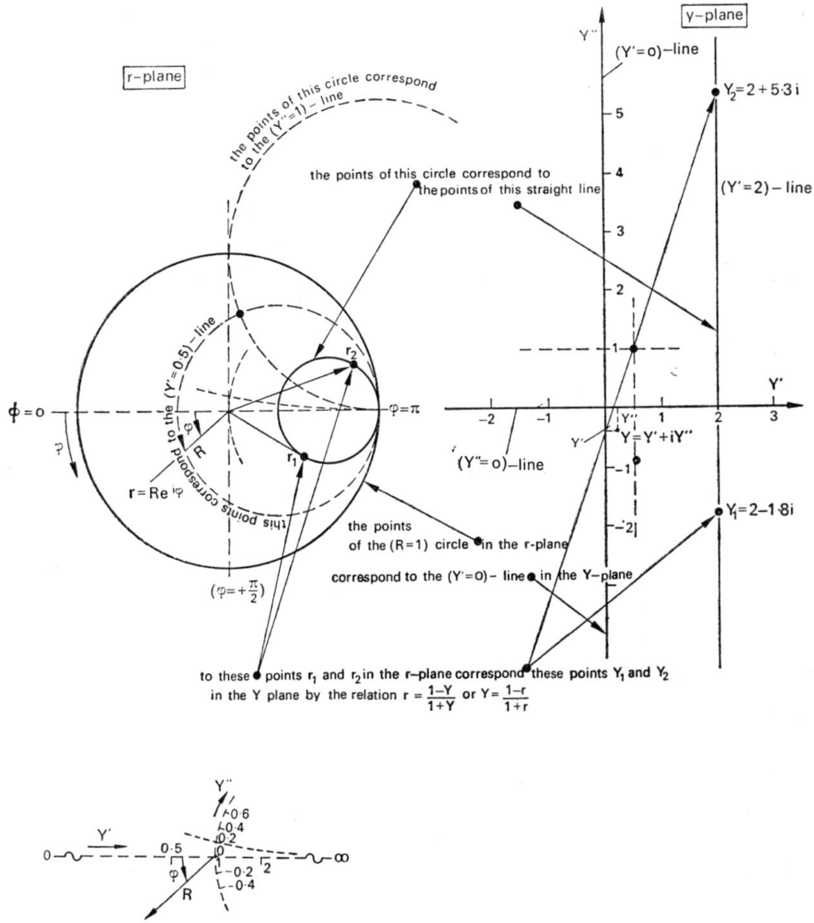

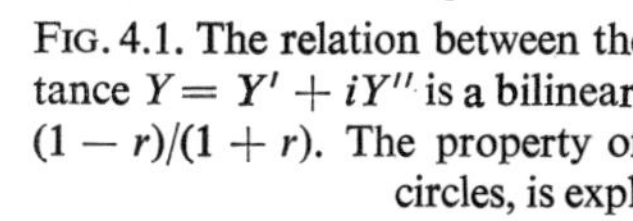

Centre part of main figure

FIG. 4.1. The relation between the reflection coefficient $r = \mathscr{R}^{i\varphi}$ and the admittance $Y = Y' + iY''$ is a bilinear transformation $r = (1 - Y)/(1 + Y)$ or $Y = (1 - r)/(1 + r)$. The property of such transformations, circles transform into circles, is explored in the Smith diagram.

a reference radius, respectively. On the other hand, each point also has two Y-coordinates, given by the curved lines $Y' =$ constant and $Y'' =$ constant, the circles for Y drawn on the diagram. To a given point $r_1 = R_1 e^{i\varphi_1}$, located in the diagram (an r-plane) at R_1 from the centre and on a radius vector which makes an angle φ_1 with the base line, corresponds a point $Y_1 = Y_1'. + iY_1''$ in the Y-plane, through the relation $Y_1 = (r_1 - 1)/(r_1 + 1)$. This point lies on the intersection of the straight line $Y' = Y_1'$ and the straight line $Y'' = Y_1''$ in the Y-plane. To this point corresponds, by eq. (5), the point r_1 in the r-plane situated on the intersection of the circle which corresponds to $Y'' = Y_1''$ and the circle which corresponds to $Y' = Y_1'$. On a Smith diagram each physical point (you can mark one with a pencil) has two sets of coordinates. One set, R and φ (its own coordinates in the plane), define a complex number $r = \mathscr{R}^{i\varphi}$ and another set (coordinates transposed from the Y-plane) given by the values Y' and Y'' of the circles drawn in it, that intersect at that point, define a complex number $Y = Y' + iY''$. For any point, the numbers r and Y are related by $r = (1 - Y)/(1 + Y)$.

In practice, $R \leqq 1$ so that a Smith diagram will be a circular map. Such a map, as commercially available, is reproduced in Fig. 4.2. A consequence of $R \leqq 1$ is that $Y' \geqq 0$. Indeed $Q_0^{-1}/Q_e^{-1} \geqq 0$.

We have drawn less lines in Fig. 4.1 in order to clarify the explanation. Around the point $Y = 0$ the Y-lines in the r-plane are not too distorted (see the detail in the figure). This may be helpful in order to remember what is positive and what is negative. They appear as in the rectangular diagram. In the upper half of the plane, Y'' is positive. The values of Y'' are labelled along the great circumference. The circles Y' = constant have their centres on the horizontal base line $\varphi = \pi$. The circles Y'' = constant have their centres on a line tangential to the great circle at $Y = 0$ (or $r = -)1$. The base line for r points towards $Y' = 0$, and thus to the left. φ is as usual measured anticlockwise. Hence $\mathscr{R}r > 0$ on the left and $\mathscr{I}r > 0$ on the lower half of the plane. In electronics, the relation between $Z = 1/Y$ and r is often used. Now

$$\frac{1 - Z}{1 + Z} = -r \tag{6}$$

so that we may use the same diagram putting Z for Y on the circles, and with the base line for r pointing to the right, toward $Z = \infty$ and φ pointing anticlockwise. We shall only use admittance diagrams.

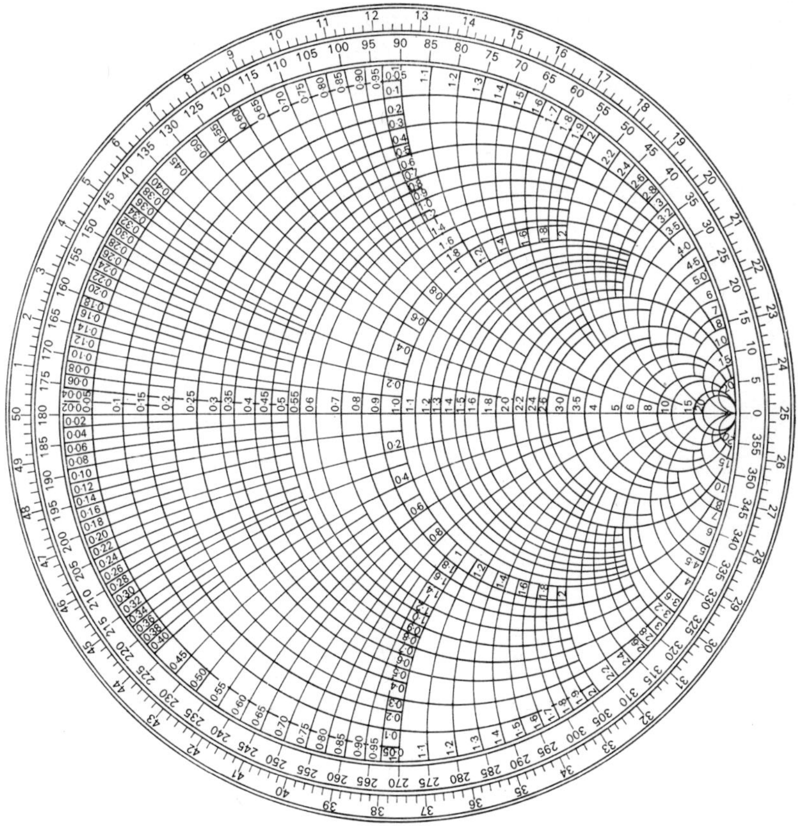

FIG. 4.2. A Smith diagram as it is available commercially.

(b) *The cavity in the Smith diagram*

A cavity with a certain eigendamping $1/Q_0$ and a certain eigenfrequency ω_a which is coupled to a waveguide through a certain external Q_e and excited at a frequency ω may be represented on a Smith diagram by a point, its admittance Y_0.

$$Y_0 = \frac{1/Q_0}{1/Q_e} + i\,\frac{2\,\dfrac{\omega - \omega_a}{\omega_a}}{1/Q_e}. \tag{7}$$

When the exciting frequency is changed, this point travels in the diagram along the circle $Y' = Y_0' = (1/Q_0/(1/Q_e)$, called "the locus of the cavity". The amplitude R of the reflection coefficient will pass through a minimum for $\omega = \omega_a$ or $Y'' = 0$ and this may be useful for determining experimentally the ω_a of a cavity. R passes through zero only if $1/Q_0 = 1/Q_e$. In this case, we say that the cavity is matched. No wave is reflected when $r = 0$. If the coupling of the cavity to the guide is different, one distinguishes between an overcoupled cavity, where

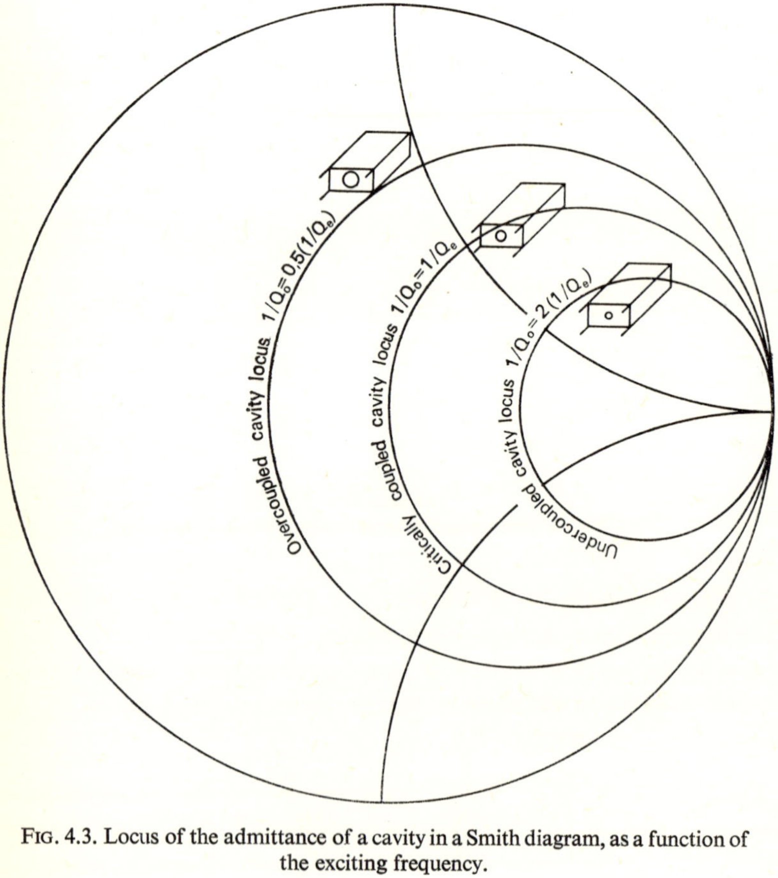

FIG. 4.3. Locus of the admittance of a cavity in a Smith diagram, as a function of the exciting frequency.

$1/Q_e > 1/Q_0$, and an undercoupled cavity, where $1/Q_e < 1/Q_0$. The situation is represented in Fig. 4.3.

For certain simple geometric configurations of coupling, one may calculate $1/Q_e$. A useful example is a waveguide terminated by a metallic cross wall and having an iris (a metallic cross wall with a hole at its centre) at one or two half wavelengths from the end. $1/Q_e$ may be computed as a function of the diameter of the hole. The diameter of the hole required for matching (i.e. $1/Q_0 = 1/Q_e$) depends on $1/Q_0$ and $1/Q_0$ may depend strongly on the temperature of a given cavity, since it depends on the conductivity of the wall. Therefore cavities are sometimes designed with variable coupling. It is not the diameter of the hole that is made variable. Such a "diaphragm" would introduce many losses and instabilities. There are other types of coupling; for example, one can introduce a metallic or dielectric pin in the hole or just before it.

(c) *E.s.r. in the Smith diagram*

Let us now study a cavity coupled to a waveguide and containing a paramagnetic sample inside. Let $\langle\chi\rangle = 0$ first. The cavity has a certain eigendamping $1/Q_0$ and an eigenfrequency ω_a. It may be operated at a frequency ω slightly different from ω_a. Then the impedance is

$$Y_0 = \frac{1/Q_0}{1/Q_e} + \frac{2i(\omega - \omega_a)/\omega_a}{1/Q_e}.$$

This is a certain point in the Smith diagram, Fig. 4.4. We have delimitated a region in this diagram where

$$0{\cdot}1 < \frac{1/Q_0}{1/Q_e} < 10 \quad \text{and} \quad \left|\frac{2(\omega' - \omega_0')/\omega_0'}{1/Q_e}\right| < 2. \qquad (8)$$

The point $Y_0 = 0{\cdot}5 + 0{\cdot}6i$ is marked. Now we vary the static magnetic field $B_s = B_0 + B_d(t)$ through resonance. Then $\langle\chi\rangle$ will change and Y will describe a curve in the diagram, as a function of the parameter

B_d, starting from Y_0 and finishing at Y_0. Let us consider the case when $\langle\chi\rangle$ has a Lorentzian shape:

$$\langle\chi\rangle = \frac{K_1}{B_d + i\delta} \quad \text{or} \quad -i\frac{\langle\chi\rangle}{1/Q_0} = \frac{\Delta Y}{Y_0'} = \frac{K}{\delta - iB_d}. \tag{9}$$

A property of bilinear transformations is that points that lie on a circle in one plane correspond to points that lie on a circle in the other plane; e.g. the circles $Y' =$ constant and $Y'' =$ constant; circles of infinite radius

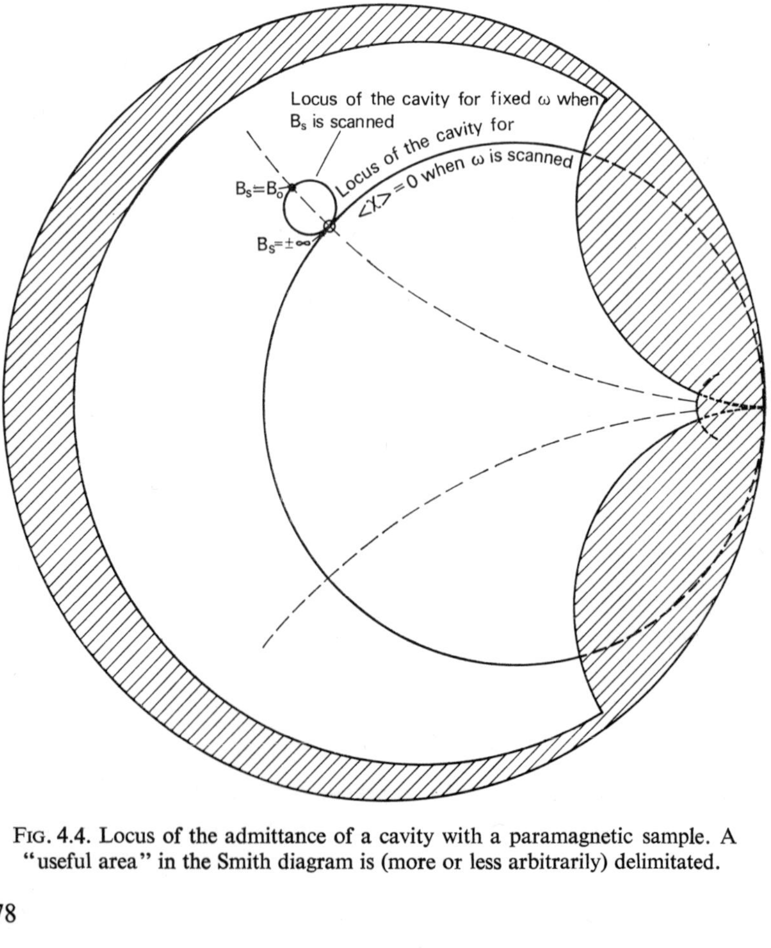

FIG. 4.4. Locus of the admittance of a cavity with a paramagnetic sample. A "useful area" in the Smith diagram is (more or less arbitrarily) delimitated.

in the Y-plane correspond to circles in the r-plane. We may eliminate B_d from

$$\Delta Y' = \frac{Y_0' K\delta}{B_d^2 + \delta^2} \quad \text{and} \quad \Delta Y'' = \frac{Y_0' K B_d}{B_d^2 + \delta^2}$$

and verify directly that the points in the Y-plane lie on a circle. It follows that the corresponding points in the r-plane also lie on a circle. A more elegant proof is to consider a Z-plane with the bilinear transformation

$$Z = 1/\Delta Y \quad \text{or} \quad \frac{1}{Z} = Y - Y_0. \tag{10}$$

Since the points for each B_d lie on a straight line or a circle with infinite radius in the Z-plane, $Z = (\delta - iB_d)/KY_0'$, they lie on a circle in the Y-plane and hence in the r-plane.

We may easily draw this circle for the Lorentzian line in the diagram. It lies between the $Y' = Y_0'$ circle and the

$$Y' = Y_0' + \frac{\langle\chi\rangle''_{max}}{1/Q_e}$$

circle since $\langle\chi\rangle''_{max} \geqq \langle\chi\rangle'' \geqq 0$. Also, it is tangential to these circles at $Y'' = Y_0''$ since for $Y'' = Y_0''(B_d = \pm\infty$ and $B_d = 0)$ we have $\partial Y_m'/\partial B_d = 0$. Such a circle is drawn in Fig. 4.4. If $\langle\chi\rangle$ (B_d) is not a Lorentzian curve, the locus in the Smith diagram may no longer be a circle but it will still be a closed curve, lying between $Y' = Y_0'$ and

$$Y' = Y_0' + \frac{\langle\chi\rangle''_{max}}{1/Q_e},$$

tangential to $Y' = Y_0'$ at $Y'' = Y_0''$ in any case, and to

$$Y' = Y_0' + \frac{\langle\chi\rangle''_{max}}{1/Q_e}$$

at $Y'' = Y_0''$ if the line is symmetric. For our further discussion, we shall use a circle for the locus of $\langle\chi\rangle$ because it is easier to deal with. The considerations, however, are valid for any practical resonance line. The circle is described while the static field is scanned.

4.3. Microwave circuit elements

(a) *Traffic regulating components*

Before dealing with spectrometer systems, we must say something about microwave components. Until now, we have dealt extensively with a cavity and a waveguide coupled to this cavity. Of course we need more than this in order to make a microwave measurement. We need a microwave source, a device that generates microwave energy flux into a waveguide. We need a detector, a device that transforms the microwave flux into a quantity accessible to further analysis. (We cannot see or hear the microwave energy flux.) And we need devices that regulate the traffic of microwave flux. All these components joined together form a microwave circuit. The source and the detector will be discussed separately below. We first deal with traffic regulating components.

A very simple spectrometer is drawn in Fig. 4.5 (a). The *circulator* is a device that separates a forward wave from a backward wave in the guide which is connected to the cavity. Power which enters a circulator through one port is not reflected but transmitted entirely through the next port, i.e. from 1 to 2 or from 2 to 3 or from 3 to 1. (One can also have a four-port circulator.) A microwave power source, here a klystron, sends power by a travelling wave that goes to the cavity through the circulator, and the wave reflected from the cavity goes through the circulator to the detector.

Instead of a circulator we could also use a *magic tee*. The scheme would be as in Fig. 4.5 (b). A magic tee is a passive junction of waveguides with such a symmetry that a wave which enters a branch is divided in two equal parts, going into the adjacent branches. No power goes into the opposite branch; for example, power in branch 3 is divided between branches 1 and 2. Power in 2 goes out through 3 and 4. Moreover, the phase relation is such that if a wave in branch 3 is the sum of waves from 1 and 2 then the wave in branch 4 will be their difference.

In the scheme we have put a *matched load* on arm 1, i.e. a termination with zero reflection. All the power incident on it is absorbed. With the magic tee the klystron must deliver twice as much power in order

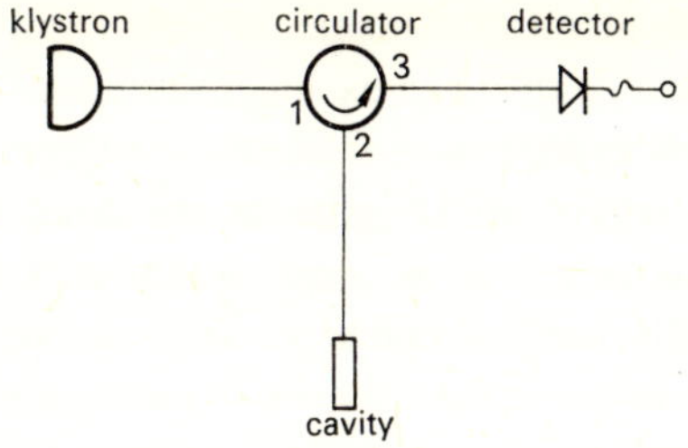

(a)

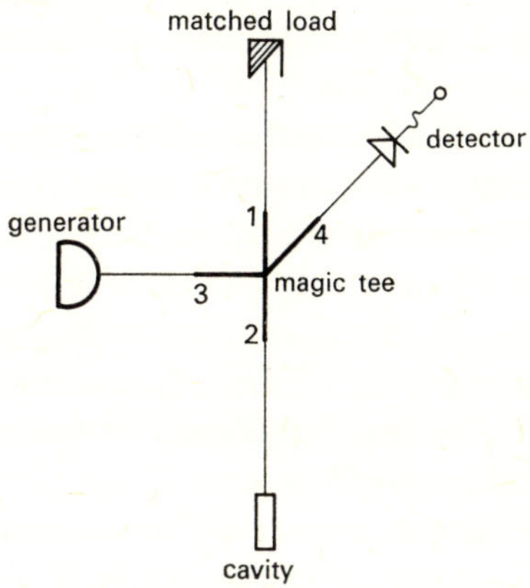

(b)

FIG. 4.5. Simple spectrometer scheme with circulator (a) and with magic tee (b).

to have the same power incident on the cavity. And the power from the cavity, with the information, is again divided by two, throwing away half of the signal power.

In general, components such as a circulator, magic tee or matched load that regulate the flow of travelling waves will not cause major problems in a spectrometer. Of course they are not ideal. For example, from the power that enters the circulator through port 1, about 5 per cent is lost in the device and about 1 per cent leaks through port 3. From the power that enters branch 3 of a magic tee only about 0·01 per cent goes through branch 4 directly. But as much as goes into the cavity goes into branch 1 and even a well-matched load still reflects about 0·01 per cent of this, half of which goes to the detector. Hence the performance of a circulator is not as good as that of a magic tee, but a circulator requires only half as much power from the klystron and does not waste signal power. In fact, the wave that leaks through from the klystron to the detector is no problem; it can be cancelled, for example, by a wave reflected from branch 1.†

In many cases one even ***needs*** power that did not "see" the cavity, in the detector, as we shall see. The important point is that such traffic-regulating devices are stable, i.e. have time-independent characteristics. For example, if they vibrate, they may cause difficulties. We call such difficulties "microphonics".

There are also other traffic-regulating devices, e.g. a simple divider, which separates a wave into two equal or unequal parts. A directional coupler may remove some percentage of a wave going from left to right, but not from a wave going from right to left (or vice versa).

Then, there are the attenuators and phase shifters, which change the complex amplitude of a wave by a fixed amount. Once again, the important point is that they should be fixed with time- and frequency-independent characteristics.

For further details about such components, we refer to the book by Poole (1967). In the following, we shall freely use circulators, magic tees, attenuators, phase shifters, dividers, etc., representing them as in Fig. 4.6. For example, we shall always separate a forward wave from a backward wave by a circulator, assumed perfect, although in practice a magic tee would be better, because of its better characteristics at the present state of technology. The numerical factor associated with a magic tee division will be taken to be exactly $1/2$ or $1/\sqrt{2}$, although in practice they are not exact and there is some leakage through forbidden ports.

† Another question is how well such a balance can be realized in practice. The frequency dependence and instability of such a balance are in fact a major limitation on the sensitivity in a classical super-heterodyne spectrometer.

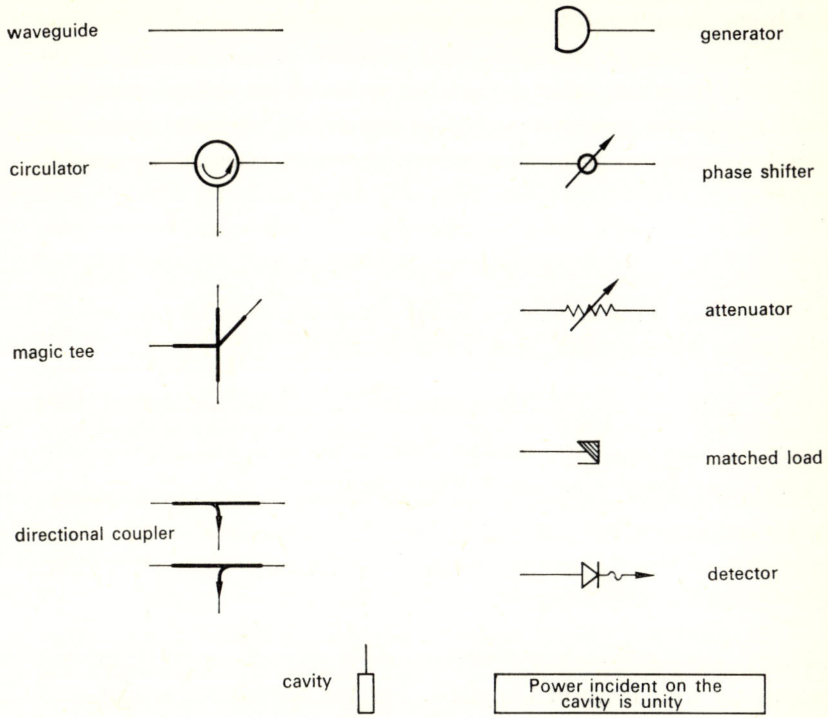

FIG. 4.6. Symbols for spectrometer schemes.

We shall also form a convention. The power incident on the cavity containing the sample is taken as a unit of power in all the spectrometer schemes. For example, in Fig. 4.5 (b) the klystron delivers slightly more than two units of power and the detector receives $|\frac{1}{2}r + \text{ a little bit}|^2$ power.

The power incident on the sample cavity is the unit of power.	Power unit convention. (11)

We must now deal with the source (e.g. a klystron) and with the detectors.

(b) *Microwave generator*

The most widely used microwave generator in spectroscopy is the klystron. There are other devices but we shall not discuss them. An ideal microwave generator would be a perfectly monochromatic and noiseless source of microwave power. It would generate a travelling wave

$$\mathcal{R} a_s \, e^{i\omega_1 t}, \tag{12}$$

the delivered power being $a_s a_s^*$, with a_s and ω_1 absolutely constant. However, this is impossible. (It would violate the basic laws of thermodynamics.) We may describe an actual source by

$$[a_s + a_n(t)] \, e^{i(\omega_s + \omega_n(t))t} \tag{13}$$

where $a_n(t)$ and $\omega_n(t)$ are random fluctuations of a and ω about their mean values a_s and ω_s. A mean value is defined as

$$a_s = \langle a \rangle = \lim_{\theta \to \infty} \frac{1}{\theta} \int_t^{t+\theta} a(t) \, dt \tag{14}$$

which is time-independent if the system is stationary. We shall deal extensively with noise in Chapter 4. For the present let us only give some definitions.

If the microwave circuit contains no frequency-dependent elements such as, for example, a cavity, then the wave incident on a detector will be proportional to a, say by a constant complex factor ϱ. The power will be

$$\varrho\varrho^*(a_s a_s^* + 2\,\mathcal{R}\, a_s^* a_n + a_n a_n^*) \tag{15}$$

and, since the mean of a_n is zero by definition, in the detector one has a certain noise power proportional to the mean power, in the ratio of $a_n a_n^*/a_s a_s^*$. This noise power will, of course, be distributed over a certain frequency range. Within a given bandwidth $d\omega/2\pi$ we shall have a noise power $N_A(\omega) \,.\, d\omega/2$ times the mean overall power of the source:

$$N_A(\omega) = \frac{\partial(a_n a_n^*)/\partial(\omega/2\pi)}{a_s a_s^*}. \tag{16}$$

This is called the *amplitude modulation noise* or AM noise. The point here is that a_n is random so that it cannot be cancelled out by another wave. The product $2\mathscr{R}a_s^* a_n$ is always zero and cannot cancel out $a_n a_n^*$.

Now, suppose a detector receives a wave $r_d + \Delta r$, where Δr is the useful information. The circuitry following the detector must have a certain bandwidth, say from ω_1 to ω_2, in order to handle this information properly. The power delivered to the detector, within this bandwidth, will be

$$(r_d + \Delta r)(r_d^* + \Delta r^*)\left(1 + \int_{\omega_1}^{\omega_2} N_A(\omega)\, d\omega/2\pi\right). \tag{17}$$

[Remember our power unit convention, eq. (11).] The variations Δr will be observable if

$$2\mathscr{R}\, r_d^* \Delta r > R_d^2\left(\int_{\omega_1}^{\omega_2} N_A(\omega)\, d\omega/2\right), \tag{18}$$

where we have assumed $|\Delta r| \ll R_d$.

The random fluctuations in frequency, ω_n, are called *frequency modulation noise* or FM noise. They manifest themselves through a detected power variation only in as much as a frequency-dependent reflection is present in the microwave circuit. By such a reflection, FM noise is transformed into AM noise and hence detected. Since the transformation depends on the admittance of the reflecting device (such as, for example, a cavity) we cannot discuss it in general terms. We only define here a frequency noise parameter as

$$n_F(t) = 2\frac{\omega_n}{\omega_s} = 2\frac{\omega - \langle\omega\rangle}{\langle\omega\rangle}. \tag{19}$$

(We use a lower-case n for this parameter in order to emphasize that n_F is not defined in the same way as N_A.)

We close this discussion of the microwave generator with the observation that the generator noise, AM noise as well as FM noise, can in general be highly reduced by appropriate circuitry, as we shall discuss below. The noise problem is more serious for detectors.

(c) *Detectors*

We must finally convert the amplitude R of a travelling wave, or, better, variations in microwave power, into a more accessible quantity.

We may, for example, transform the microwave power into heat and then measure a temperature. This is done in a bolometer. We may also rectify the voltage produced by the microwave electric field, by a semiconducting crystal. This yields a d.c. current or a current which reproduces the AM modulation of the microwave amplitude. (It may also be a voltage. This is a matter of internal impedance.) Carr and Slobodnik (1967) describe a piezoelectric detector.

The sensitivity of a detector, the variation in output (e.g. current variation) per variation in input (microwave amplitude A), is often characterized by "square-law" and "linear". "Square law" means Δ(output) $\sim \Delta A^2$ while "linear" means Δ(output) $\sim \Delta A$. Any detector is square law in the limit of zero amplitude, but crystal diodes become linear above a certain power level. Of course, if the variation ΔA is small compared to the amplitude A of the microwave, then the output (current or voltage) will always be proportional to ΔA, even in the square law region, since $\Delta A^2 = 2A\,\Delta A$. The important point is that above a certain level (about 100 microwatts of incident power) the current variation (or voltage variation) per amplitude variation of the incident wave becomes constant. $\Delta I =$ constant $\times\ \Delta A$ and no longer does $\Delta I =$ constant . A . $\Delta A = \frac{1}{2}$ constant . ΔA^2, as for a lower power level. In other words, the sensitivity $\Delta I/\Delta A$ of the diode (for $\Delta A \ll A$) is proportional to A at low power levels and becomes constant, independent of A, at higher levels. For instance, in the homodyne detection to be discussed below, one has a wave $r_b + \Delta_r$ incident on the detector, where r_b is a bias wave with amplitude R_b that may be adjusted, and Δr is the signal, $|\Delta r| \ll R_b$. The power variation incident on the detector is proportional to $R_b|\Delta r|$ and, above a certain value of R_b, the output current variation per signal amplitude, ΔR, becomes independent of R_b.

We must observe that a specification $\Delta I/\Delta A$ is really not very significant since the usefulness of ΔI depends on the impedance from which it is drawn. We can indeed amplity a current arbitrarily, using a transformer. The important question is how much signal power (given by $2A\,\Delta A$) is necessary per unit available detected signal power (given, for example, by $RI\,\Delta I$, where R is a suitable impedance). This ratio is called the conversion loss. It happens to be constant (equal to about 3·5) for a crystal detector in the linear region and increases when the incident power is lowered into the square law region.

A discussion about crystal diodes and various other types of detectors is given by Poole (1967). For our purposes, it is important to be aware of the distinction between a linear law and square law, and to know that a crystal detector will reach its highest sensitivity in the linear region without further improvement when the bias is increased.

Any detector generates its own noise power. For example, in a bolometer the variations of the resistance due to heating by microwave power are measured, and an amount $kT\,d\omega/2\pi$ of noise power in a bandwidth $d\omega/2\pi$ is available from any resistor. This is thermal noise. Its frequency spectrum is flat up to very high frequencies. If this were the only noise, then a detector at the same temperature as the microwave system would reduce the sensitivity by a factor 2, compared to a noiseless detection (and noiseless amplifier).

Semiconductors always generate a lot of noise besides the thermal noise. This additional noise is called excess noise, and depends on bias current, on incident power and on frequency. In general a *bias current* can be applied at will for minimizing noise. The *incident power*, however, also determines the gain of the detector (or the conversion loss) and a compromise has to be made. We shall describe systems which permit such a free choice of the incident power in order to obtain the best compromise between gain and noise of the detector. The *frequency dependence* is given by (excess noise) $\sim 1/f$, and this noise is therefore sometimes called $(1/f)$-noise. For good crystals in practice, this $1/f$ noise is negligible (compared to thermal noise) above some megahertz. This is the reason for frequency conversion, to be discussed below.

4.4. Spectrometer for a noiseless microwave generator

(a) *Qualitative discussion of the simplest spectrometer*

A straightforward method for measuring $\langle\chi\rangle$ is to measure the power variations in the wave reflected from the cavity. We have already given a scheme for this in Fig. 4.5. We have also already stated that $\langle\chi\rangle/Q_0^{-1}$ is a constant of the problem. Q_0^{-1} is as low as we can achieve in accordance with the sample and magnet requirements and $\langle\chi\rangle$ is a given function of B_s, the maximum being as high as possible in accordance with the planned measurement. The impedance of the cavity is

$$Y = Y_0 + \frac{i\langle\chi\rangle}{Q_0^{-1}} Y_0' \tag{20}$$

and we may choose Y_0 for the best performance, i.e. we may choose a point in the Smith diagram at which we shall locate the cavity. Y_0' is defined by the coupling and Y_0'' by the shift between the actual frequency and eigenfrequency.

By convention one unit power flows toward the cavity and hence the power incident on the detector is R^2. We may, of course, still choose the number of watts the klystron or other microwave source delivers. But this variable will be of no importance in our present, rather idealized, discussion. We shall have to relate variations in R^2 to variations in Y. Since, even apart from extra generator noise, there is always a fixed amount (kT per unit bandwidth) of thermal noise power incident on the detector, we shall have the highest sensitivity for the highest ΔR^2, at least for an ideal detector. (In fact for an actual detector, the conversion loss is also higher for low incident power and becomes constant for higher values of power.)

Let us first see in a Smith diagram how AR^2 informs us about Y' and Y'', for various locations of the cavity. In Fig. 4.7 we have drawn various points, each with its e.s.r. circle. All the circles have a diameter of $0{\cdot}2Y_0'$, i.e. $\chi''_{max}/4Q_0^{-1} = |\Delta Y|_{max}/Y_0' = 0{\cdot}2$. For a damping $Q_0^{-1} = 1/3000$ this means that we assume $\langle\chi\rangle''_{max} = 1/15{,}000$, a rather high but not impossible value. It corresponds to 20 mg DPPH at room temperature in the centre of a cavity made of one wavelength of a RG 52/U waveguide. In practice the circles are at least ten times smaller. We have drawn our e.s.r. circles of that size for clarity of the drawing, and also for showing the non-linearity of many measurements. However, we shall frequently use a first-order approximation, assuming the circles small.

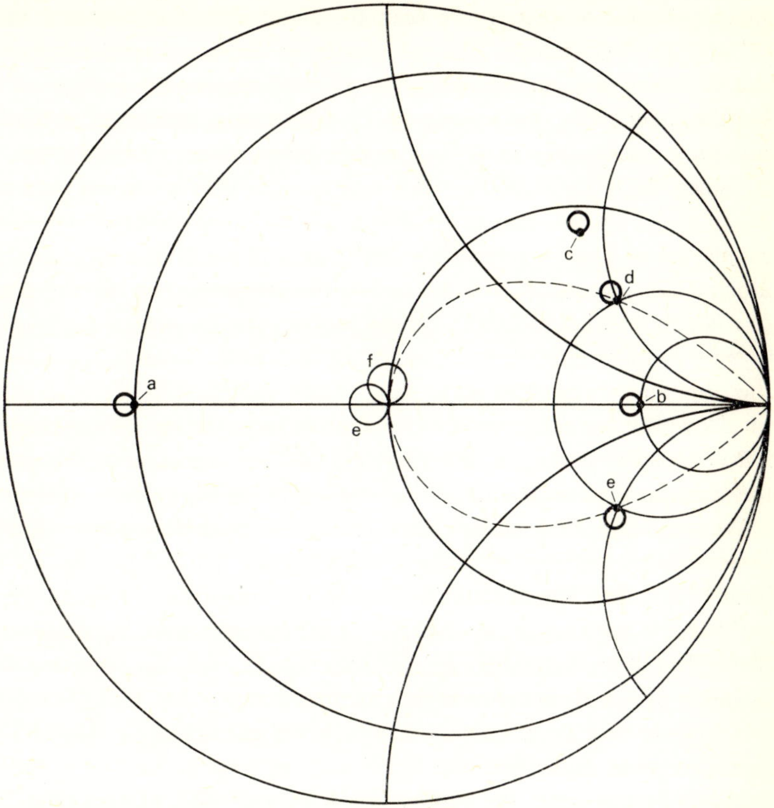

FIG. 4.7. Analysis of the spectrometer of Fig. 4.5 for different cavity admittances.

During the scanning of the field, the cavity locus travels along its e.s.r. circle. It starts (for $B_s = -\infty$) from the point Y_0, i.e. the point where the circle is tangential to the ($Y' =$ constant) circle of higher value and turns around, reaching the point opposite to Y_0, i.e. $Y_0 - |\Delta Y'|_{max}$ at resonance. It continues to travel around as B_s goes to ∞, arriving again at Y_0, the starting point. Meanwhile, we look for the changes in the length of the radius vector or better, for $R^2 = 2R\,\Delta R$.

Let us first look at circle *a*, not too close to $r = 0$. $Y_0 = 0{\cdot}2 + 0i$. The cavity is overcoupled and operated at its eigenfrequency, at least in the absence of e.s.r. If we scan the static field, the values of both Y' and Y'' will change. But the change in Y'' is perpendicular to a radius vector of r. So the change in Y'' will produce little effect on R. On the other hand, the change in Y' will cause a change in R. For a big circle, the change in R^2 will not be proportional to the change in Y', since the Y' scale on the axis $r = R$ (or $\varphi = 0$) is not linear, and the effect of Y'' on the change in R will also be a disturbance, since the radius vector does not remain normal to a ($Y' =$ constant) circle [or along a ($Y'' =$ constant) circle] during the scanning. The radius vector of r is only parallel to a ($Y'' =$ constant) line for $Y'' = 0$.

Now consider circle b at $Y_0 = 5 + 0i$. It is at the same distance from the origin as circle a and is the same size.† The effect of $\Delta Y'$ and $\Delta Y''$ on ΔR will be the same as for circle a, apart from the sign. If for circle b $\Delta R = \text{constant} \times \Delta Y'$, then for circle a, $\Delta R = -\text{constant} \times \Delta Y'$ with the same positive constant.

We may now take an arbitrary circle, for example circle c, at the same distance from $r = 0$ as a and b. It is clear that ΔR will be due to both Y' and Y''. The experimental result is a mixture of $\langle\chi\rangle'$ and $\langle\chi\rangle''$ and hence is not useful. However, if the line is Lorentzian, the maximum ΔR will still correspond to $\langle\chi\rangle''_{max}$ or to $\langle\chi\rangle'_{max} - \langle\chi\rangle'_{min}$ because the diameter of a circle is the same in any direction.

Are there any e.s.r. circles on which we can measure only $\Delta Y''$? Can we choose Y_0 so that $\Delta R \sim Y''$ only, at least in the first approximation? In this case, the radius vector of r should be tangential at Y_0 to a (constant-Y') circle just as the radius vector at $Y_0 = 0{\cdot}2$ (circle a) is tangential to the ($Y'' = 0$) circle. In this way, ΔR is independent of $\Delta Y'$. Turning a radius vector (e.g. a rule or a thin straight wire) around the Smith diagram one can easily see that we must necessarily use an undercoupled cavity. For each (constant-Y') circle with $Y' > 1$ we have two points where a radius vector is tangential, one point for $Y'' > 0$ (upper half plane) and one for $Y'' < 0$ (lower half plane).

† Circle b is slightly smaller than circle a, but another circle, also tangential to $Y'_0 = 5$ but on the other side of the ($Y' = 5$) line and also with diameter $0{\cdot}2Y_0$, would be bigger than circle a. Only infinitely small circles in $Y_0 = 0{\cdot}2$ and $Y_0 = 5$ with the same $(\Delta Y')_{max}/Y'_0$ ratio are equal. Our scale is not linear.

As an example, we have given in Fig. 4.7 the points $(2{\cdot}6 + 2{\cdot}5i)$ and $(2{\cdot}6 - 2{\cdot}5i)$ with circles *d* and *e*. They are both at the same distance from the origin as circles *a* and *b* ($R = 2/3$) and also happen to be of the same size as the circles *a* and *b*. We can draw a curve through such points, as shown (the curve is given by $Y^2 = Y''^2 + 1$). For each point of this curve, Y_0 is such so that $\Delta R \sim \Delta Y''$ only, just as for each point of the line $Y'' = 0$ we have $\Delta R \sim \Delta Y'$ only. However, *R* is parallel to $(Y'' = 0)$ but not to the curve for $\Delta R \sim \Delta Y''$ only. For $Y' < 1$ the origin of *r* lies inside the (Y' = constant) circle and there are no points where the radius vector is tangential. In this case, there are no points Y_0 for which $\Delta R \sim \Delta Y''$ only.†

Let us now come closer to the origin, along $Y'' = 0$ or along the line for $\Delta R \sim \Delta Y''$. The circles become larger. In fact, their size is proportional to $(1 - R^2)$. This will make the measurement more sensitive.

(For small signals we do not measure ΔR but ΔR^2 or $2R\Delta R$ and therefore the sensitivity is also zero at $R = 0$. The sensitivity for ΔR^2 is maximum somewhere between $R = 0$ and $R = 1$; it happens to be at $R^2 = \frac{1}{3}$. But there will be other tricks in order to overcome the difficulty and still measure on the large circle in $r = 0$. We shall discuss this below.)

A problem arises, however. For example, consider a circle with its centre at $r = 0$ ($Y_0 \neq 0$!). The circle is *not* drawn in the figure. For such an e.s.r. circle R = constant during the scanning and we measure neither $\Delta Y'$ nor $\Delta Y''$. They cancel each other out exactly. And Y_0 is

† Our diagram would perhaps be better if the circles on the $(\Delta R \sim \Delta Y'')$ curve had their centres on the curve, as the circles on the $(\Delta R \sim \Delta Y')$ line have. Or at least the circles for $(\Delta R \sim \Delta Y'')$ should have their nearest-to-origin points on the curve, and not Y_0. Then the circle (Y' = constant) that crosses the e.s.r. circle would deviate on both sides from being exactly tangential to the radius vector, just like the line (Y'' = constant) deviates on both sides from being tangential to the radius vector, for the $(\Delta R \sim \Delta Y')$ circles. Scanning the field from the point nearest to the origin through Y_0 and so forth around the circle, corresponds to scanning from the field where $\langle\chi\rangle'$ is maximum to $B = +\infty$ (Y_0) and again from $B_s = -\infty$ to the minimum of $\langle\chi\rangle'$ and then, through resonance, to $\langle\chi_{max}\rangle'$ again. In this circle Y'' or $\langle\chi\rangle'$ rises and falls only once, just as $\langle\chi\rangle''$ does in a cycle on circle *a* starting at *Y*. We shall not change our diagram, but bear this fact in mind. For small circles the difference is unimportant.

on the ($\Delta R \sim \Delta Y'$) line! But the circle is also on the ($\Delta R \sim \Delta Y''$) line. Remember that we said that Y'' causes a slight disturbance in the measurement of $\Delta Y'$ on circle a, because Y'' does not remain zero during the scanning. Here we see this effect in its most striking form. Of course, the problem will still be serious, e.g. for the circle with $Y_0 = 1$, circle e, or for circle f.

We may, by some techniques to be dealt with below, maintain $Y'' = 0$ during the scanning. By some feedback system one continuously changes the frequency, so that $2i[(\omega - \omega_a)/(\omega_a + \langle\chi\rangle')]$ remains zero. In this case one only measures $\Delta Y'$ or $\langle\chi\rangle''$. Now ΔR is independent of $\langle\chi\rangle'$. Remember, however, that ΔR is not exactly linear in ΔY, and, of course, for the circle centred at $r = 0$ the product $R\Delta R$, even with $Y'' =$ constant, is not at all proportional to $\Delta Y'$. The relation between $\Delta Y'$ and $R\Delta R$ changes not only in magnitude but even in sign when the e.s.r. circle is scanned.

(b) *Quantitative discussion*

(i) *General equation.* Let us now deal with this simple scheme in a more quantitative manner.

The wave incident on the detector is $r_0 + \Delta r$ and the power is

$$P_{\text{det}} = (r_0 + \Delta r)(r_0^* + \Delta r^*) = R_0^2 + 2\,\mathscr{R}\, r_0^*\,\Delta r + |\Delta r|^2. \tag{21}$$

We may neglect $|\Delta r|^2$ compared with the second term on the R.H.S. and hence the increment of P_{det} is

$$\Delta P_{\text{det}} \approx 2\,\mathscr{R}\, r_0^*\,\Delta r = 2R_0\,\mathscr{R}\, e^{-i\varphi}\,\Delta r. \tag{22}$$

Let us now express Δr as a function of ΔY. We shall use $\Delta Y/Y_0'$, in fact, since this is a constant in our problem of optimization. We have $|\Delta Y| \ll Y_0'$ and we assume $\Delta r \ll r$. Therefore we use differentials and drop the subscript 0. Starting from $r = (1 - Y)/(1 + Y)$ one gets

$$dr = -\frac{1}{2}(1 + r)^2\, dY = -\frac{1}{2}\, Y'\, |(1 + r)^2|\, e^{2i\varphi_{1+r}}\, \frac{dY}{Y'}. \tag{23}$$

We denote the phase of $(1 + r)$ by φ_{1+r}. A simplification is still possible:

$$|(1 + r)^2|\, Y' = (1 + r)(1 + r^*)\,\mathscr{R}\left(\frac{1 - r}{1 + r}\right)$$
$$= \mathscr{R}\,(1 - r)(1 + r^*) = 1 - R^2. \tag{24}$$

Hence

$$dr = -\frac{1}{2}(1 - R^2)\, e^{2i\varphi_{1+r}}\, \frac{dY}{Y'}. \tag{25}$$

Now we write ΔP_{det} [eq. (22)] as

$$dP_{\text{det}} = 2R\,\mathscr{R}\, e^{-i\varphi}\, dr = -R(1 - R^2)\,\mathscr{R}\, e^{i(2\varphi_{1+r}-\varphi)}\,\frac{dY}{Y'}. \tag{26}$$

The factor $R\,(1 - R^2)$ determines the sensitivity, independently of the rest of the expression, and the exponential defines the selectivity between $\langle\chi\rangle'$ and $\langle\chi\rangle''$, independently of the sensitivity. We shall first discuss the sensitivity.

(ii) *Sensitivity*. The sensitivity is given by the factor $R(1 - R^2)$ which relates the amplitude of the measured parameter ΔP_{det} to the quantity to be measured. This function is plotted in Fig. 4.8.

Observe that the sensitivity is the same for overcoupled and under-coupled cavities. The maximum occurs at $R_0^2 = \frac{1}{3}$, being $(1 - \frac{1}{3})/\sqrt{3} = 0{\cdot}385$.

This is the sensitivity for an ideal detector. It happens, however, that the gain and the conversion loss of a detector crystal depend on the

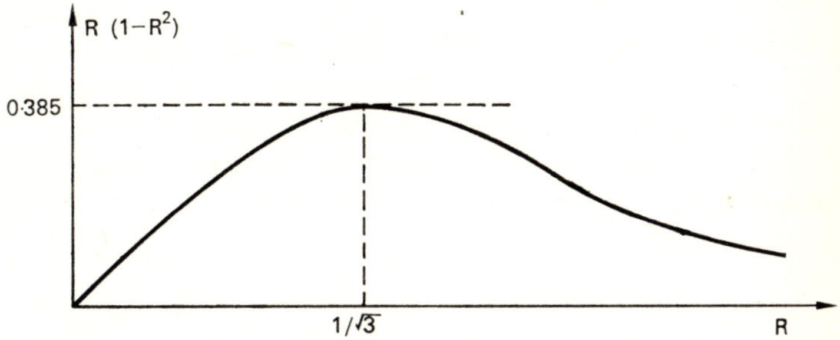

FIG. 4.8. The function $R(1 - R^2)$ has a broad maximum at $R^2 = \frac{1}{3}$.

incident power, i.e. on R^2. Actually the conversion loss becomes high when $R^2 \to 0$, and constant for $R^2 \to \infty$, so that, for suitable klystron power, the best coupling of the cavity is such that $R_0^2 = \frac{1}{3}$. The value is not critical, however, as can be seen from the graph.

The factor 0·385 may be considered as a certain loss in gain. Indeed we should prefer to measure on a large circle where ΔR is larger, i.e. for $R \to 0$. But since we only measure $2R\Delta R$, the result vanishes. We shall see below that it is possible to measure on a large circle, and still get an R, a new one, in $2R\Delta R$ that does not vanish. It is the homodyne system, important not only for obtaining greater sensitivity (by half an order of magnitude), but principally because it permits the choice of the total power incident on the crystal for the best crystal performance, without loss in ΔR. But first we have to deal with the selectivity of our actual system.

(iii) *Selectivity*. In Fig. 4.9 (lower half plane) we have drawn the angles φ_{1+r} and φ together with an auxiliary angle α for an arbitrary point. Observe that $\varphi = \varphi_{1+r} + \alpha$. Let us define

$$\psi = 2\varphi_{1+r} - \varphi = \varphi_{1+r} - \alpha. \tag{27}$$

Now the power increment may be written as

$$dP_{\text{det}} = -R(1 - R^2)\left|\frac{dY'}{Y'}\cos\psi + \frac{dY''}{Y'}\sin\psi\right|. \tag{28}$$

For $\sin\psi = 0$, we measure

$$\frac{dY'}{Y'} = \frac{\langle\chi''\rangle}{Q_0^{-1}}, \quad \text{i.e. } \textit{the absorption.}$$

This occurs only for $\psi = 0$ and $\psi = \pm\pi$. We distinguish three cases: $\varphi = \varphi_{1+r} = 0$; $\varphi_{1+r} = 0, \varphi = \pi$; $\varphi_{1+r} = \alpha = \varphi/2 \neq 0$. The third possibility is realized for points on the circumference of the Smith chart. However, the sensitivity is zero at these points. The other two possibilities are points on the $Y'' = 0$ line. For these

$$dP_{\text{det}} = -R(1 - R^2)\left(\frac{\pm dY'}{Y'}\right) = -R(1 - R^2)\left(\frac{\pm\langle\chi''\rangle}{Q_0^{-1}}\right), \tag{29}$$

the $\pm$ being the sign of $r = \pm R$.

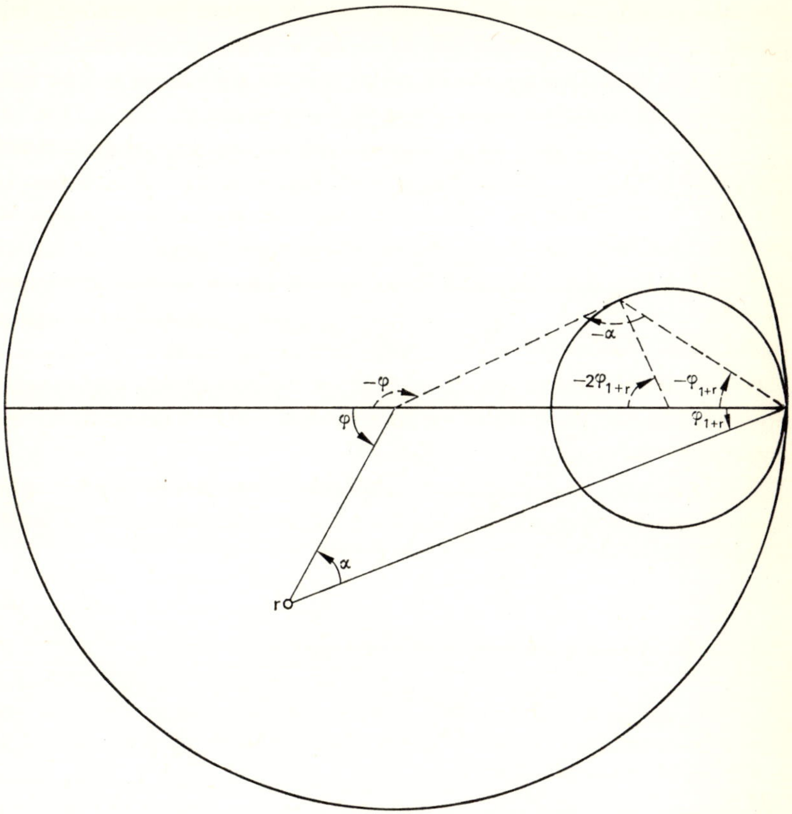

FIG. 4.9. The angle $\psi = \varphi_{1+r} + \alpha = 2\varphi_{1+r} - \varphi$ determines the selectivity. For $\psi = n\pi$, we measure absorption. For $\psi = (2n+1)\,\pi/2$, we measure dispersion.

For $\cos\psi = 0$ we measure

$$\frac{dY''}{Y'} = \frac{\langle\chi'\rangle}{Q_0^{-1}}, \quad \text{i.e. } \textit{the dispersion.}$$

This occurs for $\psi = \pm\pi/2$ or $\psi = \pm 3\pi/2$. We have drawn the angle $2\varphi_{1+r}$ for such a point in Fig. 4.9 (upper half plane).

It is the angle between the radius of the circle to which the vector r is a tangent and the base line $Y'' = 0$. This is, in fact, twice the angle

φ_{1+r} between the radius vector of $1 + r$ and the line $Y'' = 0$. (This angle has its vertex diplaced from $r = 0$ to $r = -1$.)

Now it is clear that $2\varphi_{1+r} - \varphi = \pi/2$ for the points r above the base line ($Y'' > 0$), for which the radius vector is tangential in r to the (Y' = constant) circle For these points, $\sin\varphi = \sin(\pi/2) = 1$. There is a similar collection of points under the base line ($Y'' < 0$) for which $\varphi - 2\varphi_{1+r} = \pi/2$ or $\sin\psi = \sin(-\pi/2) = -1$. For all these points,

$$dP_{\text{det}} = -R(1 - R^2)\left(\frac{\pm dY''}{Y'}\right) = -R(1 - R^2)\left(\frac{\pm\langle\chi\rangle'}{Q_0^{-1}}\right) \tag{30}$$

the $\pm$ being the sign of Y'', $+$ for the upper half plane.

It is clear that only an undercoupled cavity can be tuned to the pure dispersion mode (to "tune" means to select Y''). The points of the dispersion mode make a curve given by

$$Y'^2 = 1 + Y''^2. \tag{31}$$

This is illustrated in Fig. 4.7 (dashed curve). We require $\mathscr{R}\, e^{i(2\varphi_{1+r}-\varphi)} = 0$, or

$$\mathscr{R}\,\frac{(1 + r)^2/|1 + r^*|^2}{r/R} = 0 \tag{32}$$

or $\mathscr{R}(1 + r)^2/r = 0$. Substituting $r = (1 - Y)/(1 + Y)$ we find $\mathscr{R}\, 1/(1 - Y^2) = 0$ or $1 - Y'^2 + Y''^2 = 0$.

(iv) *Cross influence*, A point that must be discussed now is how a change in Y' may perturb a $\Delta Y''$ measurement and vice versa. The power variation incident on the detector is

$$dP_{\text{det}} = -R(1 - R^2)\left(\frac{dY'}{Y'}\cos\psi + \frac{dY''}{Y'}\sin\psi\right). \tag{33}$$

In a dY' measurement, one may in practice have some small departures from $\sin\psi = 0$. Then

$$dP_{\text{det}} = -R(1 - R^2)\left(\frac{dY'}{Y'} + \frac{dY''}{Y'}\sin\psi\right)$$

$$\cong -R(1 - R^2)\left(\frac{dY'}{Y'} \pm \Delta\psi\,\frac{dY''}{Y'}\right) \tag{34}$$

(absorption).

And for the dispersion measurement, we have in the same way

$$dP_{\text{det}} = -R(1-R^2)\left(\frac{dY''}{Y'} + \frac{dY'}{Y'}\cos\psi\right)$$

$$= -R(1-R^2)\left(\frac{dY''}{Y'} \pm \Delta\psi\frac{dY'}{Y'}\right) \quad (35)$$

(dispersion).

Various sources may contribute to a departure $\Delta\psi$ of ψ from zero or $\pm\pi$ or from $\pm\pi/2$ or $\pm 3\pi/2$. We shall no longer bother about the sign $\pm$ in eqs. (34) and (35). We analyse the perturbation

$$\Delta\psi(dY'/Y') \quad \text{on} \quad dY''/Y' \quad \text{and} \quad \Delta\psi(dY''/Y') \quad \text{on} \quad dY'/Y'.$$

This will simplify the treatment without loss of generality.

First of all, $\Delta\psi$ may have a constant component due to misalignment of the spectrometer. By "constant" we also mean with a slow drift, due, for example, to a drift in the properties of the components.

Another source of $\Delta\psi$ is noise, e.g. klystron frequency noise which changes Y'', or microphonics. Yet another source is the other component of $\langle\chi\rangle$. The measurement of $\langle\chi\rangle''$ or dY' may be perturbed by variations in φ due to $\langle\chi\rangle'$ and vice versa.

Let us first see in more detail what $\Delta\psi$ represents for *absorption* measurements. In this case $\varphi = 0, \pm\pi$. We use $d\psi$ instead of $\Delta\psi$ since $\Delta\psi \ll 1$. From Fig. 4.10 one sees that $d\varphi_{1+r} = dr''/(1+r')$ and $d\varphi = dr''/r'$. (We use $r \equiv r' + ir''$.) Hence

$$d\psi = 2d\varphi_{1+r} - d\varphi = \frac{r'-1}{r'(r'+1)}dr''. \quad (36)$$

But $r' \cong r$ and, by eq. (25),

$$dr'' = \mathscr{I}\,dr = -\frac{1}{2}(1-R^2)\mathscr{I}\,e^{2i\varphi_{1+r}}\frac{dY}{Y'} \cong -\frac{1}{2}(1-R^2)\frac{dY''}{Y'}. \quad (37)$$

Thus

$$d\psi = \frac{r-1}{r(r+1)}\left(-\frac{1}{2}\right)(1-r)(1+r)\frac{dY''}{Y'} = \frac{(1-r)^2}{2r}\frac{dY''}{Y'}. \quad (38)$$

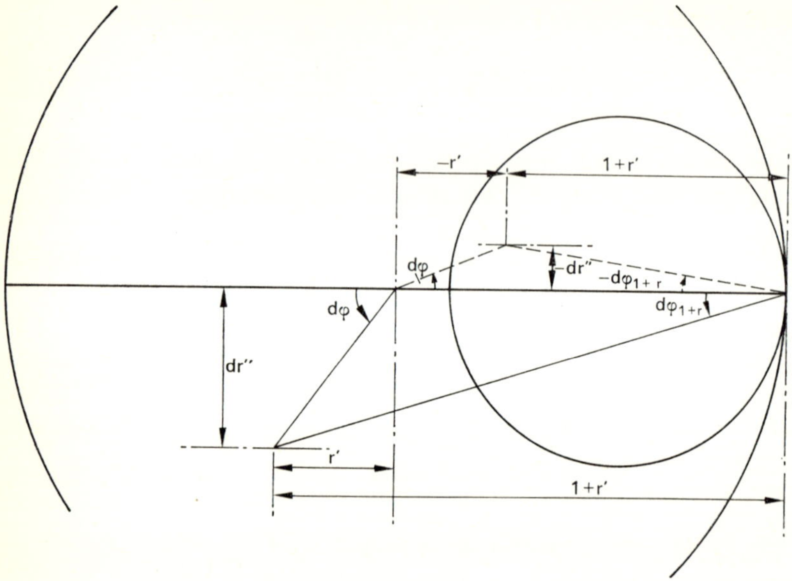

FIG. 4.10. For $\varphi \cong n\pi$, we have $d\varphi_{1+r} = dr''/(1 + r')$ and $d\varphi = dr''/r'$.

The correction is zero for $r = 1$. However, at this point the sensitivity is also zero. If $\Delta Y''$ is due only to the dispersion, we find for absorption measurements:

$$dP_{\text{det}} = \pm R_0(1 - R_0^2)\left[\frac{\langle\chi\rangle''}{Q_0^{-1}} \pm \frac{(1-r)^2}{2r}\left(\frac{\langle\chi\rangle'}{Q_0^{-1}}\right)^2\right]. \tag{39}$$

It is evident that one must not take r too close to zero. On the other hand, an overcoupled cavity is better than an undercoupled one. If there is a mismatch $\Delta Y''_{\text{error}}$ more important than this dispersion, then $\Delta\psi$ of eq. (34) is given by $[(1 - r)^2/2r]\,[\Delta Y''_{\text{error}}/Y']$ and P_{det} is proportional to

$$\frac{\langle\chi''\rangle}{Q_0^{-1}} + \frac{(1-r)^2}{2r}\,\frac{\Delta Y''_{\text{error}}}{Y'}\,\frac{\langle\chi'\rangle}{Q_0^{-1}}. \tag{40}$$

Observe that

$$\frac{\Delta Y''_{\text{error}}}{Y'} = \frac{2\,\dfrac{\omega' - \omega'_0}{\omega'_0}}{Q_0^{-1}} \tag{41}$$

is the frequency shift over the damping. If FM oscillator noise (n_F) is more important than $\langle\chi\rangle'$, then dP_{det} is proportional to

$$\frac{\langle\chi\rangle''}{Q_0^{-1}} + \frac{(1-r)^2}{2r}\left(\frac{n_F}{Q_0^{-1}}\right)^2 = \frac{1}{Q_0^{-1}}\left[\langle\chi\rangle'' + \frac{(1-r)^2}{2r}\,\frac{n_F^2}{Q_0^{-1}}\right]. \tag{42}$$

This explains why the frequency noise of the klystron may be a reason for *increasing* the damping of the sample cavity. A mismatch will, of course, enhance the effect of FM noise.

For *dispersion* measurements ($\psi = \pm\pi/2, \pm 3\pi/2$) the calculations are slightly more complicated. Also $d\psi$ now depends on Y' as well as on Y''.

We first derive a simple relation of complex calculus

$$r = \mathscr{R}\,e^{i\varphi} \rightarrow \frac{r}{r^*} = e^{2i\varphi} \rightarrow d2i\varphi = d\ln\frac{r}{r^*} = \frac{dr}{r} - \frac{dr^*}{r^*} = 2i\,\mathscr{I}\,\frac{dr}{r}.$$

Hence (43)

$$d\varphi = \mathscr{I}\,\frac{dr}{r}. \tag{44}$$

Of course, also

$$d\varphi_{1+r} = \mathscr{I}\,\frac{d(1+r)}{1+r} = \mathscr{I}\,\frac{dr}{1+r} \tag{45}$$

and hence

$$d\psi = d(2\psi_{1+r} - \psi) = \mathscr{I}\left(\frac{2}{1+r} - \frac{1}{r}\right)dr$$

$$= \mathscr{I}\,\frac{1}{r}\,\frac{r-1}{r+1}\,dr = -\mathscr{I}\,\frac{Y}{r}\,dr. \tag{46}$$

With eq. (25) for dr and with $\mathscr{R}\,e^{i\varphi}$ for r, one obtains

$$d\psi = +\frac{1}{2}\,\frac{(1-R^2)}{R}\,\mathscr{I}\,Y\,e^{2i(\varphi_{1+r}-\varphi)}\,\frac{dY}{Y'}$$

$$= \frac{1}{2}\,\frac{1-R^2}{R}\,\mathscr{I}\,e^{i(\psi-\pi)}\,Y\,\frac{dY}{Y'} = -\frac{1}{2}\,\mathscr{I}\,e^{i\psi}\,Y\,\frac{dY}{Y'}. \tag{47}$$

This holds in any case. For absorption $\psi = 0$ or $\psi = \pm\pi$ and one obtains eq. (38) after a few transformations. For dispersion
$\psi = \pm\pi/2$ or $\pm 3\pi/2$ and one gets

$$d\psi = \mp \frac{1}{2}\frac{1-R^2}{R}\left\{Y'\,\frac{dY'}{Y'} \mp Y''\,\frac{dY''}{Y'}\right\}. \tag{48}$$

Further calculus† makes it possible to reduce the expression to

$$d\psi = \pm\frac{(1+R^2)}{2R}\,\frac{dY'}{Y'} \pm \frac{dY''}{Y'}. \tag{49}$$

Comments analogous to those made in the case of absorption measurements can now be made. We leave this to the reader.

Let us only write the admixture of χ'' in a dispersion measurement

$$dP_{\text{det}} = -R(1-R^2)\left[\pm\frac{\chi'}{Q_0^{-1}} \pm \frac{(1+R^2)}{2R}\left\{\frac{\langle\chi''\rangle}{Q_0^{-1}}\right\}^2 \pm \frac{\langle\chi'\rangle\langle\chi''\rangle}{Q_0^{-2}}\right]. \tag{50}$$

(c) *Homodyne detection*

The method described above, measuring variations in the reflected power (ΔR^2), gives zero signal where the e.s.r. circle is greatest, i.e. at the origin ($R = 0$), because R is zero in $2R(\Delta R)$. We may, however, arrange things so that the R of $2R(\Delta R)$ is not zero and still have the ΔR corresponding to the greatest possible e.s.r. circle.

The trick is to combine a separate wave giving the "R" of $2R(\Delta R)$ with the wave reflected from the cavity that gives the "ΔR" of $2R(\Delta R)$. In Fig. 4.11 (b) we represent a scheme, together with the previous simplest spectrometer scheme [Fig. 4.11 (a)].

† One uses eq. (31), $Y'^2 = Y''^2 + 1$. Writing $R^2 = rr^*$ with $r = (1-Y)/(1+Y)$, one finds $R^2 = (Y'-1)/(Y'+1)$, or $Y' = (1+R^2)/(1-R^2)$. For Y'' one again uses $Y''^2 = Y'^2 - 1 = \{(Y'-1)/(Y'+1)\}/(Y'+1)^2 = R^2(1+Y')^2$. Hence $Y'' = \pm R(1+Y')$ and with the value just found for Y' this becomes $Y'' = \pm 2R/(1-R^2)$.

The klystron power is divided between a wave, with amplitude 1 (by definition), which goes into the cavity, and a "bias" wave with amplitude r_b. This amplitude r_b can be controlled in magnitude and phase

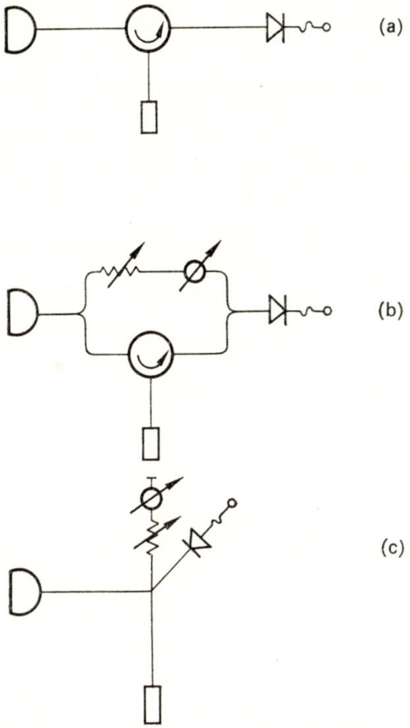

FIG. 4.11. A first improvement of the simplest spectrometer scheme (a) is shown in (b), homodyne scheme with circulator, and in (c), the homodyne scheme with magic tee.

by means of an attenuator and a phase shifter. This "bias" wave r_b and the wave r, reflected from the cavity, are added together, and form the wave $r + r_b$, which is detected. The power to be detected is

$$(r + r_b)(r^* + r_b^*).$$

Another system is shown in Fig. 4.11 (c), where a magic tee is used. The wave from the klystron is split into two equal parts. An attenuator and a phase shifter are placed in one arm. They change the wave twice, once as it enters and once after reflection at the end plate of the arm. (One could also simply use the movable end plate of the arm as a phase shifter.) If one requires $r_b > 1$, the attenuator is placed in the cavity arm. However, this also attenuates the useful signal, unless a special type of attenuator, a variable ferrite isolator, is used. This rather uncommon device attenuates only (and to a variable extent) the forward wave. Observe that some factors $\sqrt{2}$ have to be introduced here. We shall carry out our analysis for the system with a circulator. The equations can be readily adapted to the magic tee scheme.

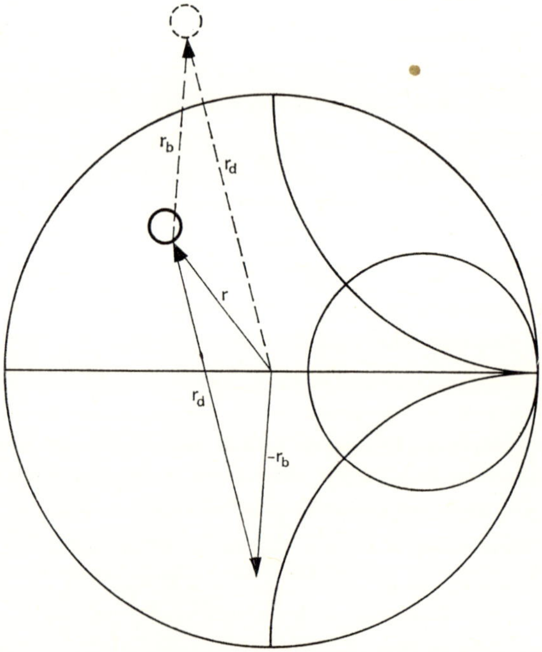

FIG. 4.12. A bias wave, r_f, is introduced in the spectrometer. We may displace the origin of the vector r_d, which represents the detected wave, over $-r_b$, instead of displacing the e.s.r. circle over $+r_b$.

We now have to make the choice of a supplementary variable. In principle the bias reflection r_b may have any value, even greater than 1. (We may divide the klystron power into unequal parts.)

We may introduce this new variable into the Smith diagram. Instead of moving our e.s.r. circles by r_b, we move the origin by $-r_b$. We choose the origin of the "detected radius vector", or the sum vector r_d, at $r = -r_b$. This involves the addition of complex numbers represented as vectors in the complex plane (see Fig. 4.12). The e.s.r. circle with its r and Y remains unchanged. The measured r_d, however, is to be computed from the origin $-r_b$ towards the e.s.r. circle. Now the variables of our spectrometer are the point Y_0 of the cavity and the "origin", $-r_b$, of the detected radius vector r_d. We measure increments in R_d or better in R_d^2 (denoted by ΔR_d^2), R_d being given by the distance from the new "origin" to the cavity-point on the e.s.r. circle. Of course, r_b is independent of field scanning.

What is now the effect of any choice of r_b? We again use the e.s.r. circles of Fig. 4.7, now drawn in Fig. 4.13. First look at circle *a*. With $r_b = 0$, we measure only $\langle\chi\rangle''$ as before. But with $r_b = e^{i0.252\pi}$, we only get $\langle\chi\rangle'$. So we can choose $-r_b$ for any circle in such a way that we measure $\langle\chi\rangle'$ or $\langle\chi\rangle''$. For example, for circle *c*, we measure $\langle\chi\rangle'$ with $(-r_b) = e^{-i0.062\pi}$ and $\langle\chi\rangle''$ with $(-r_b) = e^{i0.74\pi}$. In these examples we have chosen $R_b = 1$. We may indeed take, for the bias branch, a lossless guide with an end plate at a variable distance, so that $R_b = 1$, but the phase is variable. Now we may also measure with the e.s.r. circle at $r = 0$. This will give the most sensitive measurement. We simply take $(-r_b) = e^{\pm i\pi/2}$ for $\langle\chi\rangle'$ and $-r_b = \pm 1$ for $\langle\chi\rangle''$. The measurement by means of a bias from the same source and at the same frequency is called *homodyne* to be distinguished from *heterodyne* detection, which uses a bias at a different frequency, as we shall see later.

An interesting remark should be made. If we choose $r \approx 0$ and $r_b = \frac{1}{2} + 0i$, then the new origin of r_d will coincide with the centre of the circle $Y' = 1$. Consequently, any change in Y'' will have no influence on ΔR_d^2, not even in second-order terms. We already stressed such a fact, then only of academic interest, in eq. (38) ($r = 1$ in the simplest spectrometer).

Let us now introduce $r_b = \mathscr{R}\, e^{i\varphi_b}$ in our quantitative discussion. The wave incident on the detector is:

$$r_d = r_b + r_0 + \Delta r \equiv r_{d0} + \Delta r \tag{51}$$

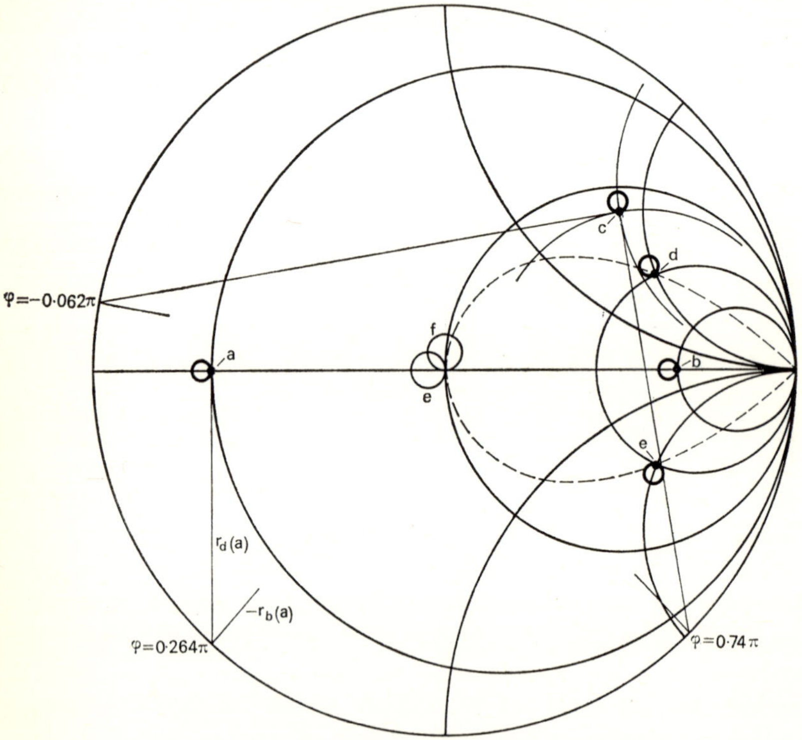

FIG. 4.13. The cavity admittances of Fig. 4.7 are now combined with a bias. In this way we can measure either $\langle\chi\rangle'$ or $\langle\chi\rangle''$ for any cavity admittance.

and the corresponding power

$$P_{\text{det}} = r_d r_d^* = R_{d0}^2 + 2R_{d0}\, \mathscr{R}\, e^{-i\varphi_d} \Delta r + |\Delta r|^2 \tag{52}$$

so that the power increment is, in the first approximation,

$$\Delta P_{\text{det}} = 2R_{d0}\, \mathscr{R}\, e^{-i\varphi_d}\, \Delta r. \tag{53}$$

We assume $|\Delta r| \ll R_{d_0} \cong R_d$ and use the expression of eq. (25) for Δr. We get

$$dP_{\text{det}} = -R_d(1 - R_0^2)\, \mathscr{R}\, e^{i(2\varphi_{1+r} - \varphi_d)} \frac{dY}{Y'}. \tag{54}$$

One now has maximum sensitivity for $R_0 = 0$. In this case, $\varphi_{1+r} = 0$ and $\varphi_d = \varphi_b$ and we have

$$dP_{\text{det}} = -R_d\left(\frac{dY'}{Y'}\cos\varphi_b - \frac{dY''}{Y'}\sin\varphi_b\right). \tag{55}$$

The situation is much simpler than in the other "simplest" spectrometer. This is because we restrict ourselves to the most sensitive condition, $r_0 = 0$.

The sensitivity is given by the factor R_d. We may choose it so as to have the best overall sensitivity, taking into account the dependence of the detector performance on R_d (or on R_d^2). In general, we shall not have to increase the bias power beyond a few tens of milliwatts.

As for the selectivity, one only has to choose the phase of r_b in order to detect $\langle\chi\rangle'$ or $\langle\chi\rangle''$. But let us analyse the cross-influences.

As in eq. (46), we find $\Delta\psi = 2\Delta\varphi_{1+r} - \Delta\varphi_b$ or

$$\begin{aligned} d\psi &= \mathscr{I}\left(\frac{2\,dr}{1+r} - \frac{dr_b}{r_b}\right) \\ &= \mathscr{I}\left[\frac{2}{1+r}\,\frac{\partial r}{\partial(r+r_b)} - \frac{1}{r_b}\,\frac{\partial r_b}{\partial(r+r_b)}\right] d(r+r_b). \end{aligned} \tag{56}$$

Variations in r and in r_b will be related to each other in the case of AM noise of the klystron power, and in the case of FM noise, if the bias arm has a frequency-dependent element similar to the cavity. But the effect of AM noise on r will be negligible compared its effect on $r + r_b$ since $R \ll R_b$, and if the bias arm is a broadband structure (not a cavity, for example) then frequency noise will have little effect on r_b' compared to its effect on r. Let us assume for the moment that dr and dr_b are independent. Then

$$d\psi = \mathscr{I}\left(\frac{2}{1+r} - \frac{1}{r_b}\right)d(r + r_b). \tag{57}$$

We choose $r \cong 0$. However, this does not mean $dr = 0$! We may only write

$$d\psi = \mathscr{I}\left(2 - \frac{1}{r_b}\right)d(r + r_b). \tag{58}$$

Let us first consider the absorption measurement. r_b is real and the only problem comes from the imaginary part of $d(r + r_b)$. Remember $(-r_b)$ is a point on the $Y'' = 0$ line.

An important remark first:

$$d\psi = \left(2 \pm \frac{1}{R_b}\right)\mathscr{I}\,d(r + r_b); \tag{59}$$

for $r_b = \frac{1}{2}$ the whole $d\psi$ vanishes! This may indeed be seen in Fig. 4.13. For $(-r_b)$ situated at $(-\frac{1}{2})$, the length of the vector $r + r_b$ is unaffected by changes in Y'' at constant $Y' = 1$. The point $r = -\frac{1}{2}$ is the centre of the circle $Y' = 1$. Let us now return to the more general case.

$\mathscr{I}(dr_b)$ may be due, for example, to microphonics which change the phase of r_b and hence introduce a component $\mathscr{I}(dr_b) \cong \pm d\varphi_b R_b$. The changes in $\mathscr{I}\,dr$ are more likely to occur. They may be due to FM noise and to the $\langle\chi\rangle'$ component. The analysis is similar to that of the "simplest" spectrometer, dealt with above. Let us just write the expression involving the influence of the $\langle\chi\rangle'$ component. $\mathscr{I}\,dr = -\Delta Y''$ and $Y' = 1$ at the origin, so that

$$d\psi = -\left(2 \pm \frac{1}{R_b}\right)\frac{dY''}{Y'} = -\left(2 \pm \frac{1}{R_b}\right)\frac{\langle\chi\rangle'}{Q_0^{-1}}. \tag{60}$$

The $\pm$ sign is the sign of $-r_b$. The effect on the measurement is given by

$$\Delta P_{\text{det}} = -r_d\left\{\frac{\langle\chi\rangle''}{Q_0^{-1}} + \left(2 - \frac{1}{r_b}\right)\frac{\langle\chi'\rangle^2}{Q_0^{-2}}\right\}. \tag{61}$$

Instead of $\langle\chi'\rangle^2$ one may put the FM noise, n_F^2, if this is important.

For the dispersion measurement, r_b is purely imaginary so that always $|2 - 1/r_b| \neq 0$. We consider only $\langle\chi\rangle''$ admixtures. So $r_b = \pm iR_b$ and the result is easily calculated:

$$\Delta\psi = -\mathscr{I}\left(2 \pm \frac{1}{R_b}\right)\left(\frac{\Delta Y'}{Y'} + i\frac{\Delta Y''}{Y'}\right)$$
$$= -\left(2\frac{\Delta Y''}{Y'} \pm \frac{1}{R_b}\frac{\Delta Y'}{Y'}\right) \tag{62}$$

and

$$\Delta P_{\text{det}} = R_d\left(\pm\frac{\langle\chi\rangle'}{Q_0^{-1}} \pm 2\frac{\langle\chi\rangle''\langle\chi\rangle'}{Q_0^{-2}} \pm \frac{1}{R_d}\frac{\langle\chi\rangle''^2}{Q_0^{-2}}\right). \tag{63}$$

Other cases of pertubation may be readily evaluated in the same manner.

4.5. Oscillator noise-suppression schemes

(a) *AM noise*

The useful signal power in the spectrometer described so far is a small change in the total power incident on the detector crystal.

$$P_{\text{det}} \cong |r_b + r_0|^2 + 2\mathscr{R}(r_b^* + r_0^*)\Delta r. \tag{64}$$

And P_{det}, practically equal to $|r_0|^2$ in the simplest scheme and to $|r_b|^2$ in the homodyne scheme, must be much greater than ΔP_{det}, because of the sensitivity requirements of the detector and because of linearity requirements. However, P_{det} is acompanied by a certain percentage of klystron noise, and the signal ΔP_{det} must be greater than this, in order to be observable. Hence this noise limits the sensitivity of the measurement. Fortunately we can reduce it in a considerable way by using appropriate microwave circuitry.

Let us first consider AM oscillator noise. Let the noise power relative to the mean power in the bandwidth of interest be given as

$$N = \int_{\omega_1}^{\omega_2} N_A(\omega)\, d\omega/2\pi. \tag{65}$$

Now

$$P_{\text{det}} = (1 + N)\,|r_b + r_0 + \Delta r|^2 \cong |r_b + r_0|^2 + N|r + r_0|^2 + 2\mathscr{R}(r^* + r_0^*)\,\Delta r. \tag{66}$$

We may, of course, neglect $N\Delta P_{\text{det}}$ before ΔP_{det} since $N \ll 1$.

The sensitivity is limited by

$$N|r_b + r_0|^2 < 2\mathscr{R}(r_b^* + r_0^*)\,\Delta r. \tag{67}$$

We have been able to reconcile a large Δr, i.e. $r \to 0$, with a high P_{det} by introducing the homodyne scheme. Can we reconcile the contradictory requirements of high power in the detector and low perturbation from klystron AM noise too? The answer is yes.

We cannot cancel the noise power on the detector, e.g. by a wave from the same source (and hence with the same noise fluctuations), because this would cancel the total bias power. But we may cancel this power after detection, by a signal from the same source that has also been detected. After detection, we no longer need the bias power. The important point is that this can be done without cancelling the signal. Let us propose a system. Its heart is the *balanced detector*. In our example we use a magic tee (Fig. 4.14), a device described in § 4.3 (a). The wave from the cavity enters arm 1 and the bias wave arm 2. The power incident on the detector of arm 3 is

$$P_{\text{det 3}} = \tfrac{1}{2}(1 + N)\,|r_b + r_0 + \Delta r|^2 = \tfrac{1}{2}\{|r_b + r_0|^2 + NR_b^2 + NR_0^2 + 2[N\mathscr{R}\, r_b^* r_0 + \mathscr{R}(r_b^* + r_0^*)\,\Delta r]\} \tag{68a}$$

and on arm 4

$$P_{\text{det 4}} = \tfrac{1}{2}(1 + N)\,|r_b - r_0 - \Delta r_0|^2 = \tfrac{1}{2}\{|r_b - r_0|^2 + NR_b^2 + NR_0^2 - 2[N\mathscr{R}\, r_b^* r_0^* + \mathscr{R}(r_b^* + r_0^*)\,\Delta r]\}. \tag{68b}$$

The output signal of each detector may be written as $G_3\Delta P_{\text{det3}}$ and $G_4\Delta P_{\text{det4}}$ respectively, where G_3 and G_4 represent the gain of the conversion. We subtract the output signals and obtain a signal $S(t)$ given by

$$S(t) = \tfrac{1}{2}(G_3 - G_4)(1 + N)(R_b^2 + R_0^2) + (G_3 + G_4)[(1 + N)\mathscr{R}\, r_b^* r_0 + \mathscr{R}(r_b^* + r_0^*)\,\Delta r]. \tag{69}$$

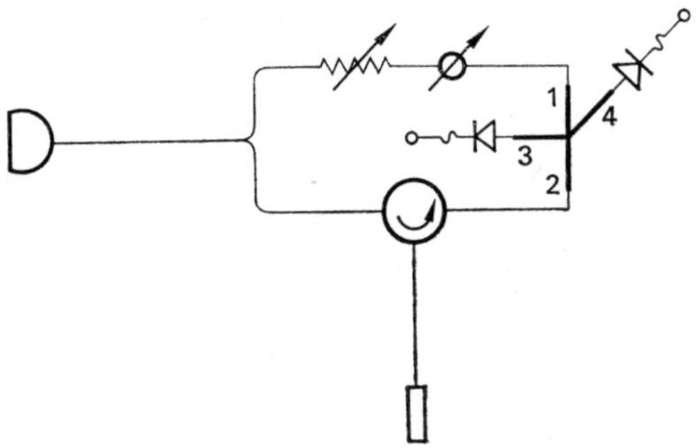

FIG. 4.14. A balanced detector is used to suppress AM **klystron** noise.

Taking $r_0 = 0$ and $G_3 = G_4 = G$ we obtain a signal free from klystron noise

$$S(t)_{\text{idealized}} = G[2\mathscr{R}\, r_b^* \,\Delta r] \tag{70}$$

just as for single homodyne detection with a noiseless klystron.

In practice one cannot obtain this result. The condition $G_3 = G_4$ can be realized fairly well by choosing a matched pair of detector crystals, and by attenuating one signal after detection and before subtraction. The major problem is the condition $r_0 = 0$. One must obtain $N|r_0| < |\Delta r|$ and for high power incident on the cavity it may be difficult to balance the microwave bridge to that extent. By microwave bridge we mean the device that separates the wave incident on the cavity from the reflected wave. In Fig. 4.14 we used a circulator, but for obtaining a low r_0 value, one must use a magic tee, so that the wave reflected from the cavity (due to $Q_e^{-1} + Q_0^{-1}$) can be cancelled out. Even with a magic tee, the ultimate sensitivity limit at high power incident on the cavity may still be due to $N|r_0| > |\Delta r|$ because of instabilities and principally because of the frequency dependence of such a bridge balance.

Some methods for eliminating r_0 have been presented in the literature. They have in common that the reflected wave r comes from a different output of the device that contains the sample. The coupling from input to output of this device is made through $\langle\chi\rangle$ itself, just as in Bloch's crossed coil arrangement for n.m.r. Such a device may be, for example, a bimodal cavity as used by Teaney, Klein and Portis (1961). A brief discussion is given by Poole (1967, p. 508). The junction spectrometer of Brodwin and Burgess (1963) is a similar solution. Dering (1964, p. 33) claimed that a correction should be made to their theory.

The "selective-transmission" technique (Lewis and Carver, 1964) is another possibility, applicable in some cases.

This is an opportunity we have to point out that other devices, different from a reflex cavity, may eventually be used for particular reasons. One may, for example, use a transmission cavity, with separate input and output connections but both coupled to the same mode of vibration of the electromagnetic field. Another device which could be employed is the helix. In any case, one has to deduce the relation between the susceptibility χ of the sample and the fluctuations of the output wave, Δr per unit input wave. The relation between the incident power and the HF field intensity at the sample may also be important; with these two relations at hand, one can apply the given theory to the device. For our reflection cavity the relation between Δr and χ is given by eq. (25) which, for a matched cavity ($Q_e^{-1} = Q_0^{-1}$), leads to

$$\Delta r = \frac{1}{2} \frac{\langle \chi \rangle}{Q_0^{-1}} \tag{71}$$

apart from a phase factor. The relation between $\langle \chi \rangle$ and χ, as well as the field intensity at the sample, depends on the particular field configuration.

(b) *FM noise*

Apart from AM noise, an oscillator will also have frequency fluctuations. We defined them by

$$n_F = 2 \frac{\omega - \langle \omega \rangle}{\langle \omega \rangle}. \tag{72}$$

They will be converted into detected power fluctuations if there is a frequency-dependent admittance. We see from eq. (1)

$$Y = Y_0 - i \frac{\langle \chi \rangle^*}{Q_e^{-1}} = \frac{Q_0^{-1}}{Q_e^{-1}} - i \frac{2 \dfrac{\omega - \omega_a}{\omega_a}}{Q_e^{-1}} + \frac{\langle \chi \rangle''}{Q_e^{-1}} - i \frac{\langle \chi \rangle'}{Q_e^{-1}}, \tag{73}$$

that any $\langle\chi\rangle'$ measurement will be limited in the discussed schemes by:

$$n_F < |\langle\chi\rangle'|_{\max}. \tag{74}$$

Indeed, no frequency-independent bias wave can cancel this effect of n_F. On the other hand, we have seen that in general a $\langle\chi\rangle''$ measurement suffers from a second-order perturbation in $\langle\chi\rangle'$ and hence from n_F [eq. (42)]. Of course, if $n_F \ll |\langle\chi\rangle'|_{\max}$, the perturbation on a $\langle\chi\rangle''$ measurement will be negligible. But for $n_F > |\langle\chi\rangle'|_{\max}$, when a dispersion measurement is in any case impossible with the discussed schemes, one may still expect to measure $\langle\chi\rangle''$ and one will be limited here by n_F. A particular type of FM noise, slow frequency drift, may limit the sensitivity because it causes a $\Delta Y''_{\text{error}}$ [eq. (40); consider $\langle\chi\rangle'$ substituted by n_F].

We must also mention the random fluctuations in eigenfrequency of the sample cavity. This is a type of FM noise too. It will have the same effect as FM oscillator noise, as is readily seen from eq. (73). [In fact, what $\langle\chi\rangle'$ actually causes is a variation of the cavity eigenfrequency.] The fluctuations of ω_a will in general be thermal drift plus microphonics. Hence, n_F will be confined here to the d.c. – audio a.c. range.

Another fluctuation with a similar effect is a fluctuation in the phase of r_b, due, for example, to vibrations or temperature variations, which cause a variation in length of the waveguides [see eq. (2.115)] or influence a phase shifter. Remember that the phase of r_b is a phase relative to the wave that enters the cavity. Hence a spurious phase shift in either path has the same effect. A phase fluctuation $\Delta\varphi_b$ has the same effect on a $\langle\chi\rangle''$ measurement as a frequency fluctuation $\Delta\omega$ given by

$$\Delta/\varphi_b = \left(2 - \frac{1}{r_b}\right) \frac{2\dfrac{\Delta\omega}{\omega}}{Q_0^{-1}} \tag{75}$$

as can be seen from eq. (60). Indeed $\Delta\varphi_b = \Delta\psi$ in this case. However, one may no longer consider this $\Delta\varphi_b = 0$ for $r_b = \frac{1}{2}$, because the fluctuation is also on r_b itself.

Can we now once again construct an appropriate circuitry in order to minimize FM effects? Let us first consider the strongest restriction, eq. (74),

$$n_F < \langle\chi\rangle'.$$

How can we prevent n_F from masking $\langle\chi\rangle'$?

Observe that $\langle\chi\rangle'$ causes, in fact, a change in the cavity eigenfrequency, while the noise n_F is mostly present in the actual frequency of the oscillator. Hence we must find a system that separates the oscillator frequency fluctuations from the cavity eigenfrequency changes. It is because both are coupled in eq. (73) that we arrive at the requirement $n_F < \langle\chi\rangle'$. This separation may be realized with a second cavity, inserted in the bias branch (Redhardt, 1961). Indeed this cavity, exposed to the same FM noise, may produce the same amplitude fluctuation as our sample cavity and be subtracted from it. There remain only the amplitude changes due to fluctuations in the eigenfrequency of our sample cavity. And even the last ones, due to thermal drift or to microphonics, may be compensated by constructing the two cavities—the sample cavity and the bias cavity—so that they have the same temperature fluctuations and the same vibrations (e.g. one may make a double cavity from the same piece of copper). In this case, only the amplitude increments due to $\langle\chi\rangle'$ are not cancelled. A scheme is given in Fig. 4.15. Let us represent

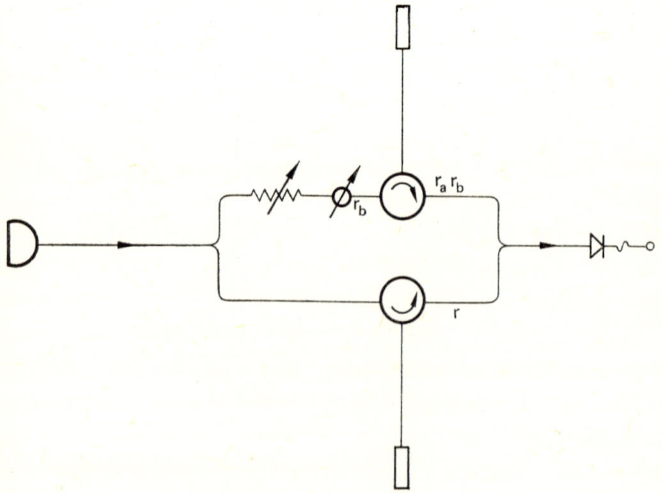

FIG. 4.15. FM klystron noise may be suppressed by a second cavity.

by r_a the reflection coefficient of this second cavity with eigenfrequency $\omega_{aa'}$ eigendamping Q_{0a}^{-1} and external damping Q_{ea}^{-1}. The wave incident on the detector is

$$r_d = r_a r_b + r \tag{76}$$

and the rate of change of r_d with frequency noise is

$$\frac{\partial r_d}{\partial \omega} = r_b \frac{\partial r_a}{\partial \omega} + \frac{\partial r}{\partial \omega}. \tag{77}$$

Let r_a and r depend on the same factor $2(\Delta\omega/\omega) = x$. Now

$$\frac{\partial r_d}{\partial x} = r_b \frac{\partial r_a}{\partial x} + \frac{\partial r}{\partial x} = r_b \frac{\partial r_a}{\partial y_a}(i/Q_{ea}^{-1}) + \frac{\partial r}{\partial y}(i/Q_e^{-1}). \tag{78}$$

Using eq. (25) for $\partial r/\partial y$ we get

$$dr_d = \left\{ \frac{-\frac{1}{2}(1 - R_a^2)\, R_b}{Q_{ea}^{-1}} e^{i(2\varphi_1 + r_a + \varphi_b)} + \frac{-\frac{1}{2}(1 - R^2)}{Q_e^{-1}} e^{i2\varphi_1 + r} \right\} \frac{2\Delta\omega}{\omega}. \tag{79}$$

It is obvious that, by a suitable choice of r_b and r_a, one can make the factor in brackets zero. One chooses, for example, r_a nearly equal to r, and adjusts the difference by means of r_b. Remember that $\Delta\omega/\omega$ means the common deviation, not the deviation due to $\langle\chi\rangle'$, in only one cavity. One can now treat this r_d as an ordinary r of a single cavity, and complete the spectrometer, for example, as in Fig. 4.16 to be compared with Fig. 4.15.

In order to eliminate the second-order influence of FM noise in $\langle\chi\rangle''$ measurements, one can of course use the same circuit. But there are also other, simpler, tricks.

Really, the simplest way is to choose $r_b = +\frac{1}{2}$ in a simple homodyne spectrometer or, in general, $(-r_b)$ in the centre of the cavity locus circle in the Smith diagram. This has been stressed after eq. (59) and no further comment is needed. One must, however, deal with microphonics, eq. (75), but this is simplified by the fact that the spectrometer has only a small number of components.

However, this method fails if one has to use balanced detection, since one eliminates the noise in only one of the detectors. Also, there

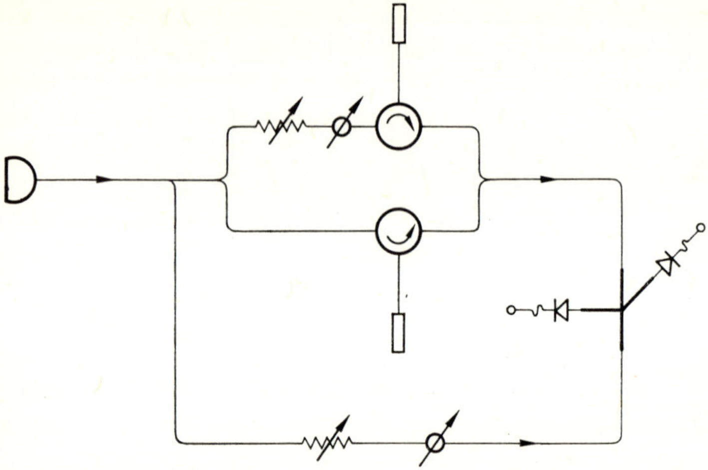

FIG. 4.16. Combination of AM and FM noise suppression.

are sometimes other features, such as, for example, detector crystal characteristics, which do not permit this choice of r_b. In these cases one can only try to minimize the variations in $(\omega - \omega_a)$. We say variations in $(\omega - \omega_a)$ and not variations in ω. Indeed, it is useless to have, for example, a perfectly stable oscillator frequency if the cavity eigenfrequency drifts away.

We distinguish between rapid variations in $\omega(t)$, say above some tens of kHz, and slow variations, including drift.

Rapid variations in practice occur only in the oscillator frequency. Hence the only solution here is to have it with a low FM noise. This is a well-defined problem, which has nothing to do with e.s.r. In general it is easier to have an oscillator with low FM noise at low power. One may, for example, multiply the frequency of a quartz crystal, oscillating at 5 MHz, up to 150 MHz and then select the 60th harmonic by a microwave cavity tuned at 9 GHz. The oscillator at higher power level may be phase-locked electronically to such a low-power oscillator. The FM noise (and drift) of a klystron may also be reduced by locking it electronically to the eigenfrequency of a stable-high-Q cavity, which is temperature stabilized.

In modern microwave oscillators, FM noise at higher frequencies is in general less important than slow variations or drift in frequency. Remember that $\Delta Y''_{\mathbf{error}}$ in eq. (40) causes more trouble than n_F if $\Delta Y''_{\mathbf{error}} > n_F/Q_0^{-1}$ since $\Delta Y''_{\mathbf{error}}$ emphasizes the effect of n_F. Hence, the important thing is to maintain $\omega - \omega_a$ at a low value. The solution here is to electronically lock the oscillator frequency to the eigenfrequency of the sample cavity. Frequency stabilization is discussed extensively by Poole (1967, p. 194). Let us simply remark that in principle the obvious solution would be to use the sample cavity as a tank circuit of the oscillator, as in a r.f. marginal oscillator. However, the undamping of the circuit by a triode is limited to below $\sim$1 GHz and the undamping by velocity modulated electrons, as in a klystron, is not practical. An extremely stable oscillator, in principle suitable for this purpose, has been constructed by Nguyen Tuong Viet (1967). It consists of a superconducting cavity, undamped by an external circuit with a travelling wave tube microwave amplifier. Perhaps a tunnel diode might also supply a practical solution in the near future.

4.6. Frequency conversion

The schemes given in the former section may help to reduce some of the noise influences. In order to reduce the noise power further, one may perhaps search for a frequency band in which the noise power is weaker than at other frequencies. This is, of course, impractical for thermal noise, but many other noise sources, such as microphonics or a crystal detector, have a frequency-dependent noise spectrum.

We must "transfer" the signal to the desired frequency band. If the original signal is $s = S(t)$ then the signal $S(t) \cos \omega t$, with $\omega \gg (\partial s/\partial t)/S$, is a signal at frequency ω with amplitude modulation $S(t)$. The "d.c." signal is transferred to the frequency band around ω. In the same way, for example, a signal $s = S_m \cos \Omega t$ may be converted into a signal $S_m \cos \Omega t \cos \omega t = \frac{1}{2} S_m \cos (\Omega + \omega) + \frac{1}{2} S_m \cos (\Omega - \omega) t$; $(\Omega \ll \omega)$.

We shall now see how to transfer a signal by microwave frequency conversion. Another similar topic, "signal modulation", will be discussed in Chapter 4. In principle it is rather simple to obtain a frequency conversion in the microwave system. One only has to use a different frequency for the bias wave r_b of the homodyne system (e.g. using a second microwave oscillator, called the *local oscillator*). Such a system is called heterodyne. Let us consider the form it takes. We use the system shown in Fig. 4.11 (b) above, reproduced here in a modified way (Fig. 4.17). r_b now has a different frequency. Let us write the time dependence explicitly. The waves are respectively given by

$$\mathscr{R}[re^{i\omega t}] \quad \text{and} \quad \mathscr{R}[r_b\, e^{i(\omega+\omega_b)t}]$$

$$= \mathscr{R}[r_b\, e^{i\omega_b t}\, e^{i\omega t}] = \mathscr{R}[R_b\, e^{i(\varphi_b+\omega_b t)}\, e^{i\omega t}].$$

Hence we may repeat the analysis of the homodyne system, but substituting $r_b\, e^{i\omega_b t}$ for r_b or introducing a time-dependent phase $(\varphi_b + \omega_b t)$ instead of the time independent φ_b. This is correct in as much as $\omega_b \ll \omega$

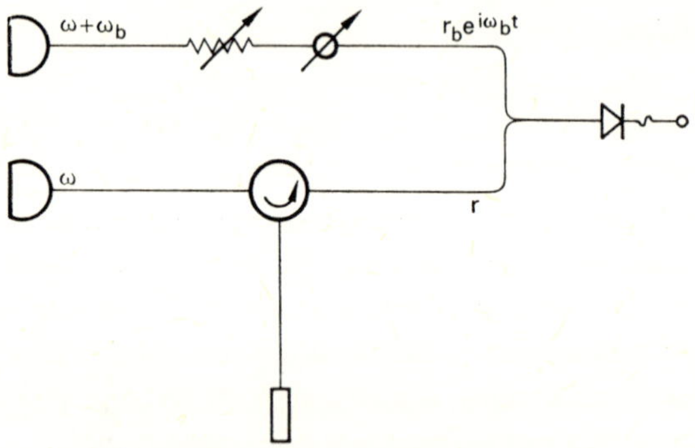

FIG. 4.17. A heterodyne spectrometer.

and the time means are taken over a few periods $2\pi/\omega$, so that, for example, the "time mean" of the power incident on the detector is still time dependent. In fact, the detection process always takes this "time mean" over a few periods $2\pi/\omega$, but fluctuations at a frequency ω_b are reproduced in the detected signal if ω_b is less than the response frequency of the detector. For common microwave diodes, $\omega_b/2\pi$ may be up to 60 MHz without any difficulty. In an X-band spectrometer, this is still less than

1 per cent of $\omega/2\pi$ (≈ 10 GHz). We add that ω_b is called the intermediate frequency (IF).

For a balanced bridge ($r \cong 0$) one now has [see eq. (55)]

$$\Delta P_{\text{det}} = -R_b \mathscr{R}\, e^{i(\varphi_b+\omega_b t)} \frac{dY}{Y'}$$
$$= -R\left\{\frac{dY'}{Y'}\cos(\varphi_b - \omega_b t) - \frac{dY''}{Y'}\sin(\varphi_b - \omega_b t)\right\}. \tag{80}$$

It appears that this result is rather poor with respect to selectivity. Indeed $\langle\chi\rangle'$ and $\langle\chi\rangle''$ are completely mixed. If one were to analyse the amplitude S_m of the signal of frequency ω_b proportional to ΔP_{det}, e.g. rectifying the output, one would get

$$S_m = GR_b \frac{|dY|}{Y'} = GR_b \sqrt{\left(\frac{dY'}{Y'}\right)^2 \left(\frac{dY''}{Y'}\right)^2} \tag{81}$$

where G is the detector gain. However, one may analyse the signal proportional to ΔP_{det} in a phase selective manner. For example, one may multiply the signal $G\Delta P_{\text{det}}$ by $\cos(\varphi_b + \omega_b t)$ and then take the mean over a period $2\pi/\omega_b$, or over some periods $2\pi/\omega_b$. This gives

$$S_m = \frac{1}{2} GR \frac{dY'}{Y'} = \frac{1}{2} R \frac{\langle\chi\rangle''}{Y'} \tag{82}$$

and multiplying by $\sin(\varphi_b - \omega_b t)$ would give

$$S_m = \frac{1}{2} GR_b \frac{dY''}{Y'} = \frac{1}{2} GR_b \frac{\langle\chi\rangle'}{Q_0^{-1}} \tag{83}$$

since the mean of $\sin(\varphi_b + \omega_b t)\cos(\varphi_b - \omega_b t)$ is zero. We shall deal with phase selective detection in Chapter 4. Let us only emphasize that the factor $\frac{1}{2}$ in eqs. (82) and (83) is irrelevant for sensitivity considerations. One may first amplify the detected signal. This sensitivity question will also be discussed later, in connection with the detection problem. Another question is the phase characteristic of this IF amplifier. The phase relation between input and output has to be stable. This is also important with respect to noise, since an admixture of dY'' in an absorption (dY')

measurement [caused by a $\Delta\varphi_b$ in eq. (82)] introduces noise due to the FM noise of the klystron. For this reason the phase relation must also be frequency independent and hence the amplifier must have a certain bandwidth. One further point: observe that the phase of the intermediate frequency (ω_b) signal can be adjusted at will in the microwave circuit, as well as in the intermediate frequency signal path or in the intermediate frequency reference signal of the phase-sensitive detector. The choice depends only on technological convenience. The scheme with IF lock-in detectors requires a reference signal of frequency exactly equal to the difference between the microwave oscillator frequencies. This can be achieved by mixing these oscillator signals separately for that purpose, as for instance in Fig. 4.18 where the local oscillator, at frequency $\omega - \omega_b$, delivers 5 per cent of the power that is incident on the cavity (hence $R_b < 0{\cdot}2$) and where 0·01 power units are mixed in

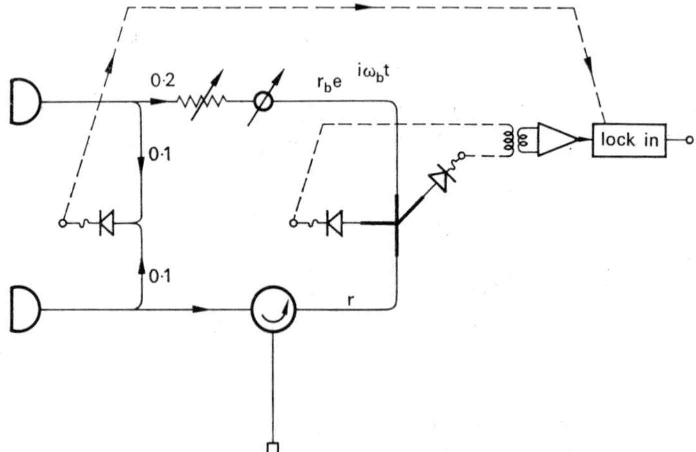

FIG. 4.18. Heterodyne spectrometer with IF phase lock for selectivity.

order to give a reference signal at IF. (We assume the components lossless.) Another possibility is to derive $r_b\, e^{i\omega_b t}$ from the signal klystron itself. A wave is modulated at ω_b and one sideband is filtered out by a cavity. The IF oscillator, which modulates the wave, then also provides the reference signal.

The method using an IF phase-sensitive detection seems straightforward in obtaining selectivity, but it substantially increases the technological complications. Fortunately, there is a simpler method, which is at least as good. We may combine the homodyne system with a very small bias, just enough to discriminate between absorption and dispersion, with heterodyne bias great enough to optimize the detection process. A scheme is shown in Fig. 4.19. A homofrequency wave r_a is mixed with Δr and the sum is mixed with a heterofrequency wave. The sum

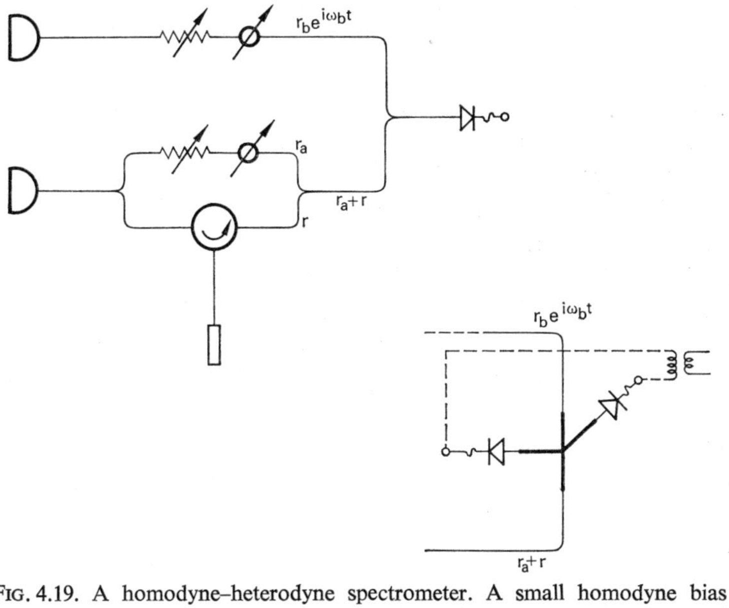

FIG. 4.19. A homodyne–heterodyne spectrometer. A small homodyne bias ensures selectivity. An appropriate heterodyne bias ensures optimum crystal performance. Balanced detection may still be used.

$r_a + r$ presents amplitude variations proportional to dY'/Y' or to dY''/Y' depending on the relative phase of r_a and r. Mixing $r_a + dr$ with a bias wave, $r_b\, e^{i\omega_b t}$, gives as in eq. (53) for dr only:

$$\Delta P_{\text{det}} = 2\,\mathscr{R}(r_a + dr)\, r_b^*\, e^{-i\omega_b t} = 2\,\mathscr{R}[R_b|r_a + dr|e^{\,i(\varphi_{a+r} - \varphi_b - \omega_b t)}] \quad (84)$$

We have indicated the phase of $r_a + dr$ by φ_{a+r}. The signal, now measured in amplitude and not phase-sensitively, is

$$S_m = GR_b|r_a + dr|, \tag{85}$$

and

$$|r_a + dr| = (R_a^2 + |dr|^2 + 2\mathscr{R}\, r_a\, dr)^{1/2} \cong R_a + \mathscr{R}\, e^{-i\varphi_a}\, dr \tag{86}$$

for $|dr| \ll R_a$. Hence, apart from a term independent of susceptibility,

$$S_m = GR_b\, \mathscr{R}(e^{-i\varphi_a}\, dr) = -\frac{1}{2} GR_b\, \mathscr{R}\left(e^{-i\varphi_a} \frac{dY}{Y'}\right)$$

$$= GR\left(-\cos\varphi_a \frac{dY'}{Y'} + \sin\varphi_a \frac{dY''}{Y'}\right). \tag{87}$$

We may now, of course, combine the klystron noise suppression schemes with this heterodyne detection. For example, in Fig. 4.18 we have introduced a balanced detector.

Let N_b be the noise of the local oscillator, defined just as N was for the signal oscillator. The variable part of the output signal may easily be written using eq. (68), but taking into account that $N \neq N_b$ and that the phase of $r_b\, e^{i\omega_b t}$ is time dependent. The result is an output like that for the direct detection, except for the noise due to N_b. For r not exactly zero, the limit is $|\Delta r| < N|r|$, due to the signal klystron noise.

The restriction $|\Delta r| < N|r|$ or, more generally, $|\Delta r|^2$ less than the total noise power which enters the same port of the balanced detector, is compatible with the fact that the total power which enters this port substantially exceeds $|\Delta r|$. Let us call this total wave r_a. It happens that

$$|r_a| \gg |\Delta r| \gg N|r_a| \tag{88}$$

is possible with modern klystrons where $N \ll 1$ for a suitable bandwidth. Hence we may also use a balanced detection in the scheme of Fig. 4.19. The result is once again the elimination (or reduction) of the noise due to N_b, i.e. the local oscillator noise.

One remark must be made. After subtracting $P_{\text{det}4}$ from $P_{\text{det}3}$, eqs. (68), there is also a constant (noiseless) part, $(G_3 + G_4)\, \mathscr{R}\, r_b^* r$, which is of frequency ω_b and may be a supplementary requirement for r, or more generally for r_a. Indeed if R_a is too big, this may saturate the intermediate frequency amplifier, even with $NR < |\Delta r|$.

A spectrometer has been built (Laffon, 1964) in which r_a and $r_b\, e^{i\omega_b t}$ are mixed in the same branch of a balanced detector and only Δr is in the other (instead of having r_a and Δr in one of the branches). This makes it possible to have selectivity (adjusting to phase between r_a and r) without unbalancing the bridge (i.e. with $r = 0$) and without lock-in detection, but at the cost of an extra IF amplifier, since the two IF signals must be detected before mixing.†

What about the FM noise suppression scheme? First of all, the FM noise limit for absorption measurements will be reduced simply by introducing the small homofrequency bias r_a, because it reduces the influence of dY''. The remaining noise, due to n_F, will behave as in the homodyne scheme. Local oscillator FM noise will not produce AM noise in the output. On the other hand, FM noise of both waves will be reproduced in the IF signal. If two different klystrons are used, the noise will be reproduced in the reference for the IF phase-sensitive detector and will not influence the detected wave. If no phase-sensitive detection is used, then this FM noise on the IF signal will not be detected if the amplifier is broadband. If both waves are produced by the same klystron, their FM noise will be coherent and cancel. Only the FM noise of the oscillator will be present, but, for the same reason as before, will not be detected.

Let us now discuss the use of a second cavity, as in Fig. 4.16. An obvious arrangement is to put it in the path of the small homofrequency bias r_a. This is as effective as in the homodyne system and requires no further comment. But we can also introduce a second cavity in the heterofrequency bias. For a two-klystron system this is, of course, meaningless,

† For details we refer to the original article. The arguments in favour (?) of this more complicated scheme are that it eliminates on one hand the noise which accompanies r and on the other hand a sensitivity loss for $r = 0$. See, however, eq. (88), bearing in mind that in any case r or $r_a \ll 1$, so that $|1 - R^2| \cong 1$, in eq. (25). In the described spectrometer, a loss of 50 per cent due to the use of a magic tee bridge rather than a circulator is admitted without comment.

since we cannot cancel the noise of one source by the noise of another incoherent source. For a bias r_b derived from the signal klystron, the amplitude variations in the IF signal, due to FM noise in the klystron, may be cancelled as in the homodyne system, and one already has a cavity in the circuit, used to filter out the $\omega + \omega_b$ component. However, the adjustment may be rather complicated.

The possibility of frequency locking in order to reduce FM noise remains. Here the IF signal offers many possibilities, but we shall deal with it in the next section.

4.7. Compensation schemes

The spectrometer schemes described in § 4.4, with the modifications discussed in § 4.5 and § 4.6, give a signal which is a more or less linear function of $\langle\chi\rangle'$ or $\langle\chi\rangle''$. We may call them "deviation" instruments. We now shall discuss another type of spectrometer, a "compensation" instrument, which uses a null method. It will be applicable for $\langle\chi\rangle'$ measurements. The principle is as follows. Since $\langle\chi\rangle'$ produces a variation in the eigenfrequency ω_a of the cavity or in $(\omega - \omega_a)$, one may compensate the variation in ω_a by changing the oscillator frequency, so as to maintain $(\omega - \omega_a)$ at null instead of measuring the deviation $(\omega - \omega_a)$.

A first method of realizing this is to observe the signal due to variations in $(\omega - \omega_a)$ obtained in a deviation spectrometer ($\langle\chi\rangle'$ measurement). This signal is considered as a null detection and one adapts the klystron frequency for $(\omega - \omega_a) = 0$. One can feed back this null detector signal to the klystron supply voltages and automatically correct the klystron frequency, so that variations in this frequency reproduce $\langle\chi\rangle'$.

Of course, no gain in sensitivity is achieved by this method. Incidentally for very small signals a null method is in general useless, since the output deviation will always be linear and more easily read than the compensation to be introduced according to the information given by the small deviation from null. This argument about sensitivity supposes that the deviation signal to be fed back is a detected one, a signal that could also be read. However, one may arrange things so that no detection is needed. One may, for instance, use the sample cavity as the tank circuit of an

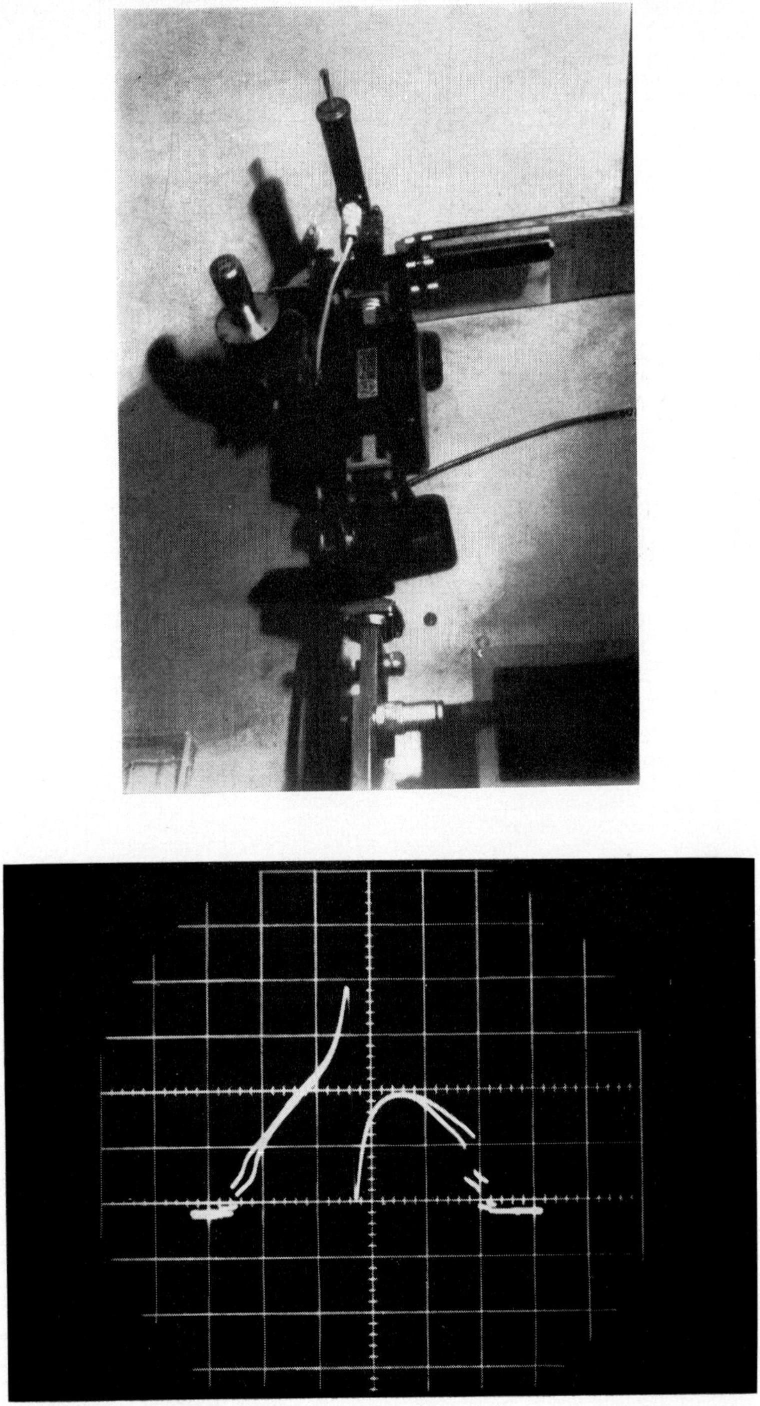

FIG. 4.20. A microwave discriminator (a) with its response curve (b).

oscillator. But this supposes the microwave signal to be amplified in some way sufficient to compensate the losses, and this amplification could also be applied to the microwave signal in a deviation spectrometer, before detection. Hence this technique also does not yield any sensitivity improvement.

On the other hand, the sensitivity of a $\langle\chi\rangle'$ measurement will generally be limited by the FM noise of the klystron unless one uses a two-cavity scheme, as in Figs. 4.18 or 4.16, but this scheme is not suitable for compensation.

In fact, compensation schemes are really useful only for large signals, when precise calibration and linearity of the signal is required,† as in measurements of static susceptibility and line shape. Indeed in such a scheme

$$2\frac{\Delta\omega}{\omega} = \pm\langle\chi\rangle' \tag{89}$$

and ω can easily be measured in an absolute way. The calibration is independent of the intensity of the HF in the cavity. (There may, however, be an admixture of $\langle\chi\rangle''$ in the same way as in a deviation spectrometer since this shifts the null position. The selectivity is not improved by a null method.)

In order to measure $\Delta\omega$ absolutely, one must use some heterodyning,‡ since ω is too high for direct counting. The relative measurement of $\Delta\omega$, for example, in order to get the line shape of $\langle\chi\rangle'$, may be done on the difference frequency after heterodyning or directly on the microwave. In the last case, one sends a sample of the wave with constant amplitude through a frequency-dependent microwave network with a high Q-cavity. Here the linearity depends on the Q of this cavity. In Fig. 4.20 (a) we have such a circuit and in Fig. 4.20 (b) the frequency response, i.e. how the frequency difference is transformed into an amplitude difference. The scope picture is obtained by scanning the frequency of a klystron at 50 Hz. Only the central part is actually used, of course.

† This is why we do not discuss compensation schemes for $\langle\chi\rangle''$ measurements. One could imagine such a scheme, but it would be more complicated than the schemes based on a frequency compensation, i.e. for $\langle\chi\rangle'$ measurements.

‡ i.e. mix with a stable known frequency and count the difference.

A very accurate method for testing the overall linearity of a spectrometer may be realized using eq. (3.30). One changes ψ by turning around $\boldsymbol{B}_s$ and then plots the signal as a function of sin ψ. (We suppose $\chi_l \ll \chi_{xx}$.)

4.8. Sensitivity

(a) *Sensitivity limit*

In a homodyne spectrometer, the current or voltage fluctuations of the signal from the detector give us $\langle\chi\rangle'$ or $\langle\chi\rangle''$, i.e. *the paramagnetic resonance signal.* This signal may be amplified and, for instance, displayed on a scope or analysed by other means. In a heterodyne spectrometer the detector current or voltage IF component is first amplified and then rectified (phase sensitively or not) so as to give a signal proportional to $\langle\chi\rangle'$ or $\langle\chi\rangle''$, at least in the first approximation. We call this, too, *the paramagnetic resonance signal*, and have to amplify and analyse. it.

In the next chapter we shall discuss the analysis of this paramagnetic resonance signal. Let us for the moment concentrate on the sensitivity with which $\langle\chi\rangle'$ or $\langle\chi\rangle''$ may be transformed into this signal.

Let us assume a homodyne or heterodyne spectrometer with ideal components and balanced bridge ($r \approx 0$). We first discuss the theoretical sensitivity limit, and here we shall consider single detection, because it is easier to discuss, although the treatment is equally valid for balanced detection (apart from klystron noise suppression). The power variation on the crystal is

$$|\Delta P_{\text{det}}| = \mathscr{R}\, r_b \frac{\Delta\, dY}{Y'} = \mathscr{R}\left[i r_b \frac{\langle\chi\rangle^*}{Q_0^{-1}} \right] \tag{90}$$

and the crystal also receives kT watts of noise power per unit bandwith or $(kT\,\Delta\omega/2\pi)$ total noise power in the bandwith of interest $(\Delta\omega/2\pi)$. T is the absolute temperature of the detector environment and k Boltzmann's constant. A wave with equal power, i.e. with

$$R_n^2 = kT\,\Delta\omega/2\pi, \tag{91}$$

would produce a detector power variation

$$P_{\text{det}n} = \mathscr{R}[2r_n r_b^* + R_n^2] \cong \mathscr{R}\, 2r_n r_b^* \tag{92}$$

since $R_n \ll R_b$. Hence the sensitivity will be limited by

$$\left|\frac{\langle\chi\rangle}{Q_0^{-1}}\right| \geqq 2R_n = 2\sqrt{kT\,\Delta\omega/2\pi}. \tag{93}$$

This limit is often referred to in the literature as the "theoretical limit".

Observe that $(kT\,\Delta\omega/2\pi)$ has to be expressed in our power units. If P is the power which flows towards the cavity, then, in any units:

$$\boxed{\left|\frac{\langle\chi\rangle}{Q_0^{-1}}\right| \geqq 2\sqrt{\frac{kT\,\Delta\omega/2\pi}{P}}} \tag{94}$$

theoretical sensitivity limit

It is obvious that one loses sensitivity if the signal is divided by 2, e.g. by a magic tee. The noise on the detector remains the same, $kT\,\Delta\omega/2\pi$, because of the black body radiation. For example, the spectrometer of Fig. 4.5 (b) is only $(2^{-\frac{1}{2}})$ times as sensitive as the spectrometer in Fig. 4.5 (a), for equal incident power on the cavity and for ideal components.† On the other hand, the klystron of Fig. 4.5 (b) delivers twice as much power as the klystron of Fig. 4.5 (a). Sometimes, such a factor of 2 or $\sqrt{2}$ must be introduced in a spectrometer because of the sensitivity, for example, because a circulator has some other defects, which a magic tee has not. Incidentally, these factors create much confusion in the literature concerning sensitivity.

Apart from this trivial effect, there are other causes which may in practice raise the sensitivity limit by about an order of magnitude. First of all, the klystron noise-suppression schemes may not work as well as planned. We stressed some of the difficulties when discussing the schemes. However, we also described some techniques to overcome these difficulties.‡

† The signal power ΔP_{det} in Fig. 4.5(b) is $(\frac{1}{2})$ times the signal power ΔP_{det} in Fig. 4.5(b) but the sensitivity is only divided by $\sqrt{2}$, because the factor $\frac{1}{2}$ is distributed between the bias and the signal amplitude $|\langle\chi\rangle/Q_0^{-1}|$. Or, in other words, the noise power which causes trouble is $R_b\sqrt{kT\,\Delta\omega/2\pi}$ which is also divided by $\sqrt{2}$.

‡ See also Poole (1967, p. 535).

The really serious limit arises from the detection. The signal-to-noise ratio in ΔP_{det} cannot be maintained when transforming it to the paramagnetic resonance signal, referred to in the introduction to this section. This is described by a noise figure. Let us only define here the relevant quantities. It involves much microwave electronics and little e.s.r. The book by Poole (1967) gives some more details.

(b) *Noise figure*

We consider a device—it may be a microwave amplifier, a crystal detector, an IF amplifier, a LF amplifier, etc.—into which a signal power S_0 and thermal noise power $N_{\mathrm{th}} = kT\Delta\omega/2\pi$, for the bandwidth $\Delta\omega/2\pi$ under consideration, enters. The device amplifies any input power by a factor G_1, the signal output power being $S_1 = G_1 S_0$, and also produces some additional noise power at the output. Without this additional noise power, the output noise N_1 would be $N_1 = G_1 N_{\mathrm{th}}$. For the actual device we define a noise factor F_1 by writing the additional noise as $(F_1 - 1)\, G_1 N_{\mathrm{th}}$, i.e. the noise at the output, *if only* N_{th} *enters*, is $F_1 G_1 N_{\mathrm{th}}$ or F_1 times the output of a noiseless amplifier. Now $N_1 = G_1 N_{\mathrm{th}} + G_1(F_1 - 1)\, N_{\mathrm{th}}$, which for this first stage happens to be $F_1 G_1 N_{\mathrm{th}}$.

Now let a second device follow the first. The input signal power is $S_1 = G_1 S_0$ and the output signal is $S_2 = G_2 S_1 = G_2 G_1 S_0$. The overall gain of the two stages is $G_{21} = G_2 G_1$. The input noise in the second device is $N = F_1 G_1 N_{\mathrm{th}}$ and the output noise is $N_2 = S_2 N_1 - (F_2 - 1) \times G_2 N_{\mathrm{th}}$. Observe that the output noise is not $F_2 G_2 N_1$. Indeed, the noise figure is defined by the excess noise produced for a thermal noise input and N_1 is already a signal, not a thermal noise input, for the second device. This signal is amplified and the result is, of course, not a useful signal but a random fluctuation. However, the device produces excess noise proportional only to the thermal input noise, not to any input noise. We may write N_2 as

$$N_2 = G_2[F_1 G_1 + (F_2 - 1)]\, N_{\mathrm{th}} = \left(F_1 + \frac{F_2 - 1}{G_1}\right) G_1 G_2 N_{\mathrm{th}}$$

so that the overall noise figure of both stages is

$$F_{21} = F_1 + \frac{F_2 - 1}{G_1} \tag{95}$$

or

$$F_{21} - 1 = (F_1 - 1) + \frac{F_2 - 1}{G_1}. \tag{96}$$

For n stages we may generalize this expression

$$F_{1n} - 1 = F_1 - 1 + \frac{F_2 - 1}{G_1} + \frac{F_3 - 1}{G_1 G_2} + \frac{F_4 - 1}{G_1 G_2 G_3}$$

$$+ \ldots - \frac{F_n - 1}{G_1 G_2 \ldots G_{n-1}}. \tag{97}$$

We may now define a signal-to-noise ratio (S/N) at different stages. The noise at the output of the n stages will be $F_{1n}G_{1n}N_{\text{th}}$ and let the signal be $G_{1n}S_0$ ($G_{1n} = G_1 G_2 \ldots G_n$). Hence the output S/N will be $1/F_{1n}$ times the input S/N, if only thermal noise is present at the input.†

Let us now return to our spectrometer. We first consider an unbiased wave Δr giving the signal

$$\frac{1}{2}\frac{\langle\chi\rangle}{Q_0^{-1}} \text{ and hence the power} \left|\frac{1}{2}\frac{\langle\chi\rangle}{Q_0^{-1}}\right|^2.$$

We assume the cavity matched, $r \approx 0$. Remember also our power unit convention. The noise power in a bandwith $\Delta\omega/2\pi$ following along it is $kT\,\Delta\omega/2\pi$ [see eq. 93)]. Hence the signal-to-noise ratio is

$$S/N = \left|\frac{1}{2}\frac{\langle\chi\rangle}{Q_0^{-1}}\right|^2 \Big/ kT\,(\Delta\omega/2\pi). \tag{98}$$

If the klystron or other noise sources affect S/N, we may express this formally by considering the spectrometer itself as an amplifier with a certain noise factor $F_{\text{system}} > 1$. The gain G_{system} of this amplifier may take into account the losses in the system; for example, using a magic tee in the signal path produces a $G_{\text{system}} = \frac{1}{2}$.

Let F_{system} and G_{system} be the F_1 and G_1 of eq. (97). It is obvious that we must first ensure that F_1 and G_1 are close to unity ($F_1 > 1$ and

† We suppose all F and G to be constant within the bandwidth $\Delta\omega/2\pi$. If not, then one must use an infinitesimal bandwith $d\omega/2\pi$ and make the appropriate integration.

$G_1 < 1$ always), since they directly effect the overall sensitivity. Sometimes, very complicated schemes are proposed in order to improve sensitivity, together with a complete lack of concern for G_{system}.

Once F_{system} and G_{system} are optimized (they can often be made close to unity) it is equally obvious from eq. (97) above that, in order to keep the overall S/N close to $(S/N)_{\text{th}}$ or F_{1n} close to unity, one must have a low $(F_2 - 1)$ value for the following stage, together with a high gain, since this gain reduces the effect of $(F_k > 1)$ in subsequent stages. This is the reason for using microwave amplification before detection (Poole, 1967, p. 571). Indeed, for a crystal detector, F is at least greater than 2 and G less than unity, while a maser may have a gain of at least an order of magnitude higher together with a noise factor close to unity. The only disadvantages in using a maser or another microwave amplifier are complexity and cost. These are, however, so important that they are only used in very specialized laboratories.

The most common technique is to start the chain after ΔP_{det} with a detector. The signal power incident on the detector in an optimized spectrometer is $S_{\text{th}} = 2R_b \cdot \frac{1}{2} \langle\chi\rangle / Q_0^{-1}$.

Using our power unit P, $P_b \equiv R_b^2 P$ is the bias power, and now $S_{\text{th}} = 2\sqrt{P_b} \frac{1}{2} \langle\chi\rangle / Q_0^{-1} \sqrt{P}$. On the other hand, the noise power in a given bandwidth $\Delta\omega/2\pi$ incident on the detector is $N_{\text{th}} = 2P_b \sqrt{kT\,\Delta\omega/2\pi}$, at least if the klystron noise has been suppressed. Hence, in this optimized spectrometer, the signal-to-noise ratio at this stage is

$$(S/N)_{\text{th}} = \frac{1}{2} \frac{\langle\chi\rangle}{Q_0^{-1}} \sqrt{P} \Big/ \sqrt{kT\,\Delta\omega/2\pi} \tag{99}$$

for the considered bandwidth. The theoretical sensitivity limit may now be defined as $(S/N)_{\text{th}} > 1$, as in eq. (94).

Because a crystal detector operates most efficiently in the linear region, the quantity

$$\frac{1}{2} \left| \frac{\langle\chi\rangle}{Q_0^{-1}} \right| \sqrt{P}$$

will be considered as the square root of the signal input power and $\sqrt{kT\,\Delta\omega/2\pi}$ as the square root of the noise input power. The detection may now formally be considered as a power "amplification", with gain G_{det} and noise figure F_{det}, substituting the microwave amplifier and hence branched directly on to the system amplifier (G_{system}, F_{system}) which takes into account klystron noise and other system noise, such as microphonics, together with system losses. In eq. (97) we set $F_{\text{system}} = F_1$, $G_{\text{system}} = G_1$, $F_{\text{det}} = F_2$ and $G_{\text{det}} = G_2$.

The "gain" of the detector is, of course, less than unity. It will be characterized by a conversion loss, the inverse of the gain. Let R_b be a wave incident on the detector. Any increment in R_b will produce a change ΔP in the rectified power delivered by the detector. The conversion loss L is defined as†

$$L = \frac{(\Delta R_b)^2}{\Delta P} = 1/G_{\text{det}} = 1/G_2 .$$

(Remember our power convention.) As for noise, the detector also produces its own noise power, t times as much as a simple resistor (t is the relative noise temperature and the output noise power is $t \,.\, kT\,\Delta\omega/2\pi$). Hence t may be identified with $F_{\text{det}}G_{\text{det}}$ or

$$F_{\text{det}} = t \cdot L. \tag{100}$$

At this point one must still introduce some real amplification, in order to increase the signal over the noise, or rather in order to make further noise contributions negligible (one cannot improve S/N by simple amplification). We need a $G \gg 1$ in eq. (97) in order to make F_{1n}, and hence S/N, independent of further $F_k > 1$. This is the role of the first signal amplifier or preamplifier, at IF. Let it have a gain $G_3 = G_{\text{amp}}$ and noise figure $F_3 = F_{\text{amp}}$. If G_{amp} is sufficiently high, say two orders of magnitude, we may neglect further noise contributions and the overall noise figure of our spectrometer will be

$$F_{1n} = F_{\text{syst}} + \frac{F_{\text{det}} - 1}{G_{\text{syst}}} + \frac{F_{\text{amp}} - 1}{G_{\text{syst}}G_{\text{det}}} = F_{\text{syst}} + \frac{tL - 1}{S_{\text{syst}}} + \frac{L(F_{\text{amp}} - 1)}{G_{\text{syst}}}$$

† And not with $\Delta(R_b)^2 = 2R_b\,\Delta R_b$ in the denominator. Only the given definition is consistent with our analysis, in which $\dfrac{1}{2}\left|\dfrac{\langle\chi\rangle}{Q_0^{-1}}\right|\sqrt{P}$ is the square root of the signal power.

or:

$$F_{1n} = F_{syst} + \frac{L\{t + (F_{amp} - 1)\} - 1}{G_{syst}}. \qquad (101)$$

In practice F_{amp} may be close to unity. A good IF amplifier may have $F < 2$ and $(F_{amp} - 1) < t$ so that one must operate the detector in such a way as to minimize (Lt). L as well as t will depend on various parameters which may be optimized; for example, t is lower at a higher frequency of the detected signal. This is the reason for using a heterodyne scheme. Also, the product Lt strongly depends on bias power, which can be optimized in the homodyne or heterodyne scheme.

References

ALZETTA, G., ARIMONDO, E., ASCOLLI, C., and GOZZINI, A. (1967), *Nuovo Cimento* **52** B, 392.

BRODWIN, M. E. and BURGESS, T. J. (1963), *I. E. E. E. Trans. Instr. Meas.* IM-**12**, 7.

CARR, P. H. and SLOBODNIK, A. J. (1967), *J. Appl. Phys.* **38**, 5153.

DERING, J. C. (1964), *Sensitivity Considerations in Paramagnetic Resonance Spectrometers* (Thesis), University of Alberta, Calgary.

GORTER, C. J. (1936), *Physica* **3**, 995.

LAFFON, J. L. (1964), *Spectrométre superhetérodyne de résonance paramagnétique électronique* (Thesis; C. E. A. rapport 2506), Université de Grenoble, Grenoble.

LEWIS, R. B. and CARVER, T. R. (1964), *Phys. Rev. Letters* **12**, 693.

MONTGOMERY, C. G., DICKE, R. H., and PURCELL, E. M. (1948), *Principles of Microwave Circuits* (M. I. T. Rad. Lab. Series No. 8), McGraw-Hill, New York.

NGUYEN TUONG VIET (1967), *Ann. Phys.* **2**, 225.

OSBORN, J. A. (1945), *Phys. Rev.* **67**, 351.

POOLE, C. P. (1967), *Electron Spin Resonance*, Interscience, New York.

REDHARDT, A. (1961), *Z. Angew. Phys.* **13**, 108.

SCHMIDT, J. and SOLOMON, I. (1966), *J. Appl. Phys.* **37**, 3719.

SŁATER, J. C. (1950), *Microwave Electronics*, D. Van Nostrand, New York.

TEANEY, D., KLEIN, M. P., and PORTIS, A. M. (1961), *Rev. Sci. Instr.* **32**, 721.

VAN GERVEN, L. (1963), *Lijnvormen in Paramagnetische Resonantie*, Interuniversitair Instituut voor Kernwetenschappen, Brussels.

CHAPTER 4

Signal Enhancement

1. Introduction

In order to improve the signal-to-noise ratio in a measurement, one may try various ways of making the signal greater and the noise smaller. One may, for example, use more sample substance, improving the filling factor, or use a cavity with lower damping. Or one may replace single detection by balanced detection in order to reduce the klystron noise (and hence the system noise figure). Suppose all this is done (or definitely not done for some reason), i.e. a signal with accompanying noise is obtained at a suitable power level, well above $kT\Delta\omega/2\pi$.

The only possible enhancement of the signal-to-noise ratio consists now in choosing an appropriate bandwidth. The noise power has a certain distribution over the frequency spectrum, which is not uniform. If one may choose the location of the signal frequency at ω_0 and if the signal is spread over a bandwidth $\Delta\omega$, one may pass signal and noise through a filter of that width centred at ω_0. The whole signal and only part of the noise appear at the output. However, the time necessary for the measurement is of the order of $1/\Delta\omega$, since the output signal changes appreciably only after that time, if the filter bandwidth is $\Delta\omega$. The final signal-to-noise ratio enhancement after a suitable choice of the centre frequency is proportional to the time needed for the measurement, since the noise is proportional to $\Delta\omega$.

Another way of stating the problem is the following. Consider a certain measurement which gives signal power S and noise power N

in a time Δt. The amplitudes (not the powers) are proportional to $\sqrt{S}$ and $\sqrt{N}$ respectively, and have $\sqrt{S}$ and $\sqrt{N}$ mixed of course. Let us now repeat the measurement n times and add the results ($\sqrt{S}$ and $\sqrt{N}$ mixed). The sum will be $n\sqrt{S} + \sqrt{nN}$. Indeed, the signal is coherent and simply adds all the n times but the noise is not coherent. Its square adds up and hence

$$N_{\text{total}} = nN.$$

In other words, $(\sum \sqrt{N_i})^2 = \sum \sqrt{N_i^2}$ + cross term, and the cross terms vanish because of the fluctuations. Thus $\sqrt{S_{\text{total}}} = n\sqrt{S}$ and $N_{\text{total}} = nN$ or $(S/N)_{\text{total}} = n(S/N)$. We again have an improvement proportional to the duration of the measurement, since it takes n times as long to make n measurements than to make one.

In this chapter we shall deal with the choice of signal frequency, the realization of a small bandwidth by lock-in detection, and sampling techniques which make it possible to add successive measurements.

2. Noise

2.1. Filter

Consider a linear system with four terminals, to be called a filter. To two of them, the input, we apply a signal voltage and from the other two, the output, we obtain another signal. For a monochromatic input signal $\mathscr{R}Se^{i\omega t}$ we get an output $\mathscr{R}g(\omega)\, Se^{i\omega t}$. This defines the gain of the system, the filter. The mean square of the output will be $|g|^2$ times the mean square of the input.

If a signal $s(t)$ of known time dependence is applied to the input we may foresee what the output signal will be. Indeed we may write the Fourier integral of $s(t)$ and multiply $e^{i\omega t}$ inside the integral by $g(\omega)$, since the system is linear. Let $s(t)$ be written as

$$s(t) = \mathscr{R} \int_0^\infty p(\omega)\, e^{i\omega t}\, d\omega/2\pi; \tag{1}$$

then the output is

$$\mathcal{R} \int_{0}^{\infty} g(\omega)\, p(\omega)\, e^{i\omega t}\, d\omega/2\pi. \tag{2}$$

On the other hand, let $R(t - t_0)$ be the output due to a delta function at the input. Then the response to a signal $\mathcal{R} S e^{i\omega t_0}$ may be written as

$$\mathcal{R}\, g(\omega)\, S\, e^{i\omega t} = \int_{-\infty}^{\infty} \mathcal{R}\, S\, e^{i\omega t_0}\, R(t - t_0)\, dt_0 = \mathcal{R} \int_{-\infty}^{\infty} S\, e^{i\omega(t_0 - t)} \times R\,(t - t_0)\, dt_0\, e^{i\omega t} \tag{3}$$

from which one deduces

$$g(\omega) = \int_{-\infty}^{\infty} R(t)\, e^{-i\omega t}\, dt. \tag{4}$$

2.2. Correlation

Now we must also examine what happens with a noise voltage $v(t)$ at the input of the filter. One might be tempted to write the Fourier series of $v(t)$ and then to analyse how each component travels through our device. This is, however, meaningless. Remember that $v(t)$ is a random function which cannot have a Fourier transform. By definition of $v(t)$ there cannot exist any mathematical expression for it because this would permit the prediction of the behaviour of $v(t)$ and hence, for instance, the cancellation of $v(t)$ by some appropriate circuitry.

We can only say something about $v(t)$ statistically; for example, we may say that the mean value is zero. We now define the mean value as

$$\langle v(t) \rangle = \lim_{\theta \to \infty} \frac{1}{\theta} \int_{t}^{t+\theta} v(t')\, dt'. \tag{5}$$

To say that $\langle v(t) \rangle = 0$ means that $v(t)$ is as likely positive as negative. For a given time t, the probability that, for example, $v(t) > 0$ is $\frac{1}{2}$, equal to the probability that $v(t) < 0$. If $\langle v(t) \rangle$ is not zero but is independent of t, we may subtract a constant. And so without any further restriction we may assume $\langle v(t) \rangle = 0$. Another statement is, for example, that $\langle v(t)^2 \rangle$ is time independent. These are statements about the system, not about the value of $v(t)$. We only say that the quoted statistical behaviour of the *system*† does not depend on time.

We may even say something more about the statistical behaviour of the system, e.g. the system may be such that: "If $v(t)$ is positive at the instant t, then it has a certain probability greater than $\frac{1}{2}$ to be positive at the instant $t + \theta$."

Consider a 1 megohm resistor and a 1 microfarad capacitor loading $v(t)$, as in Fig. 2.1 (a). If the voltage v_c over the capacitor is positive at a given instant, then it is highly probable that it will still be positive 0·1 sec later, since it takes about 1 sec to appreciably discharge the

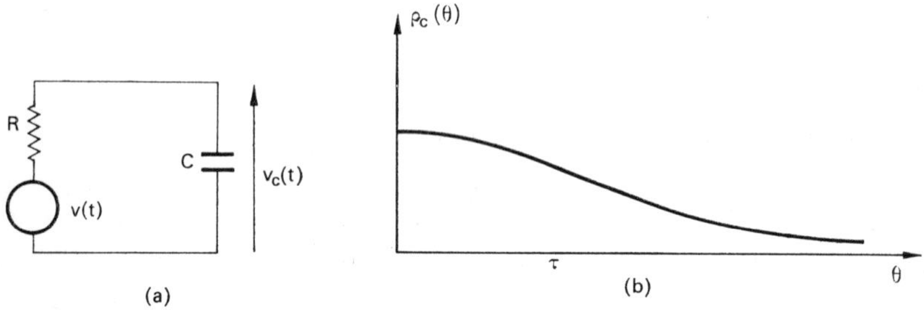

FIG. 2.1. In a RC circuit, loading a noise source $v(t)$ gives rise to a new noise voltage $v_c(t)$ appearing over the capacitor. $v_c(t)$ has a different statistical behaviour. Its correlation has a characteristic time of the order of RC. (We assume the characteristic time of $v(t)$ is much smaller than RC.)

capacitor. On the other hand, if the voltage $v(t)$ is due to very rapid motion of electrons in the resistor, it will have almost no correlation with $v(t)$ at a time 0·1 sec later. We may describe this behaviour quantitatively by a correlation function $\varrho(\theta)$, characteristic of the system and defined as

$$\varrho(\theta) = \langle v(t)\, v(t+\theta) \rangle = \lim_{\theta \to \infty} \frac{1}{\theta} \int_t^{t+\theta} v(t')\, v(t'+\theta)\, dt'. \qquad (6)$$

† e.g. a resistor at a given temperature across which we measure a voltage.

Once again we may now assume $\varrho(\theta)$ to be time independent. If $\langle v(t)\rangle$, $\langle v(t)^2\rangle$ and $\varrho(\theta)$ are time independent, we say the system is stationary to second order. For $v_c(t)$ the correlation function will be nearly $\langle v_c(t)^2\rangle$ for $\theta \ll 1$ sec and will go to zero for $\theta \gg 1$ sec. The time constant RC will be a characteristic time of the correlation function $\varrho_c(\theta)$. One may draw $\varrho_c(\theta)$ for $v_c(t)$ somewhat as in Fig. 2.1 (b).

Even if $v(t)$ is completely random, $\varrho(\theta)$ may still be a well-defined function, which may have a Fourier transform. *A priori*, one could characterize the system by even more quantities such as $\langle v(t)^3\rangle$, $\langle v(t)^4\rangle$, $\langle v(t)^2\, v(t+\theta)\rangle$, etc. But we shall limit ourselves to second-order parameters. The quantities $\langle v(t)^2\rangle$ and $\langle v(t)\, v(t+\theta)\rangle$ will be very useful later. We shall also assume $\langle v(t)\rangle = 0$. The following will also be needed:

$$\varrho(\theta) = \varrho(-\theta) \tag{7}$$

which may easily be proved from the definition for stationary systems.†

2.3. Noise through a filter

Let us now apply $v(t)$ to the input of the filter. The output $v_{\text{out}}(t)$ is completely determined by $v(t)$ and the filter characteristics. We may write this as:

$$v_{\text{out}}(t) = \int_{-\infty}^{\infty} v(t')\, R(t-t')\, dt'. \tag{8}$$

It is hopeless to try to get a better expression for $v_{\text{out}}(t)$ since $v(t')$ is by definition unknown, but we may perhaps investigate $\langle v_{\text{out}}(t)^2\rangle$. Let us use eq. (8):

$$\langle v_{\text{out}}(t)^2\rangle = \left\langle \left(\int_{-\infty}^{\infty} v(t')\, R(t-t')\, dt'\right)\left(\int_{-\infty}^{\infty} v(t'')\, R(t-t'')\, dt''\right)\right\rangle$$

$$= \left\langle \int_{-\infty}^{\infty}\int_{-\infty}^{\infty} v(t')\, v(t'')\, R(t-t')\, R(t'-t'')\, dt'\, dt''\right\rangle. \tag{9}$$

† A very clear text about random functions is presented in Angot (1961), p. 640.

Using the substitution, $\theta' = t - t'$ and $\theta'' = t - t''$, we find

$$\langle v_{out}(t)^2 \rangle = \left\langle \int_{-\infty}^{\infty} \int_{-\infty}^{\infty} v(t-\theta')\, v(t-\theta'')\, R(\theta')\, R(\theta'')\, d\theta'\, d\theta'' \right\rangle$$

$$= \int_{-\infty}^{\infty} \int_{-\infty}^{\infty} \langle v(t-\theta')\, v(t-\theta'') \rangle\, R(\theta')\, R(\theta'')\, d\theta'\, d\theta''. \tag{10}$$

In the integrand we have the expression $\varrho(\theta'' - \theta')$ and by another change of variables we get

$$\langle v_{out}(t)^2 \rangle = \int_{-\infty}^{\infty} \int_{-\infty}^{\infty} \varrho(\theta)\, R(u)\, R(u-\theta)\, du\, d\theta. \tag{11}$$

In order to use eq. (4) for $R(t)$, we replace $\varrho(\theta)$ by its Fourier transform

$$\varrho(\theta) = \int_{0}^{\infty} A(\omega)\, e^{i\omega t}\, d\omega/2\pi. \tag{12}$$

Now

$$\langle v_{out}(t)^2 \rangle = \int_{-\infty}^{\infty} \int_{-\infty}^{\infty} A(\omega)\, R(u)\, e^{i\omega u}\, R(u-\theta)\, e^{-i\omega(u-\theta)}\, d\omega/2\pi\, du\, d\theta$$

$$= \int_{0}^{\infty} A(\omega) \left[\int_{-\infty}^{\infty} R(u)\, e^{i\omega u}\, du \right] \left[\int_{-\infty}^{\infty} R(u-\theta) e^{-i\omega(u-\theta)}\, d\theta \right] d\omega/2\pi$$

$$= \int_{0}^{\infty} A(\omega)\, g^*(\omega)\, g(\omega)\, d\omega/2\pi. \tag{13}$$

Our final result

$$\langle v_{out}(t)^2 \rangle = \int_{0}^{\infty} A(\omega)\, |g(\omega)|^2\, d\omega/2\pi \tag{14}$$

may be interpreted as follows: for the range of the frequency spectrum going from ω to $\omega + d\omega$, the noise power in the source behaves as the power of a monochromatic voltage at frequency ω with mean square value $A(\omega)\, d\omega/2\pi$ (or amplitude $\sqrt{2A(\omega)\, d\omega/2\pi}$). All these contributions over the whole spectrum add without interference. Therefore we call $A(\omega)$ the noise spectrum density of the source.

3. Signal Modulation Technique

3.1. Frequency conversion

When scanning the static field (or the frequency of the microwave source) one will have a change in the output signal of the spectrometer due to $\langle\chi\rangle$. For example, the d.c. current through the detector crystal, or even the amplitude of the IF amplifier output,† changes. One may measure the output with a galvanometer and plot the result point by point as a function of the field, or scan‡ the field continuously and record the output.

However, a drift in klystron power or in cavity eigendamping produces a similar change in the output of the spectrometer. This drift must be considered as noise. We may avoid it by getting our output signal in a bandwidth around a certain frequency different from zero. Indeed, what we call drift is essentially noise in a bandwidth which goes from zero frequency up to a few cycles.

The frequency conversion of the signal has to be made in the spectrometer at a stage where the noise (here the drift) is not as yet present. For example, the heterodyne detection scheme shifts the signal only with respect to the detector noise spectrum but not with respect to cavity noise or klystron drift since these are shifted together with the signal. Heterodyning does not eliminate the effect of klystron drift. But a signal that is itself modulated will have to compete with the detector noise in the bandwidth around this modulation frequency. Incidentally, if this frequency could be of the order of several tens of megacycles, heterodyning would be completely superfluous.

There is a simple way to get the signal inside a certain bandwidth away from zero frequency, i.e. to get the signal modulated: one modulates

† If heterodyne is used we consider the time mean (over a few IF cycles) of the amplifier output power as the signal in this chapter.

‡ This scanning can be done at 60 Hz, and the output displayed on a scope. The simple integral display of the whole resonance line on a scope is considered a technique for *scanning* only. We shall discuss this below.

the static field, apart from scanning it. Let the time function i of the field be

$$B_s = B_{s0} + B_d = B_{s0} + \frac{t}{\tau} B_{d0} + B_m \cos \Omega t \tag{1}$$

with $B_{d0}/\tau \ll \Omega B_m$, i.e. with the scanning much slower than the modulation. For constant modulation amplitude very small compared to the line width (i.e. $B_m \ll \delta$) one obtains a signal output of amplitude proportional to the derivative of the resonance line. Moreover, the phase of the fundamental frequency signal, with respect to the modulation, informs us whether the derivative is positive or negative. The output is also proportional to the amplitude of modulation B_m, and hence one may prefer to use an amplitude so large that one no longer has the true derivative but has some more complicated result. For the present purpose we shall assume $B_m \ll \delta$. The output of our spectrometer is an a.c. signal, at a frequency Ω, which we must analyse and, of course, distinguish above noise.

The method of signal modulation is very useful because it introduces a frequency conversion at a very early stage. It shifts the signal frequency with respect to the overall noise spectrum of the whole spectrometer, and any drift may be avoided, except drift in the centre value of the modulated static magnetic field. (This last drift is noise, superimposed on the scanning function.) Unfortunately this technique is limited by a maximum frequency. We have shown in the second chapter that we may not change the static field at an arbitrary rate. On the other hand, in many cases this maximum frequency is at least some kHz and most noise occurs below 1 kHz, except thermal noise and detector noise. The thermal noise spectrum is flat, so that no frequency conversion can change the noise per bandwidth. Detector excess noise becomes insignificant only above some MHz. This is generally too high for field modulation, but one may use heterodyning here. In some cases, however, one may use a field modulation frequency up to half a megahertz, and here the detector excess noise, in modern crystal detectors, although not negligible, is low enough for the technique to be competitive with heterodyning (Dering, 1964).

The low-frequency noise is mostly composed of slow drift, say below 10 Hz, and microphonics due the vibrations of components or, for example, to bubbles of boiling helium or nitrogen in the cavity. A rather unexpected but possible low-frequency noise is the "hand-waving effect" quoted by Hyde (1965). "Inevitably, some microwaves leak out to fill the room and typical hand motions (usually slower than 1 metre per second) through an X-band standing wave pattern can produce modulations at 20 Hz, but not at 400 Hz."

3.2. Signal-to-noise ratio improvement

A straightforward method for enhancing the signal-to-noise ratio is, for a monochromatic signal, to pass signal plus noise through a bandpass filter with limited bandwidth and centre frequency at the signal frequency. Let us feed into a filter of gain $g(\omega)$ a monochromatic signal $s(t) = \mathcal{R}\, Se^{i\omega t}$ together with the noise $v(t)$ having a spectrum $A(\omega)$. The signal-to-noise power ratio at the output will be the mean square of the signal output, e.g. $\frac{1}{2}\,|S|^2\,|g|^2$, divided by $\langle v(t)^2\rangle$, or

$$(S/N)_{\text{power}} = \frac{S^2_{\text{r.m.s.}}|g(\omega_s)|^2}{\int_0^\infty A(\omega)\,|g|^2\,d\omega/2\pi}. \tag{2}$$

if $A(\omega)$ is constant, $A(\omega) = A_\omega$, over the frequency range where $|g|$ is Important, we may take it out of the integral. On the other hand, we shall, of course, choose the signal frequency at maximum filter gain (or adapt the filter gain to the signal frequency). Hence, $|g(\omega_s)|^2 = |g|^2_{\max}$

$$S/N_{\text{power}} = \frac{S^2_{\text{r.m.s.}}}{A_\omega \left\{\dfrac{\int_0^\infty |g|^2\,d\omega/2\pi}{|g|^2_{\max}}\right\}} \tag{3}$$

We now define a bandwidth of the filter as

$$\Delta_f \equiv \frac{\int_0^\infty |g|^2\,d\omega/2\pi}{|g|^2_{\max}}. \tag{4}$$

And we write

$$S/N_{\text{power}} = \frac{S^2_{\text{r.m.s.}}}{A_\omega \Delta_f}. \tag{5}$$

Remember the interpretation of $A(\omega)$ given after eq. (2.14). Here this suggestion may be extended to the whole filter [if $A(\omega)$ is constant over the whole frequency range of the filter].

It is now evident that one may enhance (S/N) by reducing the bandwidth Δ_f of the filter. But there are limits. Δ_f cannot be reduced arbitrarily. The technical problem of keeping the signal frequency inside the bandwidth of the filter would appear more difficult if Δ_f/ω is small. One would think that very stable oscillator and equally stable filter characteristics are required. Fortunately, there is a rather simple solution here, namely lock-in detection. We shall discuss it in the following sections.

A more fundamental limitation is the time one may take to do the measurement. This time may be limited by quite different conditions, going from magnetic field instabilities over liquid helium evaporation to the fatigue of the operator after some hours. Until now we have assumed a signal $s(t) = \mathscr{R} Se^{i\omega t}$ to be present all the time with constant S, but such a signal does not represent any real measurement. In fact the amplitude S changes as a function of time when we scan through the field. We shall see below that for changes much slower than the signal frequency ω_s, we may consider $S(t)$ applied to a low pass filter of gain $g'(\Delta\omega) = g(\omega \pm \Delta\omega)$. But if we suddenly switch on the signal at the input of a filter, such as, for example, RC circuit, a time RC elapses before the signal reaches an appreciable fraction of its final value. This time RC is proportional to $1/\Delta_f$ and hence reduction of the bandwidth Δ_f of the filter means more time for making the measurement. We shall discuss this problem when dealing with the scanning.

Another way of improving S/N is by improving S, increasing the modulation amplitude. Let us consider a dispersion or absorption line for which the maximum variation of the signal is $S_{\text{d.c.}}$. For a Lorentzian line shape it is the same for absorption and for dispersion. If we switch the field from zero to the maximum absorption value or from the dispersion minimum to the dispersion maximum we get a signal step equal to $S_{\text{d.c.}}$ in amplitude. Let us take $S_{\text{d.c.}}$ as the reference for the maximum signal value. For instance, it would be the signal amplitude for a field scanned without frequency conversion. The maximum signal-to-noise ratio is *defined* as the optimum value

$$(S/N)_{\text{power}} = \frac{S_{\text{d.c.}}^2}{A(\omega)\,\Delta_f} \tag{6}$$

and with respect to this value we shall introduce a coefficient which gives the real S/N.

The simple process of modulating the field lowers S/N with respect to this optimum value by a factor of 8 or more.

Suppose we just use δ' as the modulation amplitude on the dispersion line and set the static field centre value equal to the resonance value ($\chi' = 0$).

Considering the variation of $\langle\chi'\rangle$ linear in B_s between the maximum and minimum (a rough approximation) we get a signal of amplitude ($\frac{1}{2}\,S_{\text{d.c.}}$) and hence of mean square

$$S_{\text{r.m.s.}}^2 = \tfrac{1}{2}\,(\tfrac{1}{2}\,S_{\text{d.c.}})^2 = \tfrac{1}{8}S_{\text{d.c.}}^2\,. \tag{7}$$

Let us define a modulation efficiency M_n

$$M_n = \frac{S_{\text{r.m.s.},n}^2}{S_{\text{d.c.}}^2} \tag{8}$$

where $S_{\text{r.m.s.},n}$ is the root mean square of the nth harmonic of the signal when modulation is applied. The example shows that M_i is in any case lower than $\frac{1}{8}$. In practice M_1 will be still lower than $\frac{1}{8}$ even for optimum modulation amplitude, because the curve is not linear. There are also higher harmonics between which the available signal power has to be shared. It is clear that a modulation amplitude much greater or much less than δ' will reduce the modulation efficiency still more. For a quantitative approach we must confine ourselves to a definite line shape. The search for the modulation efficiency for various harmonics is connected to another problem, the line shape deformation due to finite modulation amplitude. Indeed, only for very small modulation amplitude does one obtain the derivative of the line shape. If we use a higher modulation amplitude, e.g. in order to improve sensitivity through M_i, one must correct for line shape deformation. These questions are studied in a great number of publications. It is a good exercise in Fourier transform calculations. We refer to the book by Van Gerven (1963). One must be aware of the fact that any claim of high precision is illusory here, since a line shape model (Lorentzian or Gaussian) is in any case only a rough approximation.

3.3. Lock-in detection. Monochromatic signals

The purpose of this and the following section is simply the analysis of a device having the same effect on the signal-to-noise ratio as a symmetrical bandpass filter with gain $g(\omega_c + \Delta\omega) = g(\omega_c - \Delta\omega)$. However, the centre frequency ω_c is automatically adjusted to the signal modulation frequency, and we use a low pass filter with gain $g'(\Delta\omega) = g(\omega_c \pm \Delta\omega)$. Such a device, called a lock-in detector, is necessary if one wishes to use a very small bandwidth, without heavy requirements on the oscillator stability, and it is often easier to construct the low pass filter than to construct the bandpass filter. The device is essentially a switch, operated synchronously with the modulation. It may be, for example, a mechanical or optical chopper or an electronic switch. Let us first see how a monochromatic signal behaves. We have a source with internal resistance R, which delivers a monochromatic signal $s(t) = S \sin \omega t$. To this source we connect a switch that inverts the connections to the load, $\omega/2\pi$ times per second. In Fig. 3.1 we show the result. If the signal $s(t)$ is in phase with the switch, one will have an output signal which is always positive. If the phase of the signal differs from the phase of the switch by π, the output will always be negative. And for a phase difference of $\pi/2$ the mean value of the output is zero.

In general let the phase relation, φ, be such that the switch goes from inverse to direct when the signal value is $S \sin \varphi$. Then the mean output will be

$$S \frac{1}{T/2} \int_0^{T/2} \sin(\omega t + \varphi)\, dt = S \frac{2}{\pi} (\cos \varphi). \tag{9}$$

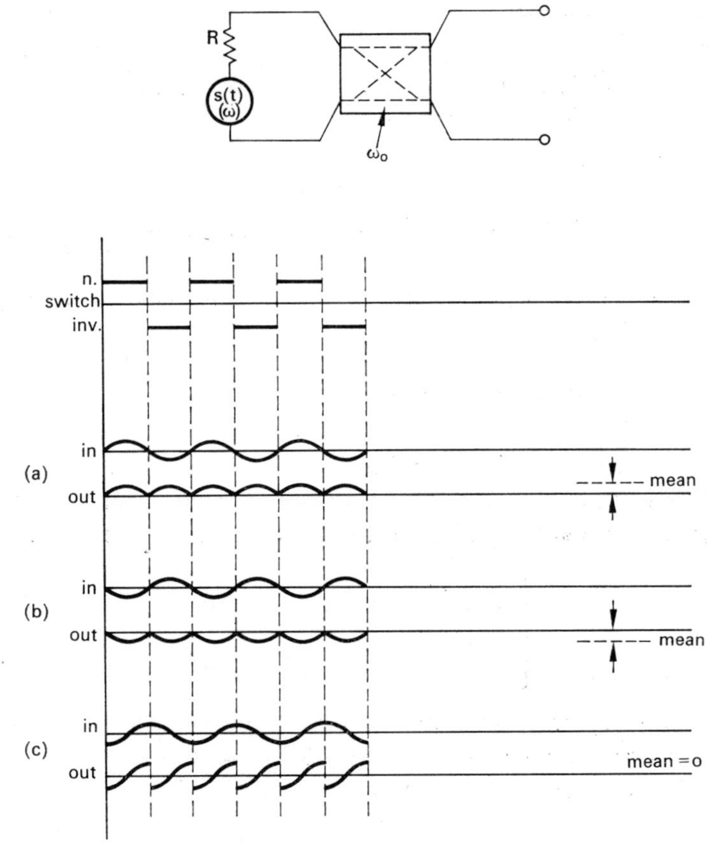

FIG. 3.1. A lock-in detector is essentially a switch that inverts the connections of a source to a load, each half cycle of an external frequency.

If the signal has a frequency $\omega + \Delta\omega$, slightly different from the switching frequency, then the mean output will follow this phase difference $(\Delta\omega t)$:

$$S\frac{2}{\pi}\cos\Delta\omega t. \tag{10}$$

Another way to get the output of the switch is to consider the switch as multiplying s by a step function. This step function can be written as the following Fourier series

$$\frac{4}{\pi}\left(\sin \omega t + \frac{1}{3}\sin 3\omega t + \frac{1}{5}\sin 5\omega t + \ldots\right) \tag{11}$$

and the result is

$$\begin{aligned} S&\left(\frac{4}{\pi}\sin(\omega + \Delta\omega)\, t \sin \omega t + \frac{1}{3}\sin(\omega + \Delta\omega)\, t \sin 3\omega t + \ldots\right) \\ &= S\frac{2}{\pi}\Bigg[\cos \Delta\omega t - \cos(2\omega + \Delta\omega)\, t + \frac{1}{3}\cos(\Delta\omega - 2\omega)\, t \\ &\quad - \frac{1}{3}\cos(\Delta\omega + 4\omega)\, t + \ldots\Bigg], \end{aligned} \tag{12}$$

which at a coarse scale compared to $1/\omega$ is $S(2/\pi)\cos \Delta\omega t$.

It is interesting to see what happens with an input signal of frequency $n\omega$, i.e. $s = \sin(n\omega t + \varphi)$. With eq. (9) or with eq. (11) one obtains

$$\begin{cases} S\dfrac{2}{\pi}\dfrac{1}{n}\cos\varphi & \text{for} \quad n \text{ odd.} \\ 0 & \text{for} \quad n \text{ even} \end{cases} \tag{13}$$

as the output. For a signal frequency $n\omega + \Delta\omega$, with $\Delta\omega \ll \omega$, one will have a coarse scale output, respectively $S(2/n\pi)\cos \Delta\omega t$ and zero.

Until now "mean value" or "coarse scale" indicated a mean over one switching period $T = 2\pi/\omega$ or

$$\frac{1}{T}\int_{nT}^{(n+1)T} \ldots\, dt = \frac{1}{T/2}\int_{nT}^{\left(n+\frac{1}{2}\right)T} \ldots\, dt. \tag{14}$$

We could also take the mean over a longer period $t \gg T = 2\pi/\omega$. For signals at the switching frequency this makes no difference. For signals of a different frequency and principally for noise, it will make a difference. In order to get the "coarse scale" output, we must integrate so that the fine scale output disappears. In order to integrate the output, let us put a capacitor across the output after the switch. This is shown in

Fig. 3.2 (a) (an impedance is drawn instead of R). $v(t)$ is an arbitrary voltage source and R its internal resistance. The voltage over the capacitor is given by

$$v_c(t) = \frac{1}{C}\int_0^{T/2} i\,dt - \frac{1}{C}\int_{T/2}^{T} i\,dt + \frac{1}{C}\int_{T}^{3T/2} i\,dt - \frac{1}{C}\int_{3T/2}^{2T} i\,dt + \dots \frac{1}{C}\int_{\dots}^{t} i\,dt \qquad (15)$$

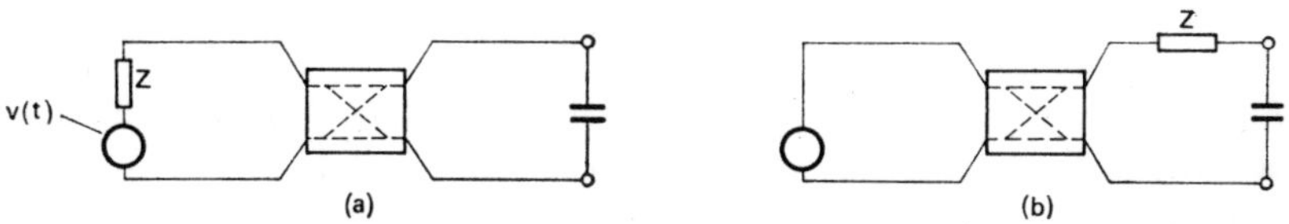

FIG. 3.2. A linear impedance in the circuit before the switch (a) may travel through the switch (b) withuot affecting the result of the analysis.

where $T = 2\pi/\omega$ is the switching period and i the current in the resistor R. This current i is, however, given by

$$i = \frac{1}{R}[v(t) - v_c(t)] \quad \text{for each first half period,}$$

$$i = \frac{1}{R}[v(t) + v_c(t)] \quad \text{for each second half period.} \qquad (16)$$

Hence

$$v_c(t) = -\frac{1}{RC}\int_0^t v_c\,dt + \frac{1}{RC}\left\{\int_0^{t/2} v(t)\,dt - \int_{T/2}^{T} v(t)\,dt + \dots \int^{t} v(t)\,dt\right\}. \qquad (17)$$

The result would be the same if we had the resistor on the other side of the switch, as in Fig. 3.2 (b). The resistor may also travel along the loop in which it is inserted, *across the switch*.† With a little thought, it

† In practice we cannot do this, because R is the internal resistance of $v(t)$. But if we know that the same result is obtained we may do it in our calculations and analysis.

is clear that the same holds for any linear passive circuit element, and for any load.

Now it is easy to get the voltage over the capacitor for an input $v(t) = s = S \sin(\omega + \Delta\omega)\, t$. We already know that the mean voltage over the resistor plus capacitor after the switch is $S\,.\,(2/\pi) \cos \Delta\omega t$. If $\Delta\omega \ll \omega$, we do not have to worry about components at frequency ω and hence we use $S\,.\,(2/\pi) \cos \Delta\omega t$ as the instantaneous voltage over the resistor and capacitor. By ordinary network theory, we obtain for the output voltage over the capacitor (using $\tau = RC$):

$$v_c = S \frac{2}{\pi} \mathscr{R} \frac{1}{1 + i\Delta\omega\tau} e^{i\Delta\omega t}. \tag{18}$$

As a check, let us calculate this voltage from eq. (17). The equation may be written, for $t = NT$, as

$$\tau v_c(NT) + \int_0^{NT} v_c\, dt = \sum_{n=0}^{2\tau-1} (-1)^n \int_{nt/2}^{\tau(n+1)T/2} v(t)\, dt$$

$$= \sum_{n=0}^{2N-1} (-1)^n \int_0^{T/2} v(t' + nT/2)\, dt' \tag{19}$$

which gives the integrated voltage at the output of the switch. We abbreviate

$$\tilde{v}(nT/2) = \frac{1}{T/2} \int_0^{T/2} v(t' + nT/2)\, dt'. \tag{20}$$

If we put $v(t) = s$ we get

$$\tilde{v}(nT/2) = \frac{1}{T/2} \int_0^{T/2} S \sin(\omega + \Delta\omega)(t' + nT/2)\, dt'. \tag{21}$$

After integration we use the fact that $\cos[x + (n/2)\,\omega T] = \cos(x + n\pi) = (-1)^n \cos x$ and we obtain

$$\tilde{v}(nT/2) = \frac{(-1)^n S}{(\omega + \Delta\omega)\, T/2} [\cos \Delta\omega\, nT/2 + \cos \Delta\omega(n + 1)\, T/2]. \tag{22}$$

Hence the integrated voltage v_c is given by

$$\tau v_c(NT) + \int_0^{NT} v_c\, dt = S \frac{T/2}{\pi(1 + \Delta\omega/2\omega)}$$

$$\times \sum_{n=0}^{2n-1} [\cos \Delta\omega\, nT/2 + \cos \Delta\omega(n+1)T/2] = S \frac{1}{\pi(1 + \Delta\omega/2\omega)}$$

$$\times \left[1 + 2\left\{\sum_{n=1}^{2t/T} \cos \Delta\omega\, nT/2\right\} + \cos \Delta\omega\, NT\right]. \tag{23}$$

If we neglect details at a time scale T, we may put $NT = t$ and differentiate so as to obtain:

$$\tau \frac{\partial v_c}{\partial t} + v_c(t) = S \frac{2 \cos \Delta\omega t}{\pi(1 + \Delta\omega/2\omega)} \cong S \frac{2}{\pi} \cos \Delta\omega\tau. \tag{24}$$

The second member is indeed the output voltage if no capacitor is shunted ($t = 0$). The complete equation also gives the voltage over the capacitor. Since now $\partial/\partial t = i\Delta\omega$, we obtain eq. (18).

We may describe the whole situation formally as follows. An input signal $s = \mathscr{R} S e^{i(\omega_0 + \Delta\omega)t}$ is applied to the device.

First the frequency is shifted from $\omega_0 + \Delta\omega$ to $\Delta\omega$ and then the result is "attenuated" by $2/\pi$ and "filtered" by a filter with gain $g(\omega) = 1/(1 + i\Delta\omega t)$:

$$S e^{i(\omega_0 + \Delta\omega)t} \to \frac{2}{\pi} S e^{i\Delta\omega t} \to \frac{2}{\pi} S \frac{1}{1 + i\Delta\omega\tau} e^{i\Delta\omega t}. \tag{25}$$

The r.m.s. value or, more generally, the time mean defined as

$$\langle f(t) \rangle = \lim_{\theta \to 0} (1/\theta) \int_0^{\theta} f(t)\, dt \tag{26}$$

may be defined for the input as well as for the output of the whole device

$$\langle s_{\text{out}}^2 \rangle = \frac{4}{\pi^2} |g|^2 \langle s_{\text{in}}^2 \rangle = \frac{4}{\pi^2} \frac{1}{1 + (\Delta\omega)^2 \tau^2} \langle s_{\text{in}}^2 \rangle. \tag{27}$$

Thus the power gain of the device is $(4/\pi^2)\,|g(\Delta\omega)|^2$. Here the frequency shift is irrelevant.

Let us generalize our result. We have a monochromatic signal $\mathscr{R}Se^{i\omega t}$ from a source with internal impedance Z connected to a filter. We may formally consider Z as belonging to the filter. This being done, let $g(\omega)$ be the gain of the new filter as a function of the frequency $\omega = \omega_0 + \Delta\omega$. The output signal is now $\mathscr{R}g(\omega)\,Se^{i\omega t}$. The output power is $|gS|^2$, or $S^2|g|^2$ if we choose the time origin so that S is real. We now ask what is the effect of introducing a switch at a frequency ω_0 between source and filter. We first observe that the impedance Z may travel through the switch in our diagram without affecting the result of the analysis. This holds because Z is linear and has no intrinsic polarity (contains no rectifier, for instance). Hence we may write the input of the filter (including Z) as $(\mathscr{R}Se^{i\omega t})$ × step function (ω_0) or $(2/\pi)\,S|\cos \Delta\omega\, t - \cos{(2\omega_0 + \Delta\omega)}\ldots|$; the output will be

$$(2/\pi)\,S\{g(\Delta\omega)\,e^{i\Delta\omega t} - g(2\omega_0 + \Delta\omega)\,e^{i(2\omega+\Delta\omega)t} + \tfrac{1}{3}\,g(2\omega_0 - \Delta\omega)\,e^{i(2\omega_0-\Delta\omega)t} + \ldots\}. \tag{28}$$

Now let $g(\omega)$ be a low pass filter, with a bandwidth much less than ω_0. In this case only the first term in the expansion of the step function is important. The mean output power is half the squared output amplitude or

$$\frac{1}{2}\,\frac{4}{\pi^2}\,S^2|g(\Delta\omega)|^2, \tag{29}$$

i.e. $(4/\pi^2)\,|g(\Delta\omega)|^2$ times the input powe

If we only had a filter, without a switch, of gain

$$|g'(\omega_0 \pm \Delta\omega)| = |g(\Delta\omega)| \tag{30}$$

the output power would be

$$\mathscr{R}\,Se^{i(\omega_0+\Delta\omega)t}\,g'(\omega_0 + \Delta\omega) = s^2|g(\Delta\omega)|^2. \tag{31}$$

Hence the switch, at frequency ω_0, plus a filter, with gain $g(\Delta\omega)$, has the same effect on the output power as a voltage attenuator of $2/\pi$ plus a filter, with a gain shifted over the frequency axis by ω_0.

We may also describe the effect of the switch by a voltage attenuation of $2/\pi$ plus a frequency shift of ω_0 of the signal frequency:

$$Se^{i(\omega_0+\Delta\omega)t} \to \frac{2}{\pi} Se^{i\Delta\omega t}. \tag{32}$$

3.4. Lock-in detection. Noise

A switch + filter with gain $g(\Delta\omega)$ gives for the signal $4/\pi^2$ times the power attenuation of a single filter of gain $g'(\omega_0 \pm \Delta\omega) = g(\Delta\omega)$. Does he same hold for the n oise? The power attenuation by a filter $g'(\omega)$ is

$$\langle v(t)^2 \rangle \to \int_0^\infty A(\omega)\, |g'|^2\, d\omega/2\pi. \tag{33}$$

What is the attenuation produced by a switch + filter of gain $g(\Delta\omega) = g'(\omega + \Delta\omega)$?

We already know that we may slide the internal impedance of the noise through the switch. Hence, let us include this impedance in the filter circuit and consider a noise source with zero internal impedance, a switch, and a filter of gain $g(\Delta\omega)$.

The input to the filter is now $v_{\omega_0}(t) = [v(t) \times \text{square wave}]$:

$$v_{\omega_0}(t) = \frac{4}{\pi} \sum_{n=1}^{\infty} \frac{\sin{(2n-1)\,\omega_0 t}}{(2n-1)}\, v(t) \tag{34}$$

where ω_0 is the switching frequency. And the correlation function of $v_{\omega_0}(t)$ is

$$\varrho_\omega(\theta) = \langle v_{\omega_0}(t)\, v_{\omega_0}(t-\theta) \rangle = \left(\frac{4}{\pi}\right)^2 \sum\sum_{nm} . \lim_{\theta \to \infty} \frac{1}{\theta} \int_0^\theta$$

$$\times \frac{\sin{(2n-1)\,\omega t}\, \sin{(2m-1)\,\omega(t-\theta)}}{(2n-1)(2m-1)}\, v(t)\, v(t-\theta)\, dt. \tag{35}$$

We expand the product of sines. This gives cosines and we retain only the cosines that are independent of t, since for the others the integral vanishes because of the randomness of $v(t)$. Hence we obtain, after a little manipulation

$$\varrho_{\omega}(\theta) = \left(\frac{4}{\pi}\right)^2 \sum_n \frac{1}{2} \frac{\cos (2n - 1)\, \omega_0}{(2n - 1)^2} \varrho(\theta) . \tag{36}$$

The Fourier transform of $\varrho_{\omega}(\theta)$ may be found by replacing $\varrho(\theta)$ by its transform [eq. (2.12)]

$$\begin{aligned}
\varrho_{\omega} &= \left(\frac{4}{\pi}\right)^2 \sum_n \frac{\cos (2n - 1)\, \omega_0}{2(2n - 1)^2} \frac{1}{2} \int\limits_{-\infty}^{\infty} A(\omega')\, e^{i\omega'\theta} \frac{d\omega'}{2\pi} \\
&= \mathscr{R}\left(\frac{4}{\pi}\right)^2 \sum_n \frac{1}{2(2n - 1)^2} \frac{1}{2} \int\limits_{-\infty}^{\infty} A(\omega')\, e^{i[\omega' + (2n-1)\omega]\theta} \frac{d\omega'}{2\pi} \\
&= \mathscr{R}\left(\frac{4}{\pi}\right)^2 \sum_n \frac{1}{2(n - 1)^2} \frac{1}{2} \int\limits_{-\infty}^{\infty} A[\omega'' - (2n - 1)\, \omega]\, e^{i\omega''\theta} \frac{d\omega''}{2\pi} .
\end{aligned} \tag{37}$$

And by definition

$$\varrho_{\omega} = \tfrac{1}{2} \int\limits_{\infty}^{\infty} A_{\omega}(\omega'')\, e^{i\omega''\theta}\, d\omega''/2\pi . \tag{38}$$

Hence the noise spectrum density after the switch, $A_{\omega_0}(\omega)$ is given as a function of the original noise spectrum $A(\omega)$ by

$$A_{\omega_0}(\omega) = \sum_n \left(\frac{4}{\pi}\right)^2 \frac{1}{2(2n - 1)^2} A[\omega'' + (2n - 1)\, \omega_0] . \tag{39}$$

The noise power at the output of a filter with gain $g(\omega)$ will be

$$\int\limits_0^{\infty} A_{\omega_0}(\omega')\, g^2(\omega')\, d\omega'/2\pi = \sum_n \left(\frac{4}{\pi}\right)^2 \frac{1}{2(2n - 1)^2}$$

$$\times \int\limits_0^{\infty} A[\omega' + (2n - 1)\, \omega_0]\, |g(\omega')|^2\, d\omega/2\pi \tag{40}$$

and only for $[\omega - (2n - 1)\,\omega_0]$ within the bandwidth of the filter, supposed much less than ω_0, will there be an output noise power. Hence this noise power is

$$\left(\frac{2}{\pi}\right)^2 2 \int_0^\infty A(\Delta\omega' + \omega_0)\,|g(\Delta\omega')|^2\, d\Delta\omega'/2\pi. \tag{41}$$

If we assume $A(\omega_0 + \Delta\omega') = A(\omega_0 - \Delta\omega')$ and define $g(\Delta\omega) = g(-\Delta\omega)$ for $\Delta\omega < 0$, we may write this as

$$\left(\frac{2}{\pi}\right)^2 \int_\infty^\infty A(\omega_0 + \Delta\omega')\,|g(\Delta\omega')|^2\, d\Delta\omega/2\pi. \tag{42}$$

It is $(2/\pi)^2$ times the noise power which would be delivered from $v(t)$ through a filter of gain $|g'(\omega_0 \pm \Delta\omega)| = |g(\Delta\omega)|$.

Let us summarize our conclusions. We have a signal voltage $s = \mathscr{R}Se^{i\omega t}$ at a frequency $\omega = \omega_{ch} + \Delta\omega$ and noise voltage $v(t)$, with a correlation function $\varrho(\theta)$ and noise spectrum density $A(\omega)$, from a source with internal impedance $Z(\omega)$. If we connect a chopper [frequency $\omega_{ch}/2\pi$] to this source it is irrelevant whether we consider Z to be located before or after the chopper. We may slide Z through the chopper. Hence we consider it together with a network branched to a source with zero impedance, and we are free to insert a chopper between this zero impedance source and the network containing Z. We now have two schemes:

(a) source + symmetric bandpass filter $g_1(\omega)$

$$|g_1(\omega_{ch} + \Delta\omega)| = |g_1(\omega_{ch} - \Delta\omega)|,$$

(b) source + chopper at frequency ω_{ch} + lowpass filter with gain $g(\Delta\omega)$

$$|g(\Delta\omega)| = |g_1(\omega_{ch} \pm \Delta\omega)|.$$

The signal of the source is $\mathscr{R}Se^{i\omega t}$ and the source noise has a spectrum $A(\omega)$.

The signal outputs are respectively (coarse scale)

$$\text{(a)}\quad \mathscr{R}\,[Se^{i(\omega_{ch}+\Delta\omega)t}\, g_1(\omega_{ch} + \Delta\omega)], \tag{43}$$

$$\text{(b)}\quad (2/\pi)\,\mathscr{R}\, Se^{i\Delta\omega t} \times g(\Delta\omega).$$

The output signal power is

$$\text{(a)}\quad \tfrac{1}{2} S^2 |g(\omega)|^2 = \tfrac{1}{2} S^2 |g(\Delta\omega)|^2 \tag{44}$$

(b) $(2/\pi)^2$ times the output in (a).

The output noise power is

$$\text{(a)}\quad \int_{-\infty}^{\infty} Ag(\omega)|^2\, d\omega/2\pi, \tag{45}$$

(b) $(2/\pi)^2$ times the ouptut in (a).

Hence the signal-to-noise ratio is the same for a chopper plus filter with gain $g(\Delta\omega)$ as for a filter with gain $g_1(\omega_{ch} \pm \Delta\omega) = [g(\Delta\omega)]$. In practice, $A(\omega_{ch} + \Delta\omega)$ is nearly constant over the range where $[g(\Delta\omega)]$ is important.

$$\int_{-\infty}^{\infty} A(\omega_{ch} + \Delta\omega)\, |g(\Delta\omega)|^2\, d\Delta\omega/2\pi = A_{\omega ch}\, 2 \int_{0}^{\infty} |g(\Delta\omega)|^2\, d\Delta\omega/2\pi.$$

We may define a bandwidth of the filter with gain $|g(\Delta\omega)|^2$ as

$$\Delta_{ch} \equiv \frac{2\int_0^{\infty} |g|^2\, d\Delta\omega/2\pi}{|g_{max}|^2}$$

the same as the bandwidth of $g_1(\omega)$ if $|g_1(\omega_{ch} \pm \Delta\omega)| = |g(\Delta\omega)|$. Now the signal-to-noise ratio is

$$\frac{S^2_{r.m.s.}}{A_{\omega ch}\Delta_{ch}}.$$

One could in principle enhance S/N by decreasing Δ_{ch}. However, Δ_{ch} is limited because we must observe variations in S and the time it takes to observe them goes to infinity if Δ_{ch} goes to zero.

4. Signal Accumulation Technique

4.1. Time of measurement

Let us now consider a signal $S(B_s)$ fed into a low pass filter of gain $g(\Delta\omega)$. $S(B_s)$ may be the direct output of the spectrometer, or the r.m.s.

value of the modulated signal. In the latter case we assume of course a filter of gain $g'(\omega_0 \pm \Delta\omega) = g(\Delta\omega)$ or the equivalent arrangement with a lock-in detector.

In order to measure $S(B_s)$ we vary the field with time. A first method is to scan the field up and down linearly, through the line; the function of the field is then

$$B_s(t) = B_{s0} + \frac{t}{\tau} B_{d0}. \tag{1}$$

[See eq. (3.1).] Another method, used principally for oscilloscope display, is the harmonical scanning of B_s. In any case $S(t)$ becomes a periodic function of time and this time function must pass through the filter $g(\Delta\omega)$. We may write the Fourier transform of this time function $S(t)$ and require that the lowest harmonics are of such a frequency that they pass through the filter.

Let us, for clarity, define a particular situation. We scan through a line, from n linewidths below to n linewidths above the centre of a symmetric absorption line. The linear scanning rate is α seconds for one linewidth. We choose the linewidth as the unit of field and α as the unit of time. Let us emphasize this by using x for the field and θ for the time, with $x = 0$ and $\theta = 0$ at the line centre. Of course, $S(x) = S(\theta)$. We may constantly repeat the scanning and the Fourier components of this periodic function are given by

$$\int_{-n}^{n} S(\theta) \cos k \frac{\pi\theta}{n} \, d\theta = \frac{n}{\pi} \int_{-\pi}^{\pi} S\left(\frac{n\sigma}{\pi}\right) \cos k\sigma \, d\sigma. \tag{2}$$

The question now is how rapidly do the Fourier components decrease with k. Indeed, the filter with bandwidth $\Delta\omega$ must be such that the important Fourier components pass, i.e.

$$k_1 \frac{2\pi}{2n} \lesssim \Delta\omega \tag{3}$$

if k_1 is the highest component we like to retain.

Because $S(\theta)$ is essentially limited to a linewidth above and below the centre, we may put 1 for the cosine, in the integral in eq. (2), for the harmonics for which the time for scanning two linewidths is much less than half a period of the cosine, i.e. if

$$2 \ll \frac{n}{k}. \tag{4}$$

All the harmonics up to $k \ll n/2$ will simply be

$$\int_{-n}^{n} S(\theta)\, d\theta.$$

The harmonic $k = n/2$ will still be important. Let us say that most of the information is contained in the harmonics up to

$$k_s \lesssim \frac{n}{2}. \tag{5}$$

Hence the bandwidth of the filter must be such that $\Delta\omega \gtrsim \pi/2$ in units α^{-1} or the time used to cross one linewidth must be

$$\alpha \gtrsim \frac{\pi}{2\Delta\omega} \approx \frac{1}{\Delta\omega}. \tag{6}$$

Another question is the time spent in the measurement. It is useless to scan a line over a range $n \gg 1$ since most of the time no information is collected. For a given filter, the scanning rate α is limited by eq. (6) and any increase of n above $n \gg 1$ increases the absolute measuring time without increasing the output signal.

All these considerations are made in terms of an order of magnitude. How many harmonics one retains and how many linewidths one scans depends on line shape, required accuracy, noise level, shape of the filter gain function, etc. The line itself is in general unknown before the measurement. Repeating the measurement of a perfectly known line in order to do it in the least possible time is in any case a waste of time. Let us therefore state, as a rough estimation, that we need a time $2\pi/\Delta\omega$ for measuring a line:

$$\boxed{\text{measuring time} \gtrsim 2\pi/\Delta\omega.} \tag{7}$$

In a typical low pass filter $\Delta\omega/2\pi$ is roughly the bandwidth, in hertz, specified by the "3 dB points".

4.2. Noise suppression by accumulation

Let us make n measurements of the same event; for example, we record a resonance line as a function of the static field B_s, n times. We get n times a signal with noise. The signal will be the same, $S(B_s)$, for n times, but the noise will be different each time, since noise is random. However, the noise correlation function will be the same for n times, as also will be the signal-to-noise ratio. The measurements may be successively taken using the same apparatus, or simultaneously with similar apparatuses. Now we may add these n signals with their noise. For successive measurements this supposes some storage of information, and also a system that permits us to establish the equivalent points of the "independent variable" in each measurement. As for the signal, the result will be a signal power of n^2 times the individual signal power, since the total signal amplitude is n times the signal S. In order to see what happens to the noise, let us analyse the mean (signal and noise) power. Since

$$\left\langle \sum_{i=1}^{n} v_i \right\rangle = \left\langle \sum_{i \neq j} v_i v_j \right\rangle = 0$$

and

$$\left\langle \sum_{i=1}^{n} v_i^2 \right\rangle = \sum_{i=1}^{n} \langle v_i^2 \rangle = n \langle v_i^2 \rangle$$

we get

$$\left\langle \left(nS + \sum_{i=1}^{n} v_i \right)^2 \right\rangle = n^2 S^2 + n \langle v_i^2 \rangle .$$

Hence the signal-to-noise power ratio is enhanced by a factor of n.

Of course, it takes n times as long to make n measurements and, in principle, the same S/N enhancement could be obtained by making the filter bandwidth n times smaller.

Stating it in another way, the effect of the addition is to divide the bandwidth by n, or to multiply the integration time by n.

In fact the use of a low pass filter is also a kind of addition, an integration. In a filter the line is added point by point, while in the addition technique one records the whole line and adds successive records. The principal advantage of the addition technique is that it permits much longer measuring times. Indeed, the bandwidth of a low filter is in practice achieved by a RC circuit, and RC = 1 min requires, for example, a capacitor of 1 μF with a leak resistance higher than 10 MΩ. Thus the integration time is limited to a few minutes.

The addition over long times is usually made by digital techniques. For instance, after ΔB_s of the field scanning, the paramagnetic resonance signal, eventually transformed by an analog digital converter, is fed into one of a series of counting channels. The *n*th channel accumulates the signal corresponding to $B_{s,\mathrm{ref}} + n \,.\, \Delta B_s$. The intervals ΔB_s may be, for example, taken as time intervals, if a linear scanning is provided. After each cycle, one may again adjust the value of the reference field $B_{s,\mathrm{ref}}$ by starting the time base of the channels by a reference signal derived from a field measurement. For example, a n.m.r. signal at a fixed frequency may give a pulse each time B_s passes over its resonance value.

For total measuring times shorter than a few seconds, there exists a very simple addition technique, in fact the oldest technique used in e.s.r. measurements: the *oscilloscope display*. One scans the static field to and fro with an amplitude greater than the line width, and centre value at the line centre. If a synchronous signal is applied to the horizontal deflection of the scope and the output of the spectrometer to the vertical deflection, one obtains a graph of the signal as a function of the static field as a scope pattern. Figure 5.1 of Chapter 2 shows a picture from a dualbeam oscilloscope giving $\chi'(B_s)$ and $\chi''(B_s)$. The field scanning may be made with any time function $B_s(t)$, provided the horizontal deflection is synchronous, and the fastest $\partial B_s/\partial t$ is still below the limit discussed in Chapter 2. Incidentally, if the limit is exceeded this fact will manifest itself by hysteresis, visible on the scope because the trace for $\partial B_s/\partial \tau > 0$ will no longer coincide with the trace for $\partial B_s/_d\tau < 0$.† The bandwidth

† Observe that an apparent hysteresis will also appear if the bandwidth of the spectrometer is not large enough. At 30 Hz a 0·1 mF condenser in series with the 1 MΩ scope input impedance may produce a visible apparent hysteresis.

of the scope has to be a few times the scanning frequency. Using a 60 Hz scanning frequency, one obtains a convenient trace and, at the cost of some deformation, one may cut down some low-frequency noise (e.g. drift) below 60 Hz, without the "field modulation technique", and hence without a modulation loss factor [this factor is always below $\frac{1}{8}$; see eq. (3.8)]. The addition is automatically made because the trace of the scope has some remanence; e.g. noise is seen as a broadened straight line with small fluctuations in the width. These fluctuations in the width (and not the width itself) are the noise which must be less than the signal. In order to increase the measuring time, one may take a photograph of the scope trace. The measuring time will be the time of exposure, and this time determines the final S/N ratio, practically independently of the modulation frequency, if we adapt the filter bandwidth to this frequency. Indeed, a higher modulation frequency means a greater bandwidth but also a greater number of records added and the two effects cancel.

Integral display is very easy, but the technique has two important limitations. First it is technically difficult to produce an a.c. field of frequency above 10 Hz and amplitude above some tens of mT in the gap of a large laboratory magnet; on the other hand, the measuring time is limited to a few seconds.

References

Angot, A. (1961), *Complements de Mathematiques*, Ed. de la Revue d'Optiques, Paris.

Dering, J. C. (1964), *Sensitivity Considerations in Paramagnetic Resonance Spectrometers*, (Thesis) University of Alberta, Calgary.

Hyde, J. S. (1965), *Ninth Annual NMR–EPR Workshop*, Varian, Palo Alto.

Van Gerven, L. (1963), *Lijnvormen in Paramagnetische Resonantie*, Interuniversitair Instituut voor Kernwetenschappen, Brussels.

Index

Index

OTHER TITLES IN THE SERIES IN NATURAL PHILOSOPHY

Vol. 1. DAVYDOV—Quantum Mechanics
Vol. 2. FOKKER—Time and Space, Weight and Inertia
Vol. 3. KAPLAN—Interstellar Gas Dynamics
Vol. 4. ABRIKOSOV, GOR'KOV and DZYALOSHINSKII—Quantum Field Theoretical Methods in Statistical Physics
Vol. 5. OKUN'—Weak Interaction of Elementary Particles
Vol. 6. SHKLOVSKII—Physics of the Solar Corona
Vol. 7. AKHIEZER *et al.*—Collective Oscillations in a Plasma
Vol. 8. KIRZHNITS—Field Theoretical Methods in Many-body Systems
Vol. 9. KLIMONTOVICH—The Statistical Theory of Non-equilibrium Processes in a Plasma
Vol. 10. KURTH—Introduction to Stellar Statistics
Vol. 11. CHALMERS—Atmospheric Electricity (2nd edition)
Vol. 12. RENNER—Current Algebras and their Applications
Vol. 13. FAIN and KHANIN—Quantum Electronics
Vol. 1. Basic Theory
Vol. 14. FAIN and KHANIN—Quantum Electronics
Vol. 2. Maser Amplifiers and Oscillators
Vol. 15. MARCH—Liquid Metals
Vol. 16. HORI—Spectral Properties of Disordered Chains and Lattices
Vol. 17. SAINT JAMES, THOMAS and SARMA—Type II Superconductivity
Vol. 18. MARGENAU and KESTNER—Theory of Intermolecular Forces
Vol. 19. JANCEL—Foundations of Classical and Quantum Statistical Mechanics
Vol. 20. TAKAHASHI—An Introduction to Field Quantization
Vol. 21. YVON—Correlations and Entropy in Classical Statistical Mechanics
Vol. 22. PENROSE—Foundations of Statistical Mechanics
Vol. 23. VISCONTI—Quantum Field Theory—Vol.1
Vol. 24. FURTH—Fundamental Principles of Theoretical Physics
Vol. 25. ZHELEZNYAKOV—Radioemission of the Sun and Planets
Vol. 26. GRINDLAY—An Introduction to the Phenomenological Theory of Ferroelectricity
Vol. 27. UNGER—Introduction to Quantum Electronics
Vol. 28. KOGA—Introduction to Kinetic Theory. Stochastic Processes in Gaseous Systems
Vol. 29. GALASIEWICZ—Superconductivity and Quantum Fluids
Vol. 30. CONSTANTINESCU and MAGYARI—Problems in Quantum Mechanics
Vol. 31. KOTKIN and SERBO—Collection of Problems in Classical Mechanics
Vol. 32. PANCHEV—Random Functions and Turbulence